THE NA

A strategy fo

THE NATION'S HEALTH
A strategy for the 1990s

A report from an Independent Multidisciplinary Committee
chaired by Professor Alwyn Smith

Edited by Alwyn Smith and Bobbie Jacobson

SPONSORED BY
The Health Education Council (to April 1987)
The Health Education Authority (from April 1987)
King Edward's Hospital Fund for London
The London School of Hygiene and Tropical Medicine
The Scottish Health Education Group

King Edward's Hospital Fund for London

© 1988 Health Education Authority, London School of Hygiene and
Tropical Medicine and King Edward's Hospital Fund for London

Typeset by Tradespools Ltd
Printed and bound in England by Hollen Street Press

Distributed for the King's Fund by Oxford University Press

ISBN 0 19 724647 8 (paperback)
ISBN 0 19 724648 6 (cased)

King's Fund Publishing Office
14 Palace Court
London W2 4HT

Members of Independent Multidisciplinary Committee

Professor Alwyn Smith
Former President, Faculty of Community Medicine
Department of Epidemiology and Social Oncology
University of Manchester
(Chairman)

Professor Patrick Hamilton
Department of Community Health
London School of Hygiene and Tropical Medicine
(Vice-chairman)

Dr Bobbie Jacobson
Department of Community Medicine
City and Hackney Health Authority
(Secretary)

Ms Celia Husband
(Administrative Assistant)
Department of Community Health
London School of Hygiene and Tropical Medicine

Dr Beulah Bewley
Specialist in Community Medicine
Wandsworth Health Authority

Professor David Donnison
Department of Town and Regional Planning
University of Glasgow

Ms Shirley Goodwin
General Secretary
Health Visitors Association

Dr J A Muir Gray
Specialist in Community Medicine
Oxford Health Authority

Dr June Huntington
Fellow in Organisational and Professional Studies
King's Fund College

Professor J N Morris
Emeritus Professor of Community Medicine
London School of Hygiene and Tropical Medicine

Professor R E Kendell
Professor of Psychiatry and Dean of the Medical School
University of Edinburgh

Dr Alan Maryon Davis
Chief Medical Officer, former Health Education Council
Consultant Medical Adviser to Health Education Authority

Baroness Masham of Ilton
Yorkshire Regional Health Authority

Professor David Metcalfe
Department of General Practice
University of Manchester

Mr Victor Morrison
King's Fund Publishing Office

Ms Usha Prashar
Director Designate,
National Council of Voluntary Organisations

Ms Jill Spratley
Lecturer in Continuing Education
Department of Community Health
London School of Hygiene and Tropical Medicine

Mr David Taylor
Director of Economic Planning and Public Affairs
Association of British Pharmaceutical Industry

Observer
Dr L B Hunt
Senior Medical Officer
Department of Health and Social Security

Acknowledgements

Our thanks to the Health Education Council, King Edward's Hospital Fund for London, London School of Hygiene and Tropical Medicine and the Scottish Health Education Group for financial support; to Celia Husband for organising the project and typing successive drafts of the report; and to Sheila Carr for the final draft.

Special thanks to Margaret Whitehead, Richard Wilkinson, Professor Richard Schilling, Tony Webb, Penny Babb, Paul Castle and Dr John Ashton for additional background research which was made possible by the Health Education Council.

Thanks to all those we consulted for help with research and comments on earlier drafts – especially Dr Valerie Beral, Dr Colin Sanderson and colleagues at the London School of Hygiene and Tropical Medicine, former Health Education Council and Scottish Health Education Group.

To the Department of Health and Social Security, the Office of Population Censuses and Surveys, the Scottish Home and Health Department, Welsh Office, Ministry of Agriculture, Fisheries and Foods, for assistance with the preparation of data.

To Dr Kimmo Leppo and Dr Ilona Kickbush and colleagues at the World Health Organization.

We are especially indebted to Sir Richard Doll for valuable comments and suggestions on the final text.

Patrick Hamilton, a major architect of this project, died suddenly while the report was in its proof stages. We shall all miss his energy and enthusiasm.

Abbreviations

AAA	Action on Alcohol Abuse
ACMD	Advisory Council on Misuse of Drugs
AFP	Alphafetoprotein
AIDS	Acquired Immunodeficiency Syndrome
ASH	Action on Smoking and Health
BMA	British Medical Association
BPA	British Paediatric Association
CDSC	Centre for Disease Surveillance and Control
COMA	Committee on Medical Aspects of Diet
CPG	Coronary Prevention Group
CRS	Congenital rubella syndrome
CVS	Chorionic villus sampling
DES	Department of Education and Science
DHSS	Department of Health and Social Security
DHA	District health authority
DMF	Decayed, missing or filled teeth
EMAS	Employment Medical Advisory Service
FPIS	Family Planning Information Service
HEC	Health Education Council
HEA	Health Education Authority
HEACW	Health Education Advisory Committee for Wales
HIV	Human Immunovirus
HSE	Health and Safety Executive
HVA	Health Visitors Association
MAFF	Ministry of Agriculture, Fisheries and Foods
MMR	Measles, mumps and rubella
MRC	Medical Research Council
MIND	National Association of Mental Health
NACNE	National Advisory Committee on Nutrition Education
NTD	Neural tube defect
OPCS	Office of Population Censuses and Surveys
RHA	Regional health authority
RCP	Royal College of Physicians
RCGP	Royal College of General Practitioners
SHEG	Scottish Health Education Group
SHHD	Scottish Home and Health Department
TACADE	Teachers' Advisory Committee on Alcohol and Drug Education

Contents

Tables

Figures

Preface

This report takes stock of Britain's health, in the sense that it examines current patterns of disease and of health-related behaviour, and asks how they can be changed for the better.

As the report shows, the nation's health continues to improve, but there is no room for complacency. While we can be justifiably proud of (for example) our relatively low rates of death among young people from accidents and violence, our road safety record, and our maternal mortality figures, that is by no means true of a number of other indicators. We are in the unenviable position of having the highest death rates from coronary heart disease in the world, with relatively high rates also for several of the cancers. The perinatal and infant mortality figures are still improving (with a controversial blip upwards in infant mortality against the trend in Scotland in 1984 and England and Wales in 1986) but at a slower rate than leading Western countries.

Some people will argue, perfectly legitimately, that mortality rates at the younger ages have dropped so much in the more affluent countries of the world that they are no longer sufficiently sensitive to act as reliable indicators of performance. But there are still such substantial differences between countries – and within the UK by region and by socioeconomic group – that a relatively low ranking frequently indicates real potential for improvement. Moreover the report discusses very fully 'living better' as well as 'living longer', and in many instances we do not have to choose between measures that ought to make an impact on one or the other of these goals. Changes in diet, drinking and smoking, exercise, environmental conditions and employment should affect both the length and the quality of our lives.

Another sterile argument is between those who maintain that people's health is in their own hands, dependent on their own behaviour, and those who take a determinist position. The latter argue that government cannot stand aloof: through legislation, economic policy, taxation and so on it shapes individual choices. The argument is sterile because both views are correct. There is much for individuals to do, and much that depends on government action, and the two are frequently interdependent and interacting.

Professor Alwyn Smith, his Steering Committee and their researcher, Dr Bobbie Jacobson, are to be congratulated on producing a balanced account that manages to avoid the pitfalls of being too polemical on the one hand, or of being so cautious and scholarly as not to be comprehensible.

The result is quite long and carefully annotated, and at the same time reasonably accessible not only to the specialist but also to the general reader. It ends by proposing a health strategy for the 1990s, identifying 17 priorities for public health action. Inevitably the 17 taken together comprise a formidable list of changes in personal behaviour and public policy, and of improvements in services. The authors recognise, however, that the evidence supporting a detailed strategy for action is stronger in some cases than in others, and they have framed their recommendations accordingly. They leave us with no valid excuse for inaction.

Robert J Maxwell
Secretary and Chief Executive Officer
King Edward's Hospital Fund for London

Introduction

The health of the nation is not simply an esoteric preoccupation of the health professions nor even an exclusive responsibility of the departments of health; there is now general agreement that it is 'everybody's business' and in 1976 the health departments of the United Kingdom published *Prevention and health: everybody's business** to emphasise that view. Although the aims of the publication seemed clearly defined – to avoid prescription and to promote discussion – there was some ambiguity in the use of the word 'everybody's' and it was possible to conclude that the responsibility for health rested with individuals. In this present volume we intend to be more explicit about where responsibilities rest as well as about what those responsibilities are. We hope that it will not only be read by individual citizens but also used by public agencies and organisations in formulating the policies and decisions that affect the public health.

In early 1985 it was felt that it would be useful both to examine progress since the issue of the 1976 document and to reconsider its general tenor and relevance to the public health problems of the present time. The then Health Education Council (subsequently the Health Education Authority), the Scottish Health Education Group, the King's Fund and the London School of Hygiene and Tropical Medicine joined in establishing a research fellowship in health promotion, and Dr Bobbie Jacobson was appointed and charged with the task of reviewing the present health issues in the light of progress since 1976. To guide the project an independent multidisciplinary committee was established which has aimed to assemble a membership reflecting a wide range of skills and experience in the sciences and professional practices with an interest in public policy relating to health. Observers from the sponsoring bodies and from the DHSS were also invited to attend.

The aims of the project were to re-examine the central problems relating to the public health, to assess the effectiveness of existing public health policies and to stimulate the development of new national strategies for the public health. The report we now issue is the product of more than two years' deliberation by the committee. It is designed to achieve these aims by analysing the issues in as accessible a language as their complexity permits, by defining some targets or priorities for public policy and, most importantly, by establishing the agenda for public and political debate about how the

*Department of Health and Social Security. Prevention and health: everybody's business. London, HMSO, 1976.

1

nation might best re-establish its pre-eminence in the pursuit of the public health.

Why re-examine the issues? The 1976 publication reflected the fashionable thinking of its time. The notion that the public health was 'everybody's business' led to a heavy emphasis being placed on the responsibility of individuals for their own health. The recognition that health depends increasingly on human behaviour resulted in the view being taken that the behaviour of individuals had replaced the quality of the environment as the key issue in the promotion of the public health. There are now good grounds for a change in that emphasis.

The earlier optimism that harmful environmental influences were relatively simple to control has given way to an increasing recognition that the environment is continuously changing – often as a result of human activities – and that many of the changes pose new threats to our health. It is also increasingly being recognised that human behaviour does not reflect individual choices alone so much as the powerful influence of the social, economic and political environments that lie substantially beyond the control of the individuals who are affected by them.

The health of the people of the United Kingdom is now almost certainly better than it has ever been and it is undoubtedly better than that of the majority of the nations of the world. Almost every index of the public health confirms the progress that has been made during the present century, and especially during the last few decades, and the people of this country enjoy a standard of health as well as a quality of health care that might well make us the envy of much of the world. However, complacency cannot be justified. Progress in the UK compares much less well with those of other countries of north western Europe, and the inequalities in health that are evident within our country make it clear that there is much more that we might have done and many challenges to which we have not so far successfully responded. Public health is a term that has traditionally embraced not simply the health of the public, but also the aims and methods of those whose concern it is to protect and promote the health of all citizens in the interests both of those individuals and of the community they comprise. It involves the promotion of health, the prevention of disease, the treatment of illness, the care of those who are disabled and the continuous development of the technical and social means for the pursuit of these objectives.

Health is very variously defined and any definition of the public health depends on current definitions of health in individuals as well as on the significance of the health of its members to the community as a whole. Health means different things at different ages and to people in different circumstances. If health is defined in terms of the state of fitness of our leading athletes then most of the rest of us would have to be considered seriously disabled. Clearly we need a definition that relates capacity to what may be legitimately expected and that applies both to young and old and to people of different physical and mental endowment. Individuals may be considered healthy to the extent that they are capable of meeting the obligations and enjoying the rewards of living in their community. A strategy for ensuring that as many people are as healthy as possible will therefore require not only measures for the promotion of health, the prevention of disease and the treatment of illness and incapacity but also the development of a society which offers a useful and rewarding role for all its members whatever the impairments from which they may suffer. We are still a long way from developing such a society and we have chosen to address a range of simpler issues. We have confined ourselves mainly to the promotion of health and the prevention of disease in the simpler senses in which these terms are generally understood.

Prevention and health promotion

Although much lip service is paid to the proposition that prevention is better than cure, we believe that for many people it is far from self-evident. Since diseases that are prevented are necessarily unreported, the success of a preventive procedure is more difficult to demonstrate than that of a therapy. To assess treatment, we compare illness and its cure in the same individuals whereas the only comparison available for the demonstration of prevention is between those who have incurred a disease and those others who have not. Since few diseases are universal it can never be certain that those not incurring the disease owe their escape to the preventive procedure under examination. Prevention therefore requires a statistical demonstration at a population level, and the frequent cynical manipulation of statistical evidence in modern society has left many people with a considerable scepticism in the face of statistics.

But there is also a sense in which prevention seems less efficient than treatment. Whereas treatment can be concentrated on those who are sick, prevention has usually to be distributed among a larger number of well persons – many of whom would probably have avoided the disease even in the absence of the preventive procedure. If we did not immunise some half a million infants against diphtheria each year it is unlikely that more than a few thousand would contract the disease. In this sense many hundreds of thousands of people receive preventive procedures unnecessarily so far as their individual health is concerned. Unfortunately, it is usually impossible to identify those who would succumb if a procedure were abandoned. Prevention is often seen as unglamorous – at least by comparison

3

with the technologically demanding procedures now prevailing in clinical medicine and surgery. The fundamental requirements for a healthy life have been known in general terms for centuries and are applied with conspicuous success in animal husbandry. All creatures need an appropriate diet, shelter from the elements, regular exercise, rewarding but not onerous work, the satisfaction of sexual drive and protection from environmental injury whether physical, chemical, biological or psychological. The human individual is also driven to extend continually the envelope of safe experience and human societies are often manipulated by some individuals to the risk of others. It is one of the functions of government to regulate such manipulation in both the best interests of collectivity and of its individual members.

A public health philosophy
No discussion of the public health or of public policy can be value-free. As health professionals and students of social policy, the committee's members inescapably function within the framework of their particular ideology. We believe it right that we should declare its principal tenets. We start from the position that health is important among the objectives and values of most individual human beings and that they expect their governments and administrations to pursue policies that will afford them the opportunity to attain lives of optimum duration and quality. We further believe that the health of its citizens is one of the most important resources needed by a nation for the pursuit of most other legitimate national objectives. We are fully aware that health is not the only, or always the most important, objective of either individuals or communities and that the cost of its pursuit is both substantial and likely to increase. Economists maintain that rational human behaviour requires some commensuration of the benefits and costs of all the options among which we seek to choose. They also recognise that such commensuration is often formidably difficult and that we are likely to do it only imperfectly for the foreseeable future. We do not wish to pre-empt the decisions which individuals and government will need to take. We have, nevertheless, considered it useful to present a review of some of the salient opportunities for health improvement that now confront us and an indication of the steps that we shall need to take if we are to seize them.

Finally, the promotion of the public health will depend crucially on whether we can survive the worst consequences of the human propensity for disputation and contrive to live at peace. The mass homicide which we call war has presented a major threat to human health throughout recorded history and, even now, hardly a day goes by without death or injury from this cause representing an important contributor to the world's ill health. Preparation for the possibility

4

of war diverts huge resources that might otherwise be directed to enhancing the quality and duration of life. Hanging over all of us is the threat that the accidental or ill-considered launch of weapons of mass-destruction will trigger an exchange of such weapons on an annihilatory scale. We have not considered ourselves competent to offer advice on how the world might learn to live at peace, but unless it does our recommendations will be in vain.

PART I: LIVING LONGER

1 Lessons from a decade of public health

What experience and history teach is
this – that people and governments
never have learned anything from
history, or acted on principles deduced
from it.

GEORG WILHELM HEGEL

Introduction   This chapter summarises the discussion and recommendations whose detailed exposition occupies the rest of the volume. In presenting this overview we have adopted a different structure from that used in developing the greater detail of the remainder of the book. We first highlight the progress (and lack of it) that has characterised the period of just over ten years since the publication of *Prevention and Health*; then, we develop the lessons to be derived from the last decade or so; finally, we summarise our recommendations for action. In this preliminary summary we have avoided detailed reference to the literature; this is dealt with in some detail in the main body of the work.

Areas where public health has improved   Improvements in health and reductions in death rates have occurred at every stage in life from birth through to old age. We live, on average, nearly as long as our counterparts in most other affluent countries.

General mortality (Chapter 2) Perinatal and infant mortality rates in each of the countries in the UK have fallen by at least 50 per cent, although we still lag behind many countries in north western Europe.

Mortality rates among young people – especially men aged 25 to 34 – are lower in the UK than almost anywhere else in the affluent world. By the age of 45, however, the expectation of further life is shorter in the UK than in many other countries.

The reduction of avoidable deaths has been impressive in the following specific areas.

Stroke (Chapter 3) Mortality rates from stroke have decreased by nearly one-third in all the UK countries, and we compare relatively well with other European countries, although there has been more progress in the USA and Japan. We do not fully understand the reasons for these trends.

Road safety (Chapter 6) The number of people killed on the roads in 1985 was the lowest for three decades. Despite a 39 per cent increase in the volume of traffic between 1975 and 1985, there was a further

9

nine per cent fall in the number of fatal and serious casualties in Great Britain. The UK has the lowest death rates from road accidents in the EEC, and one of the lowest rates in the industrialised world.

There have been important health gains in the prevention of disease and disability and in the promotion of health in the following areas.

Sexuality and unwanted pregnancy (Chapter 13) Women, especially teenagers, are exercising more effective control over their fertility: teenage conception rates decreased by nearly 14 per cent between 1974 and 1984. There has been a progressive increase in contraceptive use since 1970, and by 1983 nearly 90 per cent of sexually active people were using some form of contraception. The evidence suggests that the use of contraception applies across all social groups. Abortion rates in the UK are lower than those in most of northern Europe and north America, but have remained relatively stable. However, abortion rates among teenagers and young women rose much faster than in older age groups between 1975 and 1985.

Mental health and ill health (Chapter 10) Parasuicide has become steadily less common among women in all age groups since the mid-1970s. The reasons for this decline are unknown. Although there is no reliable information on trends in the prevalence of depression, there has been a welcome decrease in the prescription of benzodiazepine sedatives in the last decade.

Pregnancy and childbirth (Chapter 11) More effective antenatal screening, together with other unknown changes (possibly in diet), have led to a major reduction in the percentage of babies born with congenital malformations of the central nervous system between 1976 and 1985. The reported percentage of babies born with spina bifida has decreased by 63 per cent and of the related, but more severe, anencephaly by 92 per cent. Genetic counselling, antenatal screening and selective termination of pregnancy have led to a major reduction in thalassemia major within the Cypriot community. The proportion of women breast feeding at birth and at six weeks has increased, although disparity between Scotland and England, and between manual and non-manual social groups, remains.

Dental health (Chapter 12) Dental health has improved in children over the whole age range, but the improvement is most marked in five year olds where the proportion with decayed teeth fell by one third between 1973 and 1983. Evidence of improvements in the prevalence of periodental (chronic gum) disease in adults is harder to find, and the social disparity in dental health remains.

Areas where progress has been mixed The last decade has seen mixed progress in the following aspects of public health.

Infant deaths (Chapters 8 and 11) While there have been impressive reductions in overall perinatal and infant mortality, with reductions in each of the social groups, the disparity in perinatal and infant mortality rates between non-manual and manual classes remains.

Coronary heart disease (Chapters 3 and 7) There has been a small, long awaited, reduction in mortality from coronary heart disease since 1978. This has been most marked among younger and middle-aged men and women. However, the UK still has the highest death rates from coronary heart disease in the world with Northern Ireland and Scotland having higher death rates than England and Wales. Death rates from coronary heart disease among men and women from the manual classes have increased. The risk factors for coronary heart disease that have shown the biggest changes are cigarette smoking and diet. Total sales consumption of cigarettes has fallen by nearly 30 per cent in the last decade. The consumption of saturated fats has decreased over the decade, and the ratio of polyunsaturated to saturated fats has increased. Consumption of wholemeal bread has increased in all social groups, but the socioeconomic disparity in smoking rates and in many aspects of diet remains.

Lung cancer (Chapter 4) Lung cancer death rates are falling among men in all age groups and increasing among women over 55. Lung cancer death rates have fallen by almost 50 per cent among middle-aged men. These trends can largely be explained by a major decrease in tar yields. Reductions in smoking rates among women have, so far, been less impressive than among men. Smoking among children, especially among girls, is showing no sign of decline.

Suicide (Chapter 10) While suicide rates among men have steadily increased – especially among men of working age – there has been a small, overall fall in suicide rates among women – especially those aged 25–34. The reasons for these sex differences are unclear, but the increasing rate among men is closely associated with rising levels of unemployment.

Immunisation (Chapter 12) The UK compares fairly well with other affluent countries, and with European targets, in respect of uptake rates for vaccination against diphtheria, tetanus and poliomyelitis. It compares poorly with other countries, however, especially Scandinavia and the USA, in uptake levels for vaccination against pertussis (whooping cough), rubella and measles. There is wide disparity in regional and socioeconomic uptake rates within the UK. The tuberculosis immunisation programme, together with better nutrition and more effective treatment, have contributed to a continued decline of TB. Pockets of increased risk remain among the single homeless, and recent immigrants from Asia.

Physical activity (Chapter 9) Although only a minority of the population could be described as physically active, there have been small, significant improvements in participation rates for walking, swimming and athletics (including jogging). The wide sex, age and social class disparities in physical activity remain unchanged.

Areas where there has been little change over the last decade

There has been little or no progress in reducing ill health and premature death in the following areas.

Low birthweight (Chapter 11) The proportion of low birthweight births has remained at approximately seven per cent. Two-thirds of these are to women married to men in manual classes.

Congenital abnormality (Chapter 11) About one in five deaths in the perinatal period are due to congenital malformations. This proportion has remained almost unchanged over the last decade.

Postneonatal mortality (Chapters 8 and 11) has remained largely static since the mid 1970s. Sudden infant death syndrome (SIDS) (Chapter 11) has increasingly been recognised as a major, potentially avoidable cause of death during the early months of life. Although mortality from SIDS appears to have risen, this may be largely due to increased recognition and reporting of the problem.

Large bowel cancer (Chapter 4) Trends in the incidence and in the death rates from cancer of the large bowel have remained largely unchanged over the last decade. The causes of bowel cancer are not fully understood, although diet – especially one with a high fibre content – may play a protective role. Treatment has not had a major impact. There is insufficient evidence as yet to warrant a screening programme for the early detection of bowel cancer.

Breast cancer (Chapters 4 and 7) Fifteen thousand British women die of breast cancer each year. It is still the leading cause of cancer mortality among women. Although death rates have slowly risen this century, there has been no major increase in its incidence or mortality in the last decade. We do not know the cause of breast cancer, but the risk factors most closely linked with it are early age of menarche (first period) and a postponement of first pregnancy beyond the age of 35.

Cervical cancer (Chapters 4 and 7) Approximately 2,000 British women die of cervical cancer each year. This figure has remained largely unchanged over the last decade. Both the incidence and the mortality from cervical cancer among women under 35 have increased over the last decade although they remain low at these ages. Cervical cancer is most probably a sexually transmitted disease closely associated with the presence of certain types of genital wart virus. The sharp decline in the use of barrier contraception over the last two decades and earlier onset of sexual activity, together with poorly implemented cervical screening services, have almost certainly contributed to these trends.

Areas where
health is getting
worse

Social disparities (Chapter 8) Despite improvements in death rates in every age group, the gap between death rates among the non-manual and manual classes has grown wider for most causes of death in almost every age group. We estimate that annual excess avoidable deaths in the manual worker classes in men and women aged 16–74 in 1979–83 was 42,000.

Alcohol-consumption (Chapter 5) Following an 11 per cent fall in per capita alcohol consumption in the UK between 1979 and 1982, there has been a new rise of two and a half per cent between 1982 and 1985.

AIDS (Chapter 5) By July 1987 there were 935 notified cases of AIDS and over 500 deaths. The number of reported cases of AIDS has been increasing exponentially since 1982, with a doubling time of approximately 10 months in 1986. Between 30–50,000 people in the UK were estimated to have been infected with the AIDS virus in 1987. This upward trend is likely to continue over the next decade at least. AIDS is caused by human immunovirus (HIV) and can be transmitted sexually or through blood and its products.

Senile dementia (Chapter 10) Although most elderly people are not mentally ill and the age-adjusted prevalence of dementia is not increasing, the rapidly expanding *numbers* of elderly people over 75 and 85 have led to a marked rise in the total prevalence of dementia. We can expect this upward trend to continue until beyond the end of this century.

Illicit drugs (Chapter 13) The number of people taking illicit opiates (mainly heroin) has been estimated at 50,000. Although most illicit drug users experience no untoward effects, the misuse of opiates has increased substantially since the late 1970s. Other increases in illicit drug use such as amphetamines and, more recently, cocaine have also occurred.

Public health
issues which
require more
research

The causes and prevention of mental illness (Chapter 10) Although some progress has been made in determining the causes of mental handicap and certain aspects of mental illness, much more research is needed into the causes and prevention of schizophrenia and dementia. More research is needed to separate out those components of 'stress' which are environmentally and constitutionally determined. Although progress has been made in identifying 'life events' which can contribute to depression, and to a range of other health problems, more research is needed to define other aspects of stress that may contribute to both physical and mental ill health, and may prove to be more amenable to primary prevention.

The causes of physical ill health (Chapters 3, 4 and 14) We do not yet know enough about the causes of breast or bowel cancer which account for a major proportion of cancer mortality. We need to find

13

better ways of measuring work-related hazards and the relationship between environmental radiation and cancers. Although we know enough about heart disease to implement an effective strategy for prevention, we still need to know more about the way in which stress and social class influence heart disease rates.

Promoting a healthy lifestyle (Chapter 7) Although much progress has been made in assessing the different policy options in the tobacco and alcohol fields, equivalent research on nutritional policy is seriously lacking. We need carefully controlled intervention studies on the impact of social support on the elderly and their carers to guide us towards more humane policy options. Above all, we suffer from a continuing lack of reliable data on trends in risk factors affecting health, and in health-related knowledge, attitudes and practices of the nation.

Evaluation of programmes The translation of epidemiological findings into effective practice is still very incomplete. We know most about programmes aimed at reducing risk factors for heart disease. Research into factors underlying social and regional disparities in immunisation rates and cervical screening suggests relatively simple methods for more effective implementation. We need to know more about how to establish an effective organisational structure for intervention programmes, in primary care, hospital preventive services, the workplace and the wider community.

Finally, we need to develop a better understanding of the role of the communications media in the process of health promotion. We have documented some of the positive and negative influences of these media but research has focussed on evaluating the effect of short-lived, advertising campaigns. The longer term effects of editorial coverage of health deserve more attention.

The characteristics of effective public health action

Our analysis shows that there are two general approaches to public health action which are complementary.

- The 'population approach' which focuses on measures to improve health *throughout* the community.
- The 'high risk' approach which concentrates action on those who are at highest risk of ill health.

For public health problems such as coronary heart disease, alcohol-related harm and high blood pressure, there is good evidence that an exclusive focus on the 'high risk' approach is unlikely to reduce the scale of the problem.

There are eight important general principles which emerge from our analysis and are common to those public health strategies which have been most effectively implemented over the last decade.

1. Partnership between the public, professionals and policy makers

The interdependence of political, professional and public strategies is best illustrated by road safety in which long-term public debate, together with increasing professional support and ultimately legislation, ensured that compliance with the seat belt legislation has remained at 95 per cent. Moreover, numerous states in the USA were forced to repeal their seat belt legislation which had not been preceded by adequate public debate. British drinking and driving legislation has not yet received sufficient political support, and is being inadequately implemented.

The family planning strategy over the last decade illustrates how an increasingly active and well-informed public, together with adequate professional support and legislation to increase free access to family planning, has resulted in impressive increases in contraceptive use. By contrast, the relatively low professional and political commitment given to cervical screening services until the 1980s, and the absence of any obvious national attempt to inform women of the existence and value of such a service, has contributed to the poor outcomes over the last decade.

The importance of national and local agencies such as the Royal College of Physicians, ASH, the BMA and the former HEC, together with the health and local authorities, in taking a lead in the promotion of health has been clearly illustrated in the case of cigarette smoking, and in more recent initiatives to prevent the spread of AIDS.

The need to promote a willing partnership between users and professionals in the promotion of health is beginning to be recognised within primary care, and in maternity services. The increasing sensitivity to user satisfaction has prompted the establishment of patient participation groups and the use of patient-held information. Cultural and ethical objections to the use of procedures such as amniocentesis need to be better understood to maximise the efficiency of such services.

2. A good national and local organisational structure

Our analysis illustrates the importance of liaison between government departments to coordinate government policy on public health. This has so far been deliberately sought in the fields of illicit drug misuse and of AIDS for which ministerial interdepartmental committees exist. There is an equally pressing need for such liaison in other fields such as tobacco, nutrition and road safety policy. Such arrangements are already being implemented across the whole public health field in Sweden and Finland.

Unlike countries such as Canada and the USA which have discrete public health services and which have reorganised them to meet current public health challenges,[1] we have neglected the development of national and local health promotion agencies which has been

15

haphazard and uncoordinated. The loss of the post of medical officer of health, responsible to local government until 1974, has led to a relative neglect of the public health. This has been the subject of an inquiry under the chairmanship of Sir Donald Acheson.[2] The frequent reallocation and division of ministerial and departmental responsibilities for public health in the DHSS hampers communication between the DHSS and local agencies. The historical separation of the HEC, which was a quango, from health education officers, who are part of the NHS, and from local authority education departments and environmental health units has compounded these difficulties. Plans for the resolution of some of these issues should be an urgent priority for the recently created Health Education Authority which replaced the HEC in April 1987, and is part of the NHS.[3]

3. Adequate funding

It is difficult to estimate how much is spent in the UK on the promotion of health and the prevention of disease. This is partly because of genuine difficulty in deciding what constitutes 'prevention and promotion', and partly because some health authorities and the DHSS have been reluctant to provide estimates.[4,5] In the face of the need to justify all public expenditure – especially within the NHS – this is unsatisfactory, and a concerted attempt is needed to provide national and local guidelines for such allocations. The total expenditure on what was defined as prevention by one researcher in 1980/81 was estimated at £967 million.[6] This included £550 million within the NHS which represented less than five per cent of total NHS expenditure. It also included £395 million non-NHS public expenditure by all government departments and local authorities, and a further £15.5 million by private and voluntary bodies.

The current imbalance between the allocation of £17 million for the prevention of drug misuse and £20 million for the AIDS prevention campaign, compared with a total of £13 million allocated to the former HEC and SHEG for *all* other aspects of health promotion, urgently needs review.

Our specially comissioned survey of RHAs showed that some had developed a clear basis for estimating funds allocated to health promotion and disease prevention, and this formed a rational basis for future resource allocation and planning.[7] The findings of a DHSS task force in 1986 show that DHA expenditure on health education units varies from as little as £1,000 to £35,000 a year.[8]

4. The importance of long-term strategic planning

WHO has taken a lead in emphasising the need for the formulation of a clearly defined, quantified strategy for the promotion of health. As part of its campaign for Health for All by the Year 2000 it has produced a European strategy which identifies 38 targets to be achieved by the year 2000.[9]

All 33 member states – including the UK – are signatories to this strategy which had already been translated into national plans in the US,[10] Canada[11] and at least five western European countries by June 1986. The need for such a lead was endorsed at the first international conference on health promotion organised by WHO which issued the Ottawa Charter for Health Promotion.[12]

There is no such plan in the UK, although every RHA (and some DHAs) in our own survey had a strategic plan for health promotion, and about half had adopted quantified targets – many along WHO lines. The Faculty of Community Medicine has translated the WHO targets into a British context[13] and a number of metropolitan authorities have incorporated the WHO principles into a new initiative to promote Healthy Cities across the UK.[14] Successive governments have supported the idea of the promotion of health and the prevention of disease, but the emphasis has so far been on the more individualistic 'high risk' approach rather than the 'population approach'. This was the focus in *Prevention and Health: everybody's business*[15] which was reinforced in the government's health care strategy document *Care in Action* in 1981.[16] There has been more recent recognition of the need for wider action across many government departments. In evidence to the Public Accounts Committee report on preventive medicine in 1986,[17] the DHSS identified interdepartmental action on 19 health promotion and disease prevention policy areas which are broadly similar to those we identify in Chapter 15.

The increased commitment to serious planning for the prevention of the spread of AIDS, the misuse of illicit drugs and, more recently, breast cancer screening is welcome. But there is an overriding need for the development of a coherent, long-term plan for the public health. An unwillingness to plan was reflected within the HEC which did not have a clearly defined long-term strategy.[18] The creation of the new Health Education Authority offers an important opportunity for developing such a strategy which is already the stated intention of the newly formed Health Promotion Authority established by the Welsh Office.[19-21]

5. The importance of recognising barriers to the promotion of health

The barriers to the promotion of health can be formidable. The tobacco, alcohol and confectionery manufacturers together spend nearly £700 million annually on promoting products which represent hazards to health. This is more than 50 times the total annual budget for the former HEC and SHEG in 1985–86.

The Government earned nearly £11 billion in 1985 from tobacco and alcohol taxation alone. There are other, more subtle, barriers to health promotion, such as the attempts to limit the open discussion of sexuality and its health implications within the communications media and in schools. And finally, there is still a prevailing attitude within the media, and in many medical schools, and some sectors of the medical profession, that there will soon be a cure for our major health problems. While treatment has a major contribution to make, prevention has been historically more important. This is often underemphasised in glamorised reports of high technology medicine.

6. Effective mechanisms for reducing inequalities in health

While we have shown that income, housing and employment policy provide the foundation for a strategy to reduce inequalities in health, little effort has so far been directed towards finding effective mechanisms for reducing *specific* aspects of health inequality such as the social class gradient in coronary heart disease and in lung cancer. Our analysis does show, however, that the 'population approach' is likely to be more effective than efforts to reach individuals at high risk of ill health. There is evidence that measures such as fluoridation of the water supply, the wartime national nutrition policy, the mandatory use of seat belts, and legislation to provide access to free contraception and better provision of sports facilities can reduce social disparities in health and health-related practices. Preliminary research which suggests that the social disparity in smoking rates may be reduced by bigger rather than smaller increases in cigarette taxation, deserves further attention. More research into the use of food pricing mechanisms to encourage healthier eating patterns and to reduce socioeconomic differences in diet is needed.

7. Adequately funded and disseminated health education and information programmes

Our review has demonstrated the importance of educational initiatives in the promotion of health. Long-term school education programmes have been most widely adopted in the smoking and health field. Our survey of educational achievements in the health field over the last decade showed that most progress has been made in schools. By 1981, 85 per cent of English and Welsh secondary schools covered health education. Two-thirds claimed to have a planned programme, and nearly half had a designated person responsible for health education.[22] Nearly nine out of ten primary schools covered health education, although in a much less planned way. The picture for Scotland is equally encouraging. If government includes health education within the core curriculum this should reinforce these welcome trends.

The survey showed that developments in medical education were less encouraging than in nurse and teacher training. Nearly half the colleges of education in England and Wales had a compulsory 'core' of health education, and there is evidence of increasing commitment to health education within undergraduate and postgraduate nurse training.[23] Progress in undergraduate medical education has been more limited, but vocational training for GPs has taken a lead in the medical field.

8. Adequate mechanisms for research, evaluation and monitoring

Our report frequently identifies deficiencies in basic information essential to the evaluation and monitoring of public health action. This has led to a number of RHAs and DHAs conducting their own expensive and widely differing kinds of local community health survey. While this is welcome, there is a need to develop a uniform, essential database for health along the lines developed in Canada and the USA where there are regular, national health surveys which include detailed information on the health of different income and ethnic groups. The recent announcement by the government of plans to develop a 'health promotion index' in the UK are thus welcome, although they fall far short of the scope of national health surveys in north America.

Evaluation of public health action is often absent or patchy, and the tools for measuring success are inadequate. Measures designed to reduce coronary heart disease are now beginning to be systematically evaluated through reductions in risk factors, measures of the implementation process and ultimately by reductions in the incidence and mortality from the disease.[24] It is not easy, however, to devise appropriate methods for measuring the effectiveness of a health visitor working with a local community or with pensioners' groups, whose aim is to increase autonomy and community participation. These are two examples of research challenges that the community development approach presents. These challenges need to be met with new, constructive forms of evaluation, rather than blanket criticism.

Developing a strategy for the 1990s (Chapters 15–17)

We believe that a public health strategy should be directed towards the attainment of three overall health goals:

1 longevity;
2 a good quality of life;
3 equal opportunities for health.

From our analysis we have been able to identify 11 priority areas where public health action will result in major improvements in the nation's health. We have set out a plan of action for each with general objectives and quantified targets – where possible – to be achieved by the end of the century. We identify the expected health outcomes of each element of the strategy and make detailed recommendations to the following agencies.

- government;
- health promotion agencies;
- the communications media;
- training institutions;
- local authorities;
- health authorities;
- primary health care;
- employers, industry and trades unions.

The strategy has three interconnecting parts:

1 Resources for Health (Chapter 15) The first part of our strategy identifies the following elements which are essential for an effective overall strategy to promote public health:

- effective coordination and organisation at national and local levels;
- adequate funding;
- long-term commitment and programme planning;
- well-defined research and evaluation.

2 Lifestyles for health (Chapter 16) In the second part of our strategy we make detailed recommendations on the following aspects of lifestyle:

- reducing cigarette consumption;
- promoting a healthy diet;
- promoting regular physical activity;
- reducing alcohol consumption;
- promoting healthy sexuality;
- promoting road safety.

3 Preventive services for health (Chapter 17) In the third, and final part of the strategy, we make detailed recommendations on the following preventive services:

- maternity services;
- dental health;
- immunisation;
- early cancer detection;
- blood pressure reduction.

2 Statistics of mortality: the last decade

The health of the people is really the
foundation upon which all their
happiness and all their powers as a state
depend.

BENJAMIN DISRAELI

Introduction A country's health is not easily described in quantitative terms. No country could maintain a continuous record of the state of health of all its citizens and few countries attempt the systematic analysis of all records of contact between sick people and the health care services. Limited statistical analysis is usually routinely carried out on records of hospital inpatient stays and occasional surveys are conducted of outpatient contacts. Perhaps surprisingly, some of the most useful statistics of the public health are derived from medical certification of cause of death.

Most developed countries keep fairly complete and reliable records of deaths, and death is a unique, unambiguous event relating to the life and health of an individual. The certified causes of death are medical opinions and within broad categories can be relied on. Data on gender, age at death, place of death and the usual occupation followed by the deceased are generally considered to be sufficiently reliably recorded to permit useful statistical analysis which gives a broad picture of a country's health and enables comparison with other countries and with other periods. It is useful to compare present performance in the UK with that of other countries and past performance with the UK. In this chapter, we present briefly some of the salient features of recent trends in mortality because they identify some important problems that we consider in later chapters.

Mortality and longevity Statistics of deaths are usually presented as mortality rates (numbers of deaths in a period divided by the numbers in the related population or population sub-group). Since the risk of dying is very different at different ages and since different populations have different age structures it is a common practice to calculate a summary index which is so constructed that mortality at different times and places may be compared in spite of differences in population age structures. Life-tables provide a suitable summary index called the 'expectation of life'. The expectation of life at birth is essentially a current average age at death, and we can also calculate

21

Figure 1 Improvements in expectation of life in Great Britain (1972–1984)

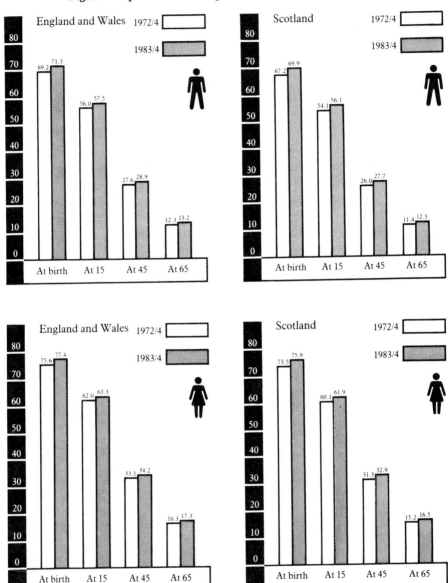

Sources: OPCS. Monitor, DH1 14. Table 22.
Registrar General for Scotland. Annual Report. Table J1.1.

expectations of further life at various ages beyond birth.

These 'expectations of life' are usually calculated from the death rates in a particular calendar year. They therefore summarise the risk of death of people born in many different years, and are thus neither a summary nor a prediction of *life expectancy* for any particular year's newborn individuals. Nevertheless, they are widely used and are useful summary statistics.

Expectation of life

Expectation of life has improved in most countries over the period for which statistics have been available. The expectations of life at birth for all countries in the UK (for 1983 deaths) are now higher than ever previously recorded. For men in England and Wales the figure was just over 71 years, and for women just over 77 years – reflecting the generally lower mortality at each age for women than for men. During the decade ending in 1983 the expectation of life at birth increased by 2.3 years for men and 1.8 years for women. Similar improvements have been recorded for Scotland (see Figure 1).

As the expectation of life at birth is essentially the average age at death, it is affected by changes in mortality rates at all ages. The great improvement that has taken place during the present century is mainly due to the considerable reductions that have occurred in mortality during infancy and childhood, but there have been improvements at all ages and mortality among older people has also improved in the last two decades. For England and Wales, the expectation of further life at age 65 increased by seven per cent for men and by six per cent for women between 1972 and 1983 (see Figure 1).

International comparisons

The duration of life in this country compares favourably with that in other comparably developed countries in Europe or elsewhere, although Japan, the Netherlands, Norway and Australia do better than the UK (see Figure 2). This is mainly because we have a relatively low infant mortality (the number of deaths in the first years of life per 1,000 live births), and a very low mortality among young adults. Our expectation of further life beyond the age of 45 is much less satisfactory, and is among the worst in north western Europe (see Figure 2).

Mortality in infancy

Mortality in infancy has traditionally been recognised as a good guide to the general quality of both health care and the standard of living in a country. In common with those of most other European countries, infant mortality rates have fallen substantially in the UK (see Figure 3), although they have fallen less rapidly than in some other countries. In 1966, England and Wales had the seventh lowest

Figure 2   Expectation of life at birth and middle age – an international comparison (1982–1984)

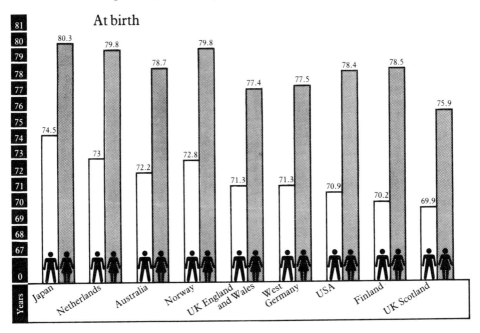

At birth

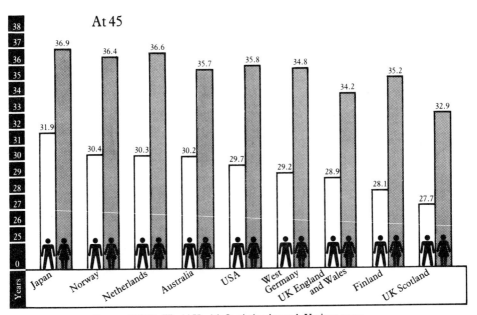

At 45

Source: WHO. World Health Statistics Annual. Various years.

24

infant mortality rate out of 14 countries in north western Europe, but by 1984 its position had dropped to ninth. Northern Ireland remained eleventh and Scotland tenth (see Table 1).

However, the overwhelming majority of deaths in the first year occur in the first week of life, and many of those early deaths occur on the first day. It is therefore useful to look at what is known as the perinatal mortality rate (the number of stillbirths and deaths in the first week of life expressed usually as a rate per 1,000 total births). Although perinatal mortality rates have fallen substantially in each of the UK countries (see Figure 4), they remain important because they now account for a large proportion of all mortality in pre-adult life, since death in childhood and adolescence is now relatively uncommon. Perinatal mortality in the UK is relatively high compared with other countries in north western Europe (see Table 1). The principal reasons for this are that the UK has a relatively high prevalence of congenital malformations at birth, as well as a higher than average proportion of babies born at low weight (less than 2500 gm – see Chapter 11). Furthermore, there seems to be much greater variation in perinatal mortality among the different regions of the UK and among the social classes than in some other countries.

Figure 3   Trends in infant mortality, England and Wales (1900–1984) and Scotland (1941–1984)

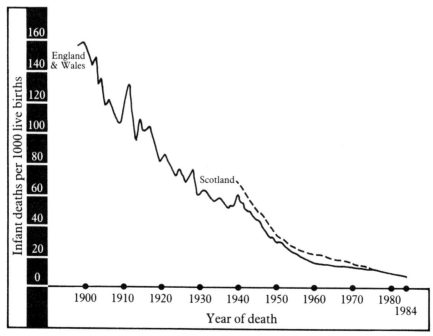

Sources: OPCS. OPCS Monitor, DH3 85/3, 13 August 1985.
Registrar General for Scotland. Annual Report. Table D1.2

Postneonatal mortality rates (deaths between age one month and one year expressed usually as a rate per 1,000 live births) offer extra insight into potentially preventable deaths in infancy, because they are sensitive to social and environmental circumstances – especially socioeconomic factors.[1] Although there has been little change in postneonatal mortality since 1980 (see Chapter 8) the longer term trend between 1969 and 1982 has been downward. Against this background there has been a dramatic rise in the mortality attributed to sudden infant death syndrome (SIDS) sometimes called 'cot deaths'. These trends have given rise to considerable concern as SIDS has now become one of the major causes of postneonatal mortality. However, much of the observed rise in SIDS may reflect increased recognition and reporting of this syndrome on death certificates.[2] Nevertheless, SIDS is clearly an important cause of loss of life in infancy. In Chapter 11, we discuss the scope for its prevention.

Mortality in adolescence and adulthood In contrast with very early life, mortality rates in adolescence and early adult life are comparatively low in the UK. This is mainly a consequence of the favourable mortality from accidents in the UK – especially traffic accidents (see Chapter 6). The UK does particularly badly however (although it is not alone in this) in expectation of

Table 1 Crude mortality rates in infancy: selected countries in north western Europe between 1966 and 1980–1984

| | Crude mortality rates /1000 total births in infancy | | | |
| | *Infant mortality* | | *Perinatal mortality* | |
	1984/5	percentage reduction 1966–1984	1980/81	percentage reduction 1966–80/81
Finland	6.5	57	9.4[1]	57
Sweden	6.7	49	8.7	54
Switzerland	7.1	58	9.2	58
Netherlands	7.9	39	10.8	52
France	8.0	62	13.0	53
Norway	8.3	43	11.0	48
Belgium	9.4	57	13.7	51
W Germany	9.6	59	10.6	62
England and Wales	10.2	46	11.8	56
Scotland	10.3	56	13.2	56
N Ireland	10.5	59	15.7	50
Luxembourg	11.7	56	10.3	56
Austria	11.4	59	12.0	60

[1] Data is for 1979
Source: World Health Statistics Annual. Geneva, World Health Organization, various years.

Figure 4   Trends in perinatal mortality, England and Wales (1928–1984) and Scotland (1941–1984)

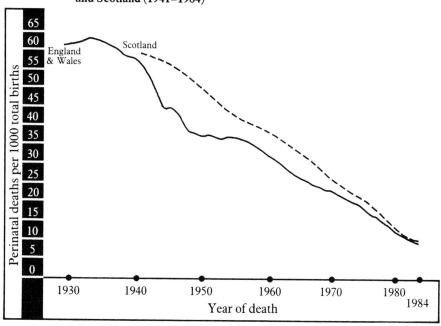

Sources: OPCS. Infant and perinatal mortality 1984. OPCS Monitor, DH3 85/3.
Registrar General for Scotland. Annual Report. Table D1.2.

further life beyond the age of 45. In these age groups mortality rates from coronary heart disease, strokes and cancers are much higher than those for many other European countries, (see Chapters 3 and 4).

Over 50 per cent of all deaths before the age of 85 are attributed to cancers and heart disease. Since there is good reason to believe that many of the deaths from these causes are potentially avoidable, we shall consider a detailed strategy for their prevention in later chapters.

Consequences of mortality trends   The substantial decline in mortality that has taken place over the past 150 years would have resulted in an even greater population increase than has taken place were it not that the annual number of live births has also substantially declined over much the same period. The net population effect of these remarkable changes has been a considerable relative increase in the proportion of older people.

This 'ageing' of the population is likely to continue beyond the end of the present century (see Chapter 14). Since the risk of developing serious illness increases with age, and the diseases characteristic of later life tend to be chronic and difficult to treat, the

27

effect of the changes in mortality and fertility has been to increase the need for health care in most industrial countries. This has distracted attention from preventive opportunities and has led to a heavier concentration on the treatment of established illness and on the care of those disabled by it. Although success in prevention tends to increase the need for caring services for an older population, there is little doubt that the average human life-span is very favourably affected by measures which not only postpone the onset of lethal and disabling conditions, but greatly enrich the quality of life overall. Despite having to abandon the older naive assumptions that success in prevention would pay for itself by reduced needs for treatment services, we can continue to argue that successful prevention enhances the quality of life over the major part of the life-span.

3 Today's epidemics: circulatory diseases

It is often necessary to make a decision
on the basis of knowledge sufficient for
action, but insufficient to satisfy the
intellect.

IMMANUEL KANT

Introduction

In Chapter 2 we identified the potential for reducing the burden of premature death in middle age by reducing the incidence of circulatory disease and cancers. In this chapter we consider the causes of coronary heart disease and stroke, and the means by which their incidence might be reduced. We compare the UK record over the last decade with that of other countries where more progress has been made. Later on, in Chapter 7, we consider in detail the evidence concerning policies needed to reduce the risk factors for heart and other diseases.

Coronary heart disease and stroke

Coronary heart disease (CHD) is the leading cause of death in the UK. In 1984 it accounted for 175,000 deaths among British men and women. Each year, 100,000 people suffer a stroke and in 1984 22,000 people in England and Wales died of stroke. Coronary heart disease and stroke have causes in common and thus common measures might be expected to reduce the incidence of both. The total cost of heart disease to the community is difficult to calculate, but estimates for 1979 suggest that CHD was responsible for the loss of 26 million working days. The Office of Health Economics estimated that in 1985–6, heart disease cost the NHS nearly £390 million.[1]

What causes heart disease and stroke?

The evidence suggests that the disease process begins early in life. Although no sector of society is immune, those with the highest death rates are men and women in the manual classes[2] (see Chapter 8), and men and women of Asian origin.[3] Although in middle age the death rate is up to five times as high for men as for women, the rates become similar in old age when heart disease is the leading cause of death for women as well as for men.

Risk factors for heart disease and stroke

A decade and a half of intensive research has clarified many of the doubts about the importance of cigarette smoking, blood cholesterol and diet, and high blood pressure – the 'classical' risk factors – in heart disease (see Table 2). Further light has also been shed on the

Table 2   Known risk factors for coronary heart disease and stroke

Risk factor	Relationship to	
	Coronary heart disease	*Stroke*
'Classical' risk factors		
Cigarette smoking	Causal	Causal in association with oral contraception
		Association recently shown for other kinds of stroke too
High blood cholesterol	Causal	Nuclear relationship
High blood pressure	Causal	Causal
Other risk factors		
Obesity	Possibly causal but acts mainly through other risk factors	Causal
Diabetes	Probably causal	Causal
Physical inactivity	Probably causal	?
Social class	Independent association	Association
Psychosocial factors	Strong independent association with lack of social support, work stress	?
Heavy alcohol consumption	Strong independent association	Strong independent association
Soft tap water	Association	?
Family history	Strong association	?

role of other risk factors such as physical inactivity, obesity and diabetes. The causes of stroke have received less attention but high blood pressure is an identifiable cause.

These conclusions are supported in numerous WHO and international expert reports on coronary heart disease in the last decade.[4-11] In the UK the Royal College of Physicians/British Cardiac Society[12] in 1976, followed by the British Cardiac Society's update in 1987,[13] the DHSS report[14] *Diet and Cardiovascular Disease* from its Committee on Medical Aspects of Diet (known as the COMA report), and the National Advisory Committee on Nutrition report[15] in 1983 (known as the NACNE report) have come to similar conclusions.

Cigarette smoking

Smoking is estimated to be responsible for one in four of all deaths from coronary heart disease.[16] The risk of developing heart disease in middle age is more than three times as great for someone who smokes more than 20 cigarettes a day as for a non-smoker. Stopping smoking is of major importance in reducing the risk of heart disease, and those who have already had a heart attack can halve their future risk of another by stopping smoking.[17] We do not know which of about 3000 identifiable components in cigarette smoke are responsible for heart disease: the case against nicotine is not entirely convincing and the case against carbon monoxide is weak.[18] The shift to lower tar cigarettes (see Chapter 4) is *not* demonstrably associated with a lower risk of heart disease.[19]

Cholesterol and diet

The higher the cholesterol level in the blood the greater the risk of heart disease.[20] The 20 per cent of people with the nation's highest cholesterol levels are three times more likely to die of heart disease than the 20 per cent with the lowest levels.[21] International trials using drugs or diet to lower blood cholesterol level have shown that there is a subsequent reduction in the risk of heart disease,[22] and the risk is commensurate with the extent to which cholesterol is lowered and the length of time over which the reduction has occurred.[23] When the results of 20 such trials of diet and drugs were statistically pooled, a 10 per cent reduction in blood cholesterol was associated with a 20–30 per cent reduction in heart disease.[24] The WHO and NACNE reports concluded that while there is no threshold level below which there is no risk of heart disease, a cholesterol level of 5.2 mmol/litre or less is associated with a low risk of heart disease in people over 30, and 4.7 mmol/litre in people under 30.

There has been uncertainty over how to define who is at high risk of heart disease according to their cholesterol levels. The available data from two British studies suggest the cholesterol levels are so high throughout the population that the *whole community* it at risk, and recent evidence shows that there is no threshold which clearly demarcates low or high risk populations.[25,26] In a study of middle aged men in 1978, cholesterol levels were generally above what American consensus holds to be a moderate or high risk.[27] In a more recent study of cholesterol levels among younger men and women, 63 per cent had levels that were above 5.2 mmol/litre.[28]

There is good evidence that the amount of saturated fat (derived mostly from animal fats) in the diet is an important determinant of cholesterol levels.[29-31] A reduction in cholesterol levels can be achieved through a reduction in total fats and saturated fats, an increase in polyunsaturated fats (mainly fat and oils of vegetable origin) and an increase in dietary fibre (roughage).[32]

By 1985, at least 65 expert groups worldwide had examined diet and disease – mostly heart disease – in the affluent world.[33] Although there is some diversity in their recommendations for diets that are commensurate with good health and the prevention of heart disease, most have the following common features:

- there should be a reduction in total energy derived from dietary fat;
- there should be a reduction in the intake of saturated fat (with some recommending small increases in the intake of polyunsaturated fats);
- there should be an increase in the intake of complex carbohydrate, starchy foods such as bread and potatoes, and fibre.

The COMA and NACNE reports differ slightly in their terms of reference: the COMA report focussed heavily on the prevention of coronary heart disease and on the role of dietary fats, while the NACNE report concerned itself with broader aspects of diet and health of which coronary heart disease was only a part. As a result, the NACNE recommendations are more comprehensive, but broadly agree with those from COMA on fats and coronary heart disease.

Table 3 shows that for those reports which have produced quantified goals there is a broad consensus concerning the reduction of total dietary fats, saturated fat, sugar and salt, and an increase in dietary fibre. The difference in amounts recommended by the NACNE and COMA reports for the reduction of energy derived from fats is partly due to the NACNE committee including calories from alcohol in its estimate.

What might be the effect of implementing such changes in the UK diet? Assuming the nation were able and prepared to comply, it has been estimated that the diet recommended by WHO might result in a 16.5 per cent reduction in average cholesterol levels and the COMA diet would result in a 12 per cent reduction.[34] This would leave 16 per cent and 38 per cent of the nation respectively with cholesterol levels that are above 5.2 mmol/litre. Although these predictions require testing, the more comprehensive recommendations of WHO (and NACNE in the UK) seem likely to achieve the most substantial health gains for the nation.

The National Food Survey is our best available guide to what the nation eats and embraces an annual estimate of all food bought for domestic consumption. In 1984, 42.6 per cent of the calories from the UK diet were derived from fat and 17 per cent from saturated fats – clearly much higher proportions than either the NACNE or COMA recommendations (see Table 3). Sugar intake was also high at 38 kg/person in 1984, and fibre low at an estimated 20 gm/person/day. Although there is no regular information on children's dietary habits, a survey of 10–14 year olds in Britain in 1983 suggested that children's diets were less healthy than those of adults and that the average proportion of energy derived from fat was 37–39 per cent, with one-third of children deriving more than 40 per cent. Moreover, school meals provide as much as 39–45 per cent of energy as fat.[35,36]

The high rate of heart disease among Asians living in the UK has led some to question whether dietary fat is a major contributory factor in heart disease. The assumption is that Asians eat a diet high in fibre, low in total fats and animal fats much like that of the average Indian in India.[37] This seemed to be the case in a survey of Asians (mostly Gujeratis) living in north west London,[38] but smaller studies in different Asian communities have shown that Bangladeshi men[39] and some Gujerati communities living in London have a high total fat intake and that fibre intake is not as high as is sometimes assumed.[40]

High blood pressure High blood pressure is a major contributory factor in both heart disease and stroke.[41,42] The higher the blood pressure, the greater

Table 3 A comparison of long-term, quantitative recommendations for dietary change

Dietary goal	Current British averages (NFS 1984)	WHO 1982	NACNE 1983	BMA 1986	COMA 1984
Percentage energy derived from total fat	42.6	30	30	30	35
Percentage energy from saturated fat	17	10	10	10	10
Sugar*	38Kg	Low	20Kg (includes hidden sugar)	20Kg (includes hidden sugar)	No increase
Salt	7–10gm/day	3.5gm/ day	reduction of 3gm/day	reduction of 3gm/day	No increase
Fibre**	20gm/day	30gm	30gm	30gm	Increase – no amount given

  * Derived from estimates of total sugar supplies for food use.
  ** Derived from 1982 estimate, COMA report.
Source: NFS National Food Survey.

the risk of heart disease. In any given population, the 20 per cent of people at the top of the blood pressure range have four times the risk of dying of heart disease compared with the 20 per cent at the bottom of the range.[43] Blood pressure patterns in the UK are such that a reduction in blood pressure of those at the highest risk end of the spectrum would have less impact than a reduction in blood pressure throughout the whole community.[44] A 10 mm decrease in the average blood pressure of the whole population might be expected to reduce the mortality attributable to heart disease by 30 per cent.[45]

Blood pressure is influenced by a combination of factors. Genetic factors, obesity, heavy drinking and a high dietary salt intake probably all play a part.[46] What we do not yet know is exactly how these factors interact with each other and with other ill-defined aspects of diet and heredity.

The WHO reports, together with the NACNE and COMA reports, have concluded that salt intake in the UK and other affluent countries is too high, and that salt is an important, potentially reducible determinant of high blood pressure. These conclusions are supported by evidence in the WHO reports and NACNE and COMA reports in the UK. They are based on incomplete evidence, however, for we have no firm information yet on whether a moderate reduction in salt intake can reduce blood pressure in otherwise healthy people. While the evidence falls short of proof, current levels of salt intake are so high that a small reduction would be without risk and likely to be of benefit. Because there is no clear difference between high and low risk groups, it is not sufficient to rely on drug treatment (secondary prevention). A reduction in salt intake throughout the population (primary prevention) if achievable, offers a more effective way of reducing the incidence of high blood pressure in the community.[47]

Blood pressure is not monitored on a national basis and is irregularly monitored in general practice. One large, individual study suggests that over one in five men (including those treated for high blood pressure) and 12 per cent of women aged 40–49 have blood pressures above the normal range.[48] These proportions were confirmed in a community survey in Wales in 1985 which showed that one in five 55–64 year olds were on drug treatment for high blood pressure.[49] There is no good evidence that people of Caribbean origin living in the UK have higher blood pressure than the white or Asian people.[50] Average daily dietary salt intake in the UK has been estimated to be at least twice as much as that recommended by WHO and NACNE.[51]

Mildly increased blood pressure

The value of treating moderate or severely increased blood pressure (systolic over 150: diastolic over 104 mm Hg) in the under 65s is not in dispute. It is less clear whether *mild* increases in blood pressure (systolic over 150 and diastolic 95–104 mm Hg) should also be treated. This question was addressed recently by the Medical Research Council (MRC) in a major randomised controlled trial of drug treatments (bendrofluazide and propranolol) in 30–64 year olds.[52] The results showed that while treatment reduced the incidence of stroke, there was no significant effect on heart disease. Despite the beneficial effect on stroke the overall consensus at present is that the benefits do not outweigh the risks[53] for the following reasons.

- It was estimated that 850 people would have to be treated for a whole year in order to prevent one stroke.
- The drugs used have troublesome side effects.
- There is a tendency of up to one-third of people with mild increases in blood pressure to return to normal *without any treatment*; moreover non-pharmacological approaches such as relaxation can in some instances be just as effective as drugs.[54]

Other risk factors: obesity and diabetes

Obesity (a weight that is 20 per cent or more above the upper limit of a standard range for a given age) and overweight (a weight that is 10–19 per cent above the upper standard range) pose a threat to health.[55] In particular, obesity is associated with heart disease, and probably contributes by increasing the risk of high blood pressure and diabetes and by raising blood cholesterol levels. For each 14 lb excess in weight there is an associated 4 mm increase in blood pressure. Levels of overweight and obesity are high among both adults and children in the UK. By the age of 11, six per cent of boys and 10 per cent of girls are overweight or obese, and this figure rises to about 12 per cent at 20. The proportion continues to rise in adulthood with about half of 50–60 year olds being overweight. Overall, 40 per cent of men and 32 per cent of women were overweight in 1981.[56]

Between one and two per cent of the population has diabetes[57,58] – about 90 per cent of which is related to overweight and obesity and is thus potentially preventable.[59] There is now renewed concern about the role diabetes might play in explaining the high death rates from heart disease among Asians. Evidence from India[60] and from Indian populations living in Trinidad[61] and the UK[62,63] has shown that the prevalence of diabetes is much higher in these communities than among people of other ethnic origins. The potential value of screening for diabetes in primary care has yet to be assessed, but dietary policies that will not only reduce blood cholesterol levels, but also obesity, and thus diabetes, offer most scope for prevention.

35

Physical activity

There is now strong evidence that physical activity is important in the prevention, not only of heart disease, but a wide range of other conditions as well – including obesity and high blood pressure. The kind of exercise needed is vigorous, aerobic exercise about two to three times a week, and we review the evidence in Chapter 9.

Socioeconomic and psychosocial factors

Working class men (there is no equivalent UK research among women) are over three and a half times more likely to die of heart disease than professional men, and this association persists after other risk factors are taken into account.[64] We do not know how the socioeconomic environment exerts its effect, but it is a relatively recent phenomenon – as the class gradient in heart disease before the 1960s was in the opposite direction. Recent research suggests that it may be in part related to the subjective levels of stress, which may in turn affect smoking rates (see Chapter 8). Past research into the nature of such stresses is difficult to interpret (see Chapter 9). In the field of heart disease, research has largely been limited to a search for the 'coronary prone' personality[65,66] which has produced equivocal findings.[67] Some promising recent research has focussed on the specific *kinds* of stress experienced in the workplace (see Chapter 14), and suggests that it may be a *combination* of high demands at work together with a lack of control over the decision-making process at work that is associated with the high rates of heart disease among manual workers.[68]

Soft water, alcohol and coffee

Soft water[69] and coffee[70] are also associated with heart disease. In the case of coffee, there is a suggestion from prospective studies in the USA that coffee increases cholesterol levels, and that the risk of heart disease rises in proportion to the amount drunk.[71] We do not know what role alcohol plays in heart disease, as research findings have been inconsistent.[72,73]

Intervention to reduce heart disease

Once a firm link between a potential factor and a disease is established, the most powerful way to demonstrate its causal contribution is to show that a reduction in this risk factor leads to a reduction of disease. This may be tested in a randomised controlled trial where the aim is to compare the outcome of an intervention in a test group with a comparison or control group which does not receive the intervention. In the case of coronary heart disease, trials are usually complex and involve multiple interventions including dietary advice or treatment, advice and support to reduce smoking, treatment of high blood pressure and the promotion of exercise. For stroke, trials have focussed mainly on the treatment of high blood pressure. Despite methodological problems, most of the major randomised controlled trials to reduce heart disease demonstrate a

Figure 5   Trends in coronary heart disease by age group, England and Wales (1974–1984)

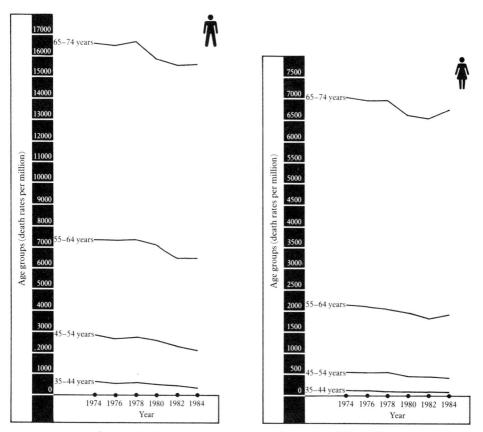

Source: OPCS Mortality statistics. Cause. Series DH2. 1974–1984.

clear relationship between risk factor reduction and reduction in the incidence or mortality from heart disease and stroke.[74]

The most carefully conducted community-based trials such as the North Karelia project in Finland[75] and the WHO Collaborative Study[76] have shown reductions in heart disease risk factors in the long term, and that the size of the reduction is proportional to the size of reduction in heart disease.

Are we meeting the challenge? There has been a long-awaited but small decrease in death rates from heart disease in men and women in England and Wales since 1978. It has occurred in all age groups (see Figure 5). The biggest reductions in heart disease since 1978 have occurred among middle-aged men, and to a lesser degree among middle-aged women. Between 1974 and 1984 death rates among 45–54 year olds fell by 22 per cent for men and 17 per cent for women.

The fall in mortality from stroke has been much more dramatic at about 30 per cent for England and Wales, Scotland and Northern Ireland between 1971–3 and 1982–3 (see Figure 6). We cannot explain this decline, but it has occurred in many other affluent countries.

The downward trend in heart disease in the UK has so far been much smaller than in the USA, Finland, Australia and elsewhere (see Figure 7). Moreover, rates in Wales have actually increased. This leaves Northern Ireland and Scotland, followed by England and Wales, with the highest death rates in the world. In the ten years to 1980, death rates from heart disease fell over three times as fast in the USA and Australia as in the UK, and nearly twice as fast in Japan. If heart disease rates in the UK had fallen at the same rate as in the USA or Australia, an estimated 25,000 deaths would have been avoided during this period.[77]

Knowledge and attitudes   Knowledge of the risks of heart disease appears to have improved, although comparative data from a decade ago are not available. A majority of Welsh men and women surveyed in 1985 (in all age groups) identified some of the risk factors for heart disease; nearly half thought too much alcohol, too little exercise and too much stress

Figure 6   International trends in stroke mortality in selected countries between approximately 1970 and 1980

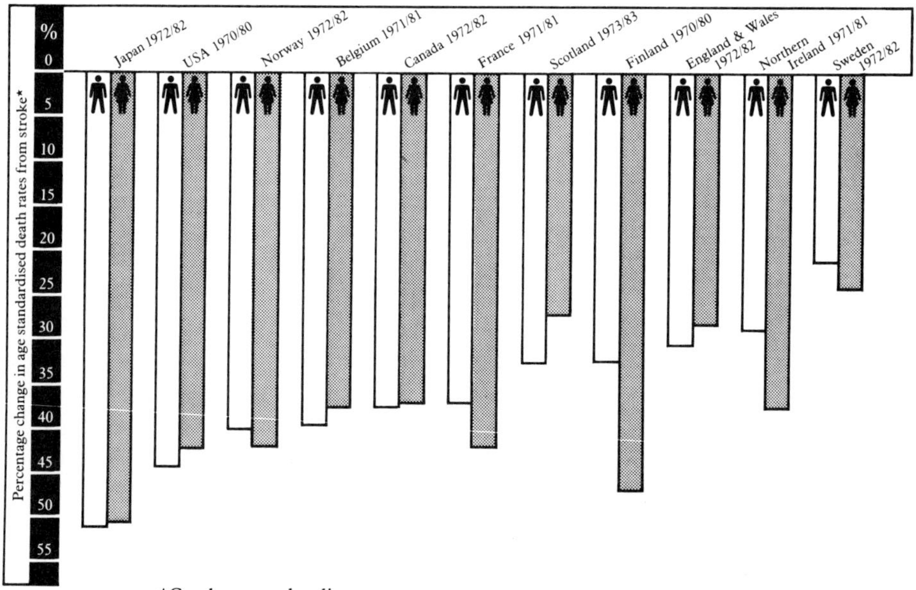

*Cerebrovascular disease
Source: Uemura K, Pisa Z. Recent trends in cardiovascular disease mortality in 27 industrialised countries. World Health Statistics Quarterly 1985, 38: 142–162.

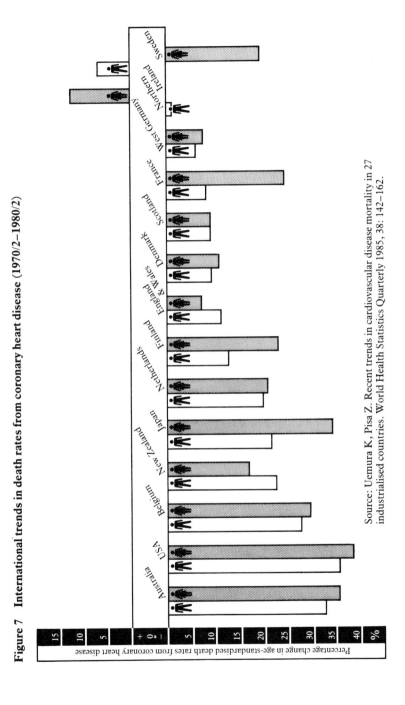

Figure 7 International trends in death rates from coronary heart disease (1970/2–1980/2)

Source: Uemura K, Pisa Z. Recent trends in cardiovascular disease mortality in 27 industrialised countries. World Health Statistics Quarterly 1985, 38: 142–162.

Figure 8   Trends in United Kingdom fatty acid intakes (1974-1984)

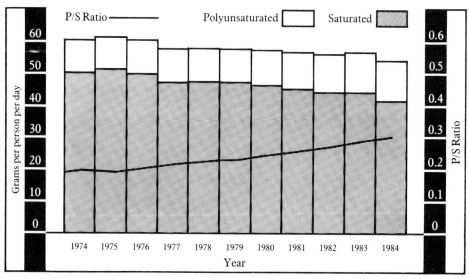

Source: Ministry of Agriculture, Fisheries and Foods. Household food consumption and expenditure. Annual Report of National Food Survey Committee. Various years.

were important. Indirect information on their doctors' activities suggested that GPs in Wales were likely to give advice on stopping smoking, but unlikely to give advice on diet, weight or alcohol consumption.[78] A UK-wide market research survey among women in 1984 confirmed the shift in attitudes towards healthier eating, suggesting that a majority took healthy eating seriously.[79]

How can the trends be explained? The impressive mortality decline in the USA is mostly due to decreasing incidence of heart attacks – as is the case in Australia and Finland too – although improved treatment has made a contribution.[80,81] Despite inadequate information, some of the available evidence links the decline in the USA to a reduction in the major risk factors:[82,83] chiefly in cholesterol decreases and in the consumption of foods containing high levels of saturated fat, and increases in sales of food high in polyunsaturated fats, together with decreases in cigarette smoking and small increases in exercise among adults.[84] The proportion of hypertensives being treated increased from 10–15 per cent of those needing treatment in the 1960s, to a majority in all socioeconomic and ethnic groups today.[85] It is estimated that 800,000 premature deaths have been prevented in the USA since 1968.[86]

The British position Unlike the USA and Canada, the UK has no comprehensive national risk factor monitoring system. We must, therefore, rely on more fragmented data sources which are often difficult to interpret over time. The continuing decline in cigarette consumption and in the prevalence of smoking may have contributed to some of the small decline in heart disease now beginning to be seen nearly everywhere in the UK. The National Food Survey shows that the British diet has improved in many respects. The ratio of polyunsaturated to saturated fat – the 'P/S ratio' – increased by 50 per cent between 1974 and 1984 (see Figure 8). This has been due to a combination of a 17 per cent decrease in saturated fat and a 20 per cent increase in polyunsaturated fat intake. Total fat consumption however has risen

Figure 9   United Kingdom per capita fat consumption (1952–1984)

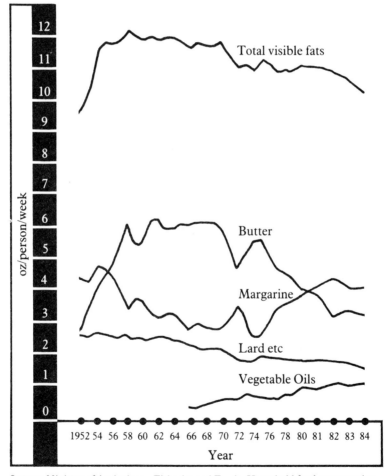

Source: Ministry of Agriculture, Fisheries and Foods. Household food consumption and expenditure. Annual Report of National Food Survey Committee. Various years.

41

as a proportion of the total energy derived from the diet. This is partly because total energy consumption has fallen.

Figure 9 shows that there has been a recent decrease in the consumption of both butter and milk which account for one-third of our total saturated fat intake. This, together with a parallel increase in the consumption of soft margarine and of skimmed milk, partly accounts for the recent increase in the 'P/S ratio' (see Figure 8).

Total sugar consumption per person (see Chapter 12) is also down by 17 per cent from 46 Kg in 1970 to 38 Kg in 1984. Although the most recent estimates (to 1982) for the total fibre content of the UK diet suggest that fibre intake has remained low at about 20 gm/ person/day, there has been a recent increase in wholemeal bread consumption (see Figure 10) which extends from the wealthy to the less well off. In 1975 white bread represented 90 per cent of total bread consumption, but had decreased to just over 50 per cent by 1986.

Although we have no systematic information, screening for high

Figure 10   Trends in white and wholemeal bread consumption in Great Britain (1975–1986)

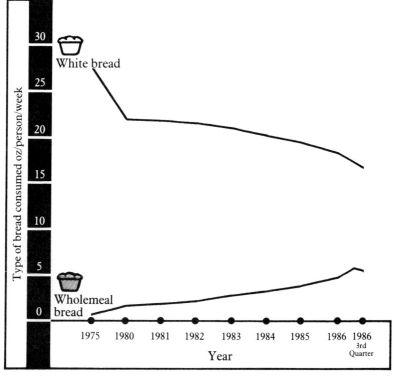

Source: Ministry of Agriculture, Fisheries and Foods. Household food consumption and expenditure. Annual Report of National Food Survey Committee. Various years.

blood pressure seems to be more commonplace. The Welsh community survey showed that two-thirds of men and over three-quarters of women had had their blood pressure checked in the last five years. Yet our most reliable evidence suggests screening and adequate treatment are far from satisfactory within primary care. A random assessment of practice notes in north west London showed that 47 per cent of those aged 30–65 had no blood pressure reading recorded in their notes; many patients were inappropriately treated after only one reading, and even more patients had no record of a follow-up blood pressure measurement.[87] Although individual commitment has shown excellent results both in disease reduction[88] and in screening levels,[89,90] the 'rule of halves' still seems to apply in general practice overall. Only half of people with high blood pressure are detected; half are treated, and only half followed up[91,92] – compared with about 80 per cent of Americans who claim to have their blood pressure checked twice a year.[93]

Long-term evidence on obesity suggests that increasing proportions of the community have become overweight in the last few decades.[94] While the General Household Survey suggests that people in this country are becoming more physically active (see Chapter 9), the changes have been small and we must await the results of the first national fitness survey for more accurate information relevant for heart disease.

4 Today's epidemics: cancers

Pessimism is a luxury we can't afford.

ANON

Introduction Having examined circulatory disease, the leading cause of death in the UK, we now turn our attention to the contribution made by cancers to overall mortality, and particularly to avoidable deaths in middle age. We consider, in more detail, what is known about the causes and potential avoidability of some cancers which account for a major proportion of mortality from cancer: lung cancer, cancer of the large bowel, breast cancer and cancer of the cervix. We then assess progress that has been made over the last decade in reducing mortality from each of these cancers. In Chapter 7 we move on to a detailed consideration of what measures might be necessary and effective in reducing the risk factors for avoidable cancers.

Cancers – how much is avoidable? Cancers are the second leading cause of death in the UK, and accounted for 24 per cent of all deaths in England and Wales in 1984. About 85 per cent of cancer is thought to be potentially avoidable.[1] Although we do not yet know enough about the causes of cancer, the two most important – cigarette smoking and diet – stand out clearly against the background of risk factors (see Table 4).

Nearly one in three cancer deaths are attributable to cigarette smoking and a further 35 per cent may be due to diet.[2] On the basis of current evidence, air pollution, food additives and other environmental causes together are unlikely to account for more than one–two per cent of all cancers (see Table 4). Although many of the compounds known to be linked to cancers are released from industry into the environment, there is no firm evidence, as yet, that they constitute a material cancer-risk *outside* the workplace.

Precise estimates for the contribution made by cancer-producing substances in the workplace to the overall burden of cancer are hard to obtain. Many registered chemicals used at work have yet to be fully tested for their carcinogenicity (cancer-producing potential). So far, relatively few workplace chemicals have been clearly linked to cancers. The best researched examples include asbestos which explains up to five per cent of deaths attributable to lung cancers, and the aromatic amines used in the rubber and dye industries have accounted for about 10 per cent of bladder cancer in men and five per cent in women.[3] Additionally, the risk of asbestos-related lung cancer is increased ten-fold by cigarette smoking.

44

Table 4   Proportion of cancer deaths attributable to different factors

Factor or class of factors	Best estimate	Range of acceptable estimates
	Percent of all cancer deaths	
Tobacco	30	25–40
Alcohol	3	2–4
Diet	35	10–70
Food additives	<1	−5–2
Reproductive and sexual behaviour	7	1–13
Occupation	4	2–8
Pollution	2	<1–5
Industrial products	<1	<1–2
Medicines and medical procedures	1	0.5–3
Geophysical factors	3	2–4
Infection	10?	1–?
Unknown	?	?

Source: Doll R, Peto R. The causes of cancer. Journal of the National Cancer Institute, 1981, 66: 1191–1308.

Is mortality from cancer rising? More than 152,000 men and women in Great Britain died of cancers in 1984. Overall cancer death rates, however, are *not* rising. Indeed, for some cancers (such as stomach cancer) they are *falling*. The overall cancer death rate offers only a limited picture of what is happening, because 'cancer' is an umbrella term for a wide range of *different* diseases – many with common causes. Total 'cancer' death

Table 5   The main causes of cancer mortality (England and Wales 1984)

	Rank	Type of cancer	Number of deaths	Proportion of cancer deaths %
MEN		All cancers	72,929	
	1	Lung	26,041	36
	2	Colorectal (large) bowel	8,291	11
	3	Prostate	6,248	9
WOMEN		All cancers	65,397	
	1	Breast	13,310	20
	2	Lung	9,698	15
	3	Colorectal	8,959	14
	4	Ovary	3,960	6
	5	Cervix	1,899	3

Source: Office of Population Censuses and Surveys. OPCS Monitor, DH2 85/3, 23 July 1985.

rates are heavily determined by a small number of the more common cancers.

Lung cancer is much the most common form of cancer (see Table 5) and contributes heavily to the overall cancer death rate. While the total cancer death rate is not rising, lung cancer rates among women are still rising rapidly and we consider the implications of these trends below.

Lung cancer –
the position
today

Among men, lung cancer rates have been falling since 1963 and are now declining in all age groups. Between 1974 and 1984 mortality from lung cancer among men in England and Wales fell by three per cent overall. Most impressive of all, however, has been the fall in lung cancer mortality among middle-aged men which halved between 1960 and 1983. The picture is different for women. Overall lung cancer death rates doubled between 1963 and 1983 although a downward trend among women under 50 has just begun (see Figure 11).

The death rates among women have accelerated so rapidly that lung cancer overtook breast cancer as the leading cause of cancer mortality among Scottish women in 1984. In England and Wales,

Figure 11   Gender difference in age-specific trends in lung cancer mortality (England and Wales)

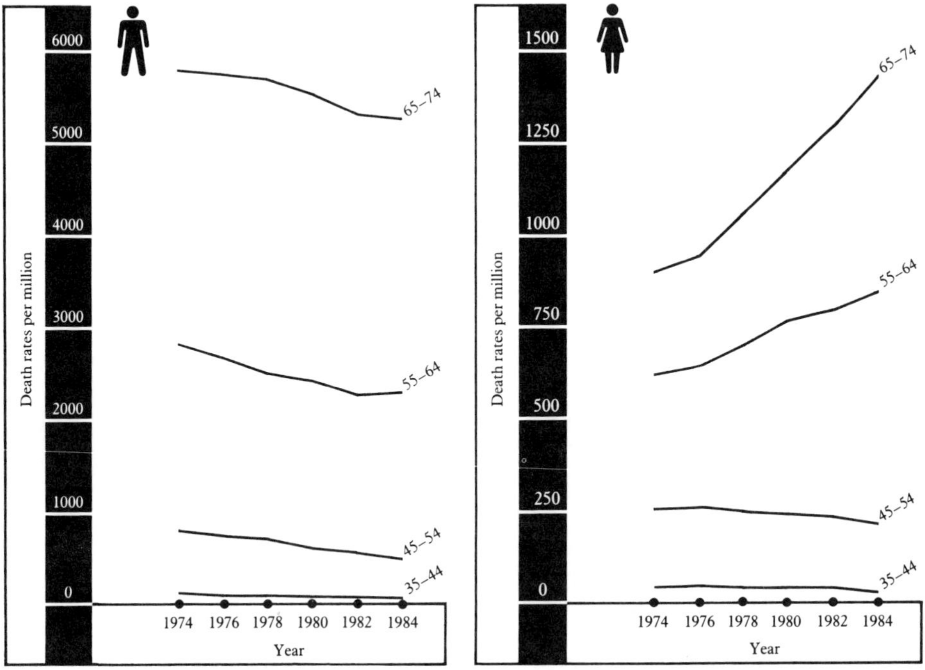

Source: OPCS. Mortality statistics. Cause. Series DH2. 1974–1984.

lung cancer rates are now approaching those for breast cancer in women over 55. Despite some encouraging changes among men, British lung cancer death rates were initially so much higher than those of most other countries that the UK – and Scotland in particular – still has the world's highest lung cancer death rates.

How can these trends be explained? Ninety per cent of all lung cancer mortality is attributable to cigarette smoking, which is also clearly linked to many other cancers, including those of the mouth, larynx, oesophagus, pancreas and bladder.[4] Since it also contributes to the deaths from coronary heart disease and chronic obstructive lung disease, smoking is estimated to kill 100,000 people in this country prematurely every year. The overall cost of cigarette smoking to the nation was estimated at £4,000 million.[5] Because it takes up to 30 years to develop lung cancer, and because the risk of developing it depends on the number of years smoked as well as on the amount smoked, past smoking trends are the main explanation for current patterns of lung cancer in men and women.

Men took up smoking in large numbers at the time of the first world war. The lung cancer epidemic we are now seeing in women occurred about a generation after that among men because the rapid

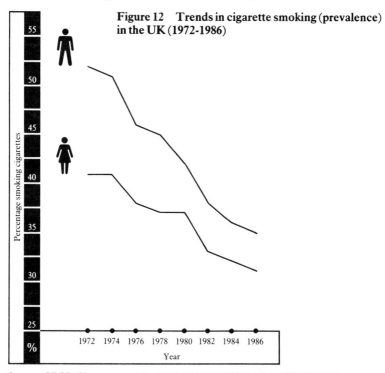

Figure 12   Trends in cigarette smoking (prevalence) in the UK (1972-1986)

Source: OPCS. Cigarette smoking 1972–1986. OPCS Monitor 1988. SS 88/1.

rise in smoking among women did not occur until during and after the second world war. The big reduction in lung cancer rates among middle-aged men is more a reflection of the changing *composition* of the cigarette over the last three decades as of changes in the *proportion* of smokers. Tar levels from cigarettes began to fall with the introduction of filters in the 1950s, but fell even more steeply (by 54 per cent) between 1965 and 1984. However, the reduction in tar levels has had *no* demonstrable effect on coronary heart disease which kills four times as many people as lung cancer.

Current smoking trends Smokers are now in a minority in every age and social group and a further decline seems probable. In the ten years to 1986 the proportion of adult smokers fell by 24 per cent among men and 18 per cent among women (see Figure 12); cigarette sales fell by 27 per cent over the same period and per capita consumption is also falling. Today's cigarettes yield over 50 per cent less tar than those of 20 years ago: average (sales weighted) tar and nicotine yields fell by 27 per cent between 1972 and 1983.

We have yet to be successful in two important matters: the socioeconomic disparity in smoking rates (see Chapter 8), and the lack of a downward trend in smoking among young people – girls in particular. In 1961, the year before publication of the Royal College of Physicians' first major report *Smoking and Health*, there were no social class differences in smoking rates. But by the 1970s, a steep, upward gradient between non-manual and manual classes was evident. Although smoking rates fell in all social groups between 1984 and 1986, the decline has been faster in the non-manual than manual classes in the last decade. In 1986, 26 per cent of men and women in the non-manual classes smoked compared with 40 per cent of men (36 per cent of women) in manual groups.

The proportion of regular smokers among secondary school children has remained stable between 1982 and 1986, although there has been a significant fall among boys since 1984 (see Table 6). There has been no similar fall among girls however, who were, for the first time, more likely to smoke than boys in all the UK countries in 1986. This narrowing of the gender gap is also reflected among adults in all groups except those age 60 or more.

New health concerns about tobacco We have focussed, so far, on the risks that cigarette smoking poses to smokers, but there is a growing body of research which suggests that passive smoking – the involuntary inhalation of other people's smoke – can cause lung cancer among non-smokers.[6,7] A review of the implications for the UK suggests that about 25 per cent of the lung cancers that occur in non-smokers (about 600 cases per year) are attributable to such passive smoking.[8]

Although other forms of tobacco use contribute less to overall tobacco-related mortality, efforts to launch a new form of sucking tobacco have caused concern as this form of tobacco is likely to cause cancers of the mouth and throat,[9,10] and evidence suggests that children are key promotional targets for this new product.[11] Proposed legislation to ban such products is thus welcome.

Why has cigarette smoking declined? The fall in cigarette smoking results from a combination of measures whose individual effects are not easy to disentangle. We analyse the determinants of consumption in more detail in Chapter 7.

Table 6   Smoking trends among secondary schoolchildren (England and Wales)

	Percentage of regular smokers[1] by school year									
	2nd		3rd		4th		5th		All years (1st–5th)	
	B	G	B	G	B	G	B	G	B	G
1982										
1984	2	2	9	7	19	15	26	28	11	11
1986	3	2	12	9	17	24	31	28	13	13
	2	2	5	6	8	18	19	30	7	12
	Total numbers interviewed									
1982	298	290	291	306	296	315	288	303	1460	1514
1984	396	364	409	338	392	341	395	340	1928	1689
1986	325	304	353	281	356	323	355	333	1676	1507

B – Boys   G – Girls

[1] Those smoking one or more cigarettes per week

Source: Goddard E, Ikin C. Smoking among secondary school children in 1986. London, HMSO, 1987.

Large bowel (colorectal) cancer In 1984, cancer of the large bowel claimed nearly 19,000 lives in Great Britain. It ranks as the second leading cause of cancer mortality among both men and women. The incidence of bowel cancer is eight times higher in this country than in southern Asia and north Africa.[12] There are wide variations within the UK itself: Scotland has higher rates than England and Wales, and there is a four-to-five-fold variation in incidence in Scotland.[13] This suggests that environmental factors may be involved – possibly dietary.

What causes cancer of the bowel? We do not know what causes bowel cancer, but some of the evidence – although it falls short of proof – suggests that diet plays an important role, as well as in other cancers and non-cancerous conditions.[14,15] A report from the Royal College of Physicians, *Medical Aspects of Dietary Fibre*, came to similar conclusions although it restricted its analysis to the role of dietary fibre.[16] The studies conducted so far show that the following aspects of diet tend to be correlated with high rates of bowel cancer:

- a diet high in total fat;
- a diet high in meat consumption;
- a diet low in fibre.

These findings have generated a series of different theories on how various dietary components might contribute to bowel cancer. In reality, it is difficult to tease out the relative contributions of meat, fat or dietary fibre, all of which are associated with an increased risk of bowel cancer, because diets low in dietary fibre tend also to be high in fats and meats.[17]

There are several kinds of evidence which suggest that a diet high in fibre may confer some protection from bowel cancer. First, fibre intake is high in many African and Asian countries where bowel cancer rates are low.[18] Second, the *pattern* of bowel cancer mortality in Britain is closely related to the daily intake of dietary fibre;[19] and third, the striking decreases in bowel cancer mortality rates which occurred in the UK between 1942 and 1962 may reflect the equally dramatic increase in dietary fibre intake during the second world war when cereal consumption more than doubled.[20] Lastly, the diet of patients with bowel cancer is generally lower in dietary fibre and higher in refined carbohydrate (mostly sugar) and fat than that of people who do not have bowel cancer.[21]

Mortality rates for bowel cancer have tended to stabilise for men since 1960, although there is evidence of a slow decline among women (see Figure 13). The incidence of bowel cancer has remained relatively unchanged, and five-year survival rates have improved little over the last decade. The reasons for the small decline in mortality among women are hard to explain, and are unlikely to be due to differences in treatment.

Early detection of bowel cancer
The principle of screening to detect early bowel cancer is attractive. The chances of long-term survival are increased from an average of 30 per cent at five years to 90 per cent if the tumour is diagnosed in its early stages.[22] There is now a test for detecting microscopic amounts of blood in the stools (occult blood tests) which is a sign of bowel cancer (but also of benign conditions). The test can be administered by people themselves or by primary care staff. Initial studies suggest that 57 per cent of patients offered such a test during a consultation can be persuaded to accept.[23] Enthusiasm for the early detection of bowel cancer has grown in the USA and numerous cancer agencies now recommend the test regularly for people over 40. These recommendations are probably premature, in the light of the available evidence.

Figure 13   Trends in mortality from bowel cancer in the UK (1910–1980)

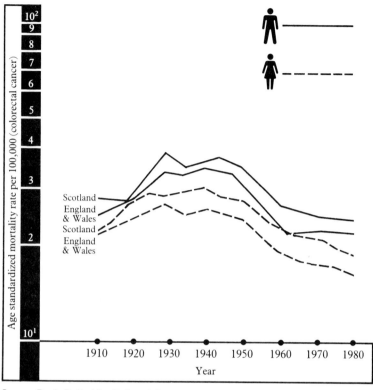

Source: Boyle P, Zaridze D G et al. Descriptive epidemiology of colorectal cancer. International Journal of Cancer 1985, 36: 9–18.

- First, there is no evidence yet that such a screening programme can reduce mortality from bowel cancer. There are major US and UK randomised controlled trials now underway.[24,25]
- It seems likely that only a small percentage of those with positive occult blood tests have bowel cancer – which makes the necessity to prove the efficacy of tests even more urgent.[26]
- Current evidence suggests that the predictive value of screening tests now available is limited.[27] Up to 30 per cent of bowel cancers may be missed, and as many as 50–80 per cent of people with positive tests do not have cancer at all.[28]
- Not enough is yet known about the natural history of progression from pre-cancer to cancer. Thus we do not yet know whether a policy of removing all pre-cancerous growths would be appropriate.
- The highest rates of bowel cancer occur in people over 70 and the ethics of imposing regular, potentially distressing procedures on

people who may later die from unassociated causes are difficult to resolve.[29]

Despite these reservations, the scope for prevention through screening may be substantial because those with a positive test who turn out to have bowel cancer are more likely to have *early* cancer which offers a much better chance of prolonged survival.

Breast cancer More British women die from breast cancer each year than from any other cancer. About 24,000 new cases are diagnosed each year and about 15,000 British women die from the disease each year. Over one-third of these deaths are among women under 65. Moreover, death rates from breast cancer are higher in the UK than elsewhere in western Europe. Although we do not yet know what causes breast cancer, there is good reason to believe that the environment plays an important role. British women are four times more likely to develop breast cancer than are Japanese women, but when Japanese women emigrate to the USA (where breast cancer rates are also high) the breast cancer death rates in their children become as high as in their counterparts in Europe.[30]

Of the numerous risk factors that have been investigated, those most strongly linked to breast cancer are: early menarche (age at first period) and first pregnancy delayed until after the age of 35.[31] These two factors, together with post-menopausal obesity, account for up to two-thirds of the difference in breast cancer rates between Japan and the USA.[32] There is also suggestive, but inconclusive, evidence linking a diet high in total fat to breast cancer.[33,34] This finding may be of considerable importance as the current tendency within the UK to derive an increasing proportion of energy from fat, rather than carbohydrate, (see Chapter 3) contributes to obesity, which is itself associated with breast cancer and early menarche.

The increasingly effective use of a number of treatments for breast cancer in which hormone receptors are blocked has led to a search for a hormonal basis for the disease. Although there is evidence that young British and American women have higher available levels of the hormone oestrogen than either Japanese or Asian women who have low breast cancer rates, we do not yet know the significance of these findings, or of how hormonal and other risk factors might interact. The impact of dietary change on the incidence of breast cancer is currently the subject of a major study in Stockholm and in the USA. More recently, attention has been concentrated on the potential relationship between the combined oral contraceptive pill and breast cancer. Research so far has largely been based on retrospective analysis and has been inconclusive. A number of studies have suggested that the pill is associated with an increased

52

risk of breast cancer among women who start taking it under the age of 25, and who continue to take it for eight or more years.[35-37] Other studies have failed to demonstrate this relationship, however,[38-40] and this includes one major prospective study among women in New Zealand who have higher rates of pill use than elsewhere.[41] The results of further prospective studies may help resolve this uncertainty.[42,43] Meanwhile, the best opportunity for reducing mortality from breast cancer lies in its earlier detection (see Chapter 7).

Breast cancer trends

Mortality from breast cancer has been increasing slowly for most of this century. Overall mortality rates for breast cancer increased by 25 per cent between 1963 and 1983. But there has been little change in either incidence or mortality in any specific age group over the last decade. The reasons for the slow increase are not known, and have not yet been shown to be associated with use of the pill. Social change that has led women to postpone their first pregnancy until a later age is thought to be important.[44]

Cervical cancer

About 2,000 British women died of cervical cancer in 1984. Although 70 per cent of deaths were among women over 55, as many as 17 per cent were among women under 44. All the evidence so far suggests that cervical cancer is essentially a preventable disease which is caused by a sexually transmitted agent. The risk is increased by early age of first intercourse, multiple sexual partners, and in the presence of sexually transmitted disease.[45]

Good evidence for the sexual transmissibility of cervical cancer comes from accumulating data which strongly suggest that variants of the human papilloma virus (HPV) – some of which cause genital warts – are the sexually transmissible agents.[46,47] Most, although not all, of the evidence supports this view.[48]

It is difficult to disentangle the relative contributions made by the various risk factors for cervical cancer, but multiple sexual partners among men and women,[49,50] cigarette smoking,[51,52] and use of the oral contraceptive pill[53] are each thought to make independent contributions. The use of the pill may increase risk in two ways. First, it does not offer a barrier to transmission of the virus in the way that the diaphragm or condom would[54] (see Chapter 7), and second, it may *specifically increase* a woman's risk of cervical cancer – although this evidence is not strong. Further research is needed to clarify the role of the pill in cervical cancer.

Trends in cervical cancer

Although overall mortality from cervical cancer is not increasing, and is decreasing in women over 40, death rates among 25–34 year olds increased between 1970 and 1982 in England and Wales and by similar proportions in Scotland and Northern Ireland. Incidence in this age group also increased over the same period. This pattern of increasing cervical cancer incidence and mortality among young women is consistent throughout the UK. If current trends continue, it has been estimated that 4,000 women will die each year of cervical cancer by the turn of the century.[55] Recent trends may reflect changes in both sexual behaviour and contraceptive practices in the last two decades (see Chapter 13), although these relationships are difficult to document. The fall in the use of barrier methods of contraception, and the growth in the use of the pill in the 1970s, are likely to have been important among young women (see Chapter 13). These trends offer scope for the prevention of cervical cancer, and also for the prevention of the spread of AIDS and sexually transmitted disease in general. We discuss these in Chapter 7.

Nuclear installations A complex problem that is now causing concern is the possible risk of cancer – especially of leukaemia – among children living near nuclear installations. There have been two broad approaches to research in this field. The first has investigated patterns of leukaemia in the vicinity of nuclear installations, and the second has analysed local radiation levels in the environment to see if they can account for the patterns observed. A DHSS enquiry[56] into the pattern of childhood leukaemia around the Sellafield nuclear plant in 1984 found a small excess of childhood leukaemia, but concluded that the amount of ionising radiation leaked or emitted from Sellafield appeared to be insufficient to account for the excess. Since then, a number of new findings have complicated these conclusions. First, there is now evidence that the emissions from Windscale (Sellafield) were 40 times greater than the evidence submitted to the DHSS enquiry had suggested.[57] Second, subsequent studies of other nuclear installations have shown similar excesses of childhood leukaemia.[58-60] The most comprehensive study so far has confirmed an increased incidence at other installations.[61,62]

The second line of research suggests that the environmental radiation levels measured at nuclear installations are generally too low to explain the excess incidence of leukaemia in the vicinity.[63] Possible explanations for these discrepant findings are that radiation levels may have been underestimated, that factors other than radiation explain clusters of leukaemia, or that repeated exposure of children to low dose radiation may be more hazardous than has previously been supposed. More research is needed to clarify these issues. Ultimately, the public health implications of nuclear energy need to be compared with those of other sources of energy such as coal – which has almost certainly been responsible for larger numbers of deaths and injuries than has nuclear power, both among those working in the industries and in the wider community.

5 Growing threats to public health

That action is best, which procures the
greatest happiness for the greatest
numbers.

FRANCIS HUTCHESON

Introduction This chapter examines alcohol-related harm and AIDS. Although
quite different problems, they have two important features in
common. Both are growing problems, and both account for a
substantial burden of premature death and suffering in early
adulthood. We first analyse the size and complexity of the challenge
presented by alcohol misuse, and the evidence for its involvement in
many health and social problems. We follow by examining trends in
alcohol consumption and in alcohol-related harm. Next we consider
the recent, rapid growth of AIDS, its causes and the pattern of its
distribution in the UK compared with other countries. We consider
predictions that have been made about future trends and the
potential impact it could have on the health of the nation. We assess
the implications of these findings for policy in Chapter 7.

**Alcohol – a
recurring threat
to public health** We have been slow, as a nation, to recognise the growing threat that
alcohol poses to health. This is partly because alcohol is an integral
part of British culture. Over 90 per cent of Britons drink (except in
Northern Ireland where 37 per cent are teetotal), and most enjoy
alcohol without apparently damaging themselves or others. In 1985
British adults over 15 drank the equivalent of 9.7 litres of pure
alcohol (over 16 pints) per head. This is the equivalent of 463 pints
of beer or 33 bottles of whisky per year for every man and woman in
the country. In 1984, more was spent on alcohol in the UK than on
clothes, and alcohol accounted for the equivalent of half of consumer
spending on food.

The range of medical, social and emotional damage caused by
alcohol is vast, but hard to quantify accurately. This is because
evidence concerning the possible contribution alcohol makes to
many health problems is still inadequate, and under-reporting of
alcohol on death certificates may lead to as much as a seven-fold
underestimate of the number of alcohol-related premature deaths.[1]
The Royal College of Physicians estimate that alcohol is responsible
for 25,000 premature deaths each year,[2] but other estimates suggest
the figure may be as high as 40,000.[3,4] In 1983 this was equivalent to
the loss of 88–144 million life years of expectation of life, and 64–
107,000 million working years.[5]

Table 7 gives an idea of the best-documented indices of alcohol-

Table 7   Alcohol misuse – some major indices of harm

Consequences of misuse	Degree of association with alcohol	Size of the problem (E & W 1984)
MEDICAL		
1 Cirrhosis of the liver	Risk proportional to daily consumption	2300 deaths
2 Cancers (Mainly digestive)	3% of all cancers alcohol-related 44-fold increased risk of oesophageal (gullet) cancer in smokers who drink heavily	c4000 deaths
3 Fatal road traffic accidents	35% alcohol-related	1500 deaths
4 High blood pressure	Risk increases with consumption	?
PSYCHOSOCIAL		
1 Alcohol dependence	100%	17,000 admissions to psychiatric hospitals (England 1983)
2 Public drunkenness	100%	108,000 convictions (1983)
3 Drinking and driving	100%	85,000 convictions (1983)

Sources: Office of Population Censuses and Surveys. OPCS Monitor, DH2 85/3, 23 July 1985.
DHSS. Mental illness hospitals and units in England: results from the Mental Health Enquiry 1983. Statistical Bulletin 1/85.
Brewers' Society. Statistical Handbook, 1984.
Home Office. Offences of drunkenness, England and Wales 1984.

related damage. In 1984, nearly 60 per cent of deaths from cirrhosis and chronic liver disease occurred before the age of 65, and up to 1,500 deaths on the roads were estimated to be alcohol-linked in 1985 (see Chapter 6). The risk of developing cirrhosis of the liver, cancer of the oesophagus (gullet) and alcohol dependence increases directly with the amount of alcohol drunk and the number of years of excessive drinking.

Although mortality from cirrhosis is neither the only, nor the most important consequence of the misuse of alcohol, it is a good indicator of trends. This is because alcohol is the most important cause of liver cirrhosis in the UK – whereas many factors must be taken into account when interpreting other alcohol-related indices. Death rates from cirrhosis of the liver also offer the most reliable way of comparing the consequences of alcohol misuse between countries. The results demonstrate that the higher the per capita alcohol

Table 8   Alcohol misuse – consequences or associations?

Problem	Per cent alcohol-related
1 General psychiatric admissions	20
2 Parasuicide	60
3 Divorce	30
4 Domestic violence	40
5 Child abuse	30
6 Assault	78
7 Criminal damage	88

Sources: Scottish Health Education Coordinating Committee. Health education in the prevention of alcohol-related problems. Edinburgh, SHECC, 1985.
Royal College of Psychiatrists. Alcohol. Our favourite drug. London, Tavistock, 1986.

consumption, the higher the death rates from cirrhosis of the liver.[6,7] Despite the high levels of alcohol-related harm that now exist in the UK, England and Wales still enjoy relatively low rates (Scottish rates are higher) compared with many other European countries.

Table 8 shows that alcohol is related to many other important medical and psychosocial problems and is one of many possible causal factors. The possible relationship between alcohol and damage to the unborn baby is one which has received more publicity than the evidence currently warrants. While heavy drinking in pregnancy is harmful to the fetus,[8] there is no good evidence yet to support recommendations for complete abstention. Indeed, the fetal alcohol syndrome is rare in the UK, and surveys suggest that most women drink very little during pregnancy.[9]

While Table 8 shows that alcohol misuse is related both to divorce and to child abuse it would clearly be an oversimplification to suggest that excessive drinking is the sole factor involved. Indeed, research is a long way from establishing the extent to which excessive drinking causes the problem, or whether marital disharmony itself (or some other problem) leads to excessive drinking.

Types of problem drinking   Problem drinking used to be seen as a practice confined to an 'aberrant' sector of the community who were known as 'alcoholics'. This is now known not to be the case as there are three identifiable kinds of problem drinking, of which alcohol dependence ('alcoholism') forms only a small proportion (see Table 9). It is important to identify the different kinds of problem drinking because they are associated with three different categories of alcohol-related harm.

- Those resulting from acute intoxication which can be either medical (such as accidents) or social such as the loss of a job or arrest for drunkenness.

- Those resulting from regular consumption over many years which are mainly medical, such as toxic damage to the liver, brain or pancreas.
- Those resulting from the development of dependence which can be a combination of medical and social problems arising in the other two categories.

Table 9   Types of problem drinking

Type	Estimate of number at risk in England and Wales	Per cent of population
Heavy drinking (showing biochemical abnormality)	3 million	8
Problem drinking (drinking which results in harm to the drinker or others)	700,000	2
Alcohol dependence	150,000	0.4

Source: Office of Health Economics. Alcohol: reducing the harm. London, OHE, 1981.

Although estimates vary according to assumptions made, Table 9 shows that three million or more people are heavy, problem drinkers. However, research confirms that while the heaviest drinkers are individually at most risk of harm, the *biggest burden* of alcohol-related ill health is to be found among those who are *less heavy drinkers*, because they are more numerous.[10] Thus, measures likely to confer maximum benefit to the community are those which reduce total alcohol consumption for the population rather than those which focus on a small, high risk minority which is often hard to reach.

The costs and benefits of alcohol

In 1983 the consequences of alcohol were estimated to have cost the nation more than £1,800 million (see Table 10). Although this estimate is based on incomplete data, it gives us an idea of the size of the total burden imposed by alcohol misuse on society. The benefits conferred by alcohol, on the other hand, are even harder, if not impossible, to quantify in monetary terms. While it is true that alcohol generated £6,346 million in tax revenue for the government in 1986–7 its misuse represents a loss to the individual. It also generates an estimated 125,000 jobs (directly or indirectly), and a trade surplus of about £500 million per year. Economists might argue that consumers must greatly value their drink if they are prepared to pay £35 million a day for it. But in our view – which is shared by WHO,[11] the Royal Colleges of Psychiatrists,[12] Physicians,[13] and General Practitioners,[14] and the BMA[15] – the magnitude of the harm caused by alcohol misuse requires urgent action.

Levels of excessive drinking

For cigarettes, all smoking – except for the tiny minority who smoke less than five cigarettes a day – is dangerous. But for alcohol, the evidence suggests that it is only damaging with excess or inappropriate use. In public health terms, it is difficult to define inappropriate drinking and who is most at risk of being harmed. This is because of inadequate information on hazardous drinking levels – we do not know enough about how alcohol affects different personal, social and biochemical factors. The risk of damage depends not only on the amount drunk, but on the body system considered, the weight and experience of the drinker, as well as the speed and the setting in which the drinking takes place. Research shows that women are at greater risk of physical damage from alcohol than men for equivalent amounts of alcohol, and experienced drinkers are better able to handle cars than young, inexperienced drinkers (see Chapter 6). We do not even know for sure whether those who drink moderately have a higher risk of coronary heart disease than teetotallers.[16,17] In essence, while we can say that drinking eight units of alcohol (four pints of beer) over a single evening may not pose a serious long-term risk to physical health, the same amount consumed by a man on an empty stomach over two hours could contribute to serious marital disharmony or a fatal road injury. The inability to designate any level of drinking as safe under all circumstances has led the WHO to conclude that there is no such thing as a threshold below which all drinking is safe.[18]

Nevertheless, we recognise the importance of trying to define

Table 10   The social cost of alcohol misuse (England and Wales 1985)

1	To industry (loss of productivity, unemployment, and so on)	£1,600 million
2	To the NHS (hospital and community)	£104 million
3	Society's response (health education and research)	£1 million
4	Material damage and criminal activities (police and court costs)	£142 million
5	Domestic disharmony and suffering	?
	TOTAL	£1,847 million

Source: Maynard A, Hardman G, Whelan A. Datanote- 9. Measuring the social costs of addictive substances. British Journal of Addiction 1987, 82: 701–706.

practical, everyday levels above which drinking becomes hazardous in particular situations – such as drinking and driving (see Chapter 6). The Royal College of Psychiatrists provided some useful guidelines[19] which are becoming widely accepted. It defined three levels of drinking: 'harmful', 'increased risk' and 'low risk' (see Table 11). Although this is helpful, we are still a long way from defining not merely the amounts, but also the specific circumstances under which drinking is risky.

Table 11 Reasonable drinking guidelines

Drinking category	Number of standard units of alcohol/week*	
	MEN	WOMEN
1 'Harmful' drinking	50 or more	35 or more
2 'Increased risk' drinking	21–49	14–34
3 'Low risk' drinking	Less than 21	Less than 14

* One standard unit of alcohol = half pint of beer, or one measure of spirits, or one glass of wine.
Source: Royal College of Psychiatrists. Alcohol. Our favourite drug. London, Tavistock, 1986.

Consumption trends

Between 1950 and 1979 alcohol consumption doubled in the UK, almost reaching the same level as that at the turn of the century. Consumption fell by 11 per cent between 1979 and 1982, and this was probably related to a combination of the economic recession and the tax increase on beer in 1981, but consumption rose again by nearly two and a half per cent between 1982 and 1985 (see Figure 14).

In recent decades national drinking patterns have changed radically. Although beer still represents nearly 60 per cent of the total market, its consumption declined by 15 per cent between 1979 and 1985. However, wine consumption more than doubled between 1970 and 1985, and consumption of spirits increased by more than 70 per cent over the same period.

While information from the General Household Survey suggests that the heaviest drinkers are concentrated among the manual workers, heavy drinking occurs in many occupational groups: publicans and journalists are among those at higher than average risk of alcohol-related harm. The heaviest drinkers are still among single men in their early to mid-twenties. But there is growing evidence that alcohol misuse, and its associated problems, may also be increasing among women. Although a 1982 DHSS survey in England and Wales suggested that women tend to be light drinkers, newer Scottish evidence suggests that alcohol consumption has risen sharply among women since 1976 but not among men.[20]

There are no good data on national drinking trends among young

Figure 14   Trends in per capita alcohol consumption in the UK (1970–1985)

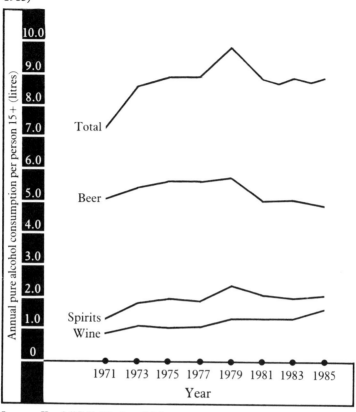

Sources: Kendell R E. The beneficial consequences of the UK's declining per capita consumption of alcohol in 1979–1982. Alcohol and Alcoholism 1984, 19, 4: 271–276. Kendell R E. Personal communication.

people. The available evidence suggests that young people are drinking more often, and starting to drink at an earlier age, but that problem drinking among adolescents does not accurately predict later difficulties in adulthood. A longitudinal study in 1983 of Scottish 15–16 year olds confirms this, and shows that average consumption among 19–20 year old boys was 24 units per week compared with nine units among girls. This represented an increase of 33 per cent for the boys, but a decrease of two per cent among the girls since 1979.[21] The Lothian study concluded that drinking was not a major or increasing problem among the majority of adolescents. A government survey of 13–17 year olds in 1984 generally confirmed the Lothian findings, but showed that consumption is higher in England and Wales than in Scotland – especially among girls. The survey also showed that the laws on under age drinking are widely flouted.[22]

Per capita alcohol consumption is clearly the best predictor of a wide range of alcohol-related harm. This conclusion is supported by evidence considered by the WHO,[23] Royal College of Psychiatrists[24] and the Government's former Central Policy Review Staff.[25] Thus, increases in per capita alcohol consumption are almost always followed by corresponding increases in death rates from cirrhosis of the liver, convictions for public drunkenness and drinking and driving, as well as first admissions to psychiatric hospitals for alcohol dependence. In the UK, as in other countries, trends in per capita consumption are closely followed by similar changes in the major indicators of alcohol-associated harm[26] (see Figure 15).

Figure 15 Alcohol consumption and trends in alcohol-related damage in the UK (1970–1982)

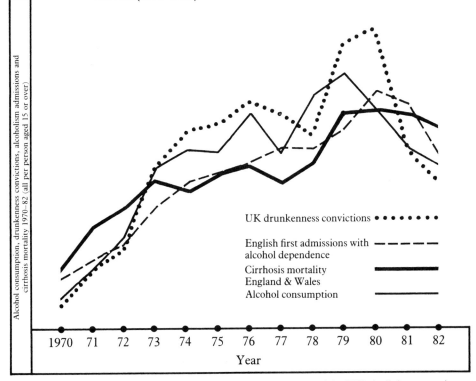

Source: Kendell R E. The beneficial consequences of the UK's declining per capita consumption of alcohol in 1979–1982. Alcohol and Alcoholism 1984, 19, 4: 271–276.

**Alcohol
consumption
and associated
damage**

Figure 15 shows that levels of damage in England and Wales increased with increasing consumption levels but, more importantly, the 11 per cent fall in per capita consumption between 1979 and 1982 was mirrored, with a lag period of one year, by a 19 per cent fall in first admissions to hospital for alcohol dependency, a 16 per cent fall in convictions for drunkenness, a seven per cent fall in drink/driving convictions, and a four per cent decline in the death rate from cirrhosis of the liver. The picture has been broadly similar for both women and men in Scotland and Northern Ireland. While trends in each indicator are influenced by a number of factors other than alcohol, when taken together it is clear that the most effective way of reducing the harm alcohol causes to society is to reduce average consumption throughout the community (see Chapter 7). As alcohol consumption is now rising again, we can expect concomitant increases in harm later this decade (see Figure 14).

AIDS: the newest challenge to public health

AIDS, or acquired immunodeficiency syndrome, is the most serious worldwide threat to public health to emerge in the last five years. In the UK alone, where the problem is still much smaller than in the USA, Africa and most other EEC countries (see Figure 16), there were more than 1,000 reported cases by Autumn 1987. Of these, nearly 57 per cent had already died. It had been estimated that the costs of hospital treatment (assuming no major advances in therapy) for AIDS patients may range between £20–30 million by 1988,[27] but this does not include costs incurred in the community.

Anxiety about AIDS stems not only from its incurable nature or from uncertainties about the growth of what is a new, and still little-

Figure 16   Cumulative incidence of AIDS in the EEC to June 1986

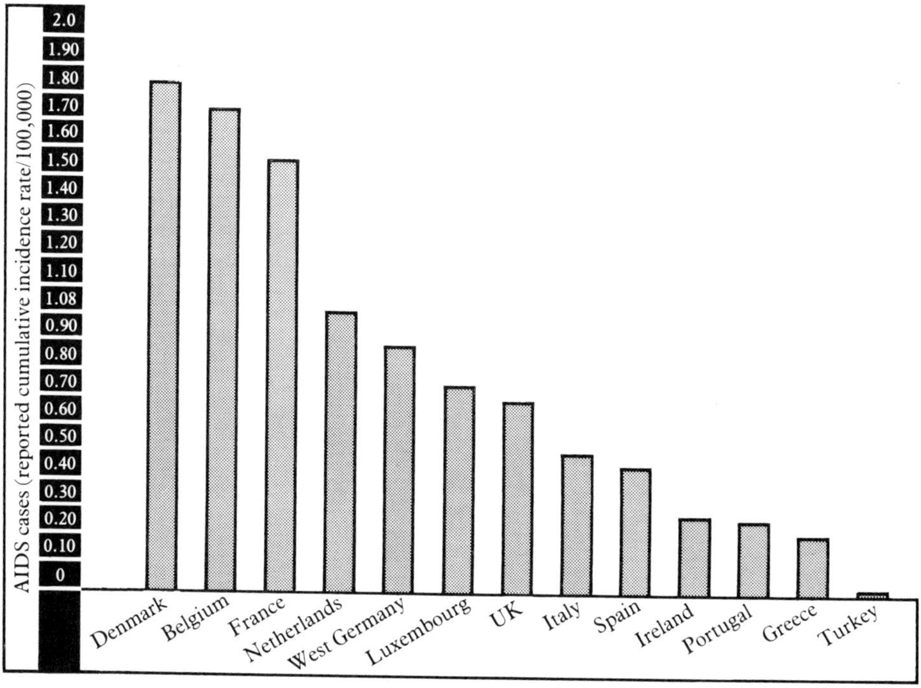

Source: Wells N. The AIDS virus: forecasting its impact. London, OHE, 1986.

63

understood epidemic, but from the realisation that its prevention requires changes in lifestyle that raise profound ethical issues. While our understanding of AIDS has grown enormously since the first case was diagnosed in 1981, there are few things that can be said with absolute certainty at such an early stage in the development of the epidemic. We are aware that many of the statements made today, may need revision in years to come.

AIDS is the end point in a wide spectrum of incompletely documented diseases caused by infection with the human immunovirus (HIV) which was first isolated in 1983. We do not yet know enough about the natural history of HIV infection to predict what proportion of people infected with HIV will go on to develop AIDS. Recent estimates (which have undergone regular upward revisions as new research is published) suggest that about one-third of those infected will develop AIDS,[28,29] but the proportion may be as high as 75 per cent.[30]

Ways of transmitting HIV infection All the evidence so far confirms that HIV cannot be transmitted by ordinary social or occupational contact.[31-34] Follow-up for periods of up to two years shows that household and non-sexual, close contacts of AIDS patients have not become HIV positive.[35] There has been no proven case of a health care worker becoming HIV positive through casual exposure associated with caring for a patient.[36] Even health care workers who have accidentally exposed themselves to HIV-infected blood run a very low risk of becoming HIV positive themselves: in studies involving more than 2,000 health care workers in Europe and the USA, only 0.25 per cent became HIV positive[37] – a much lower risk than exposure to hepatitis B virus where 6–30 per cent of staff accidentally exposed become infected.[38] In the UK study of 150 laboratory workers exposed to blood or body fluids from patients infected with HIV, none had become HIV positive themselves in the first nine months of follow up.[39]

Sexual transmission AIDS can be transmitted through semen, blood and blood products[40-42] and probably cervical and vaginal fluids.[43] The commonest route of transmission so far identified worldwide is sexual. Most AIDS cases in Europe and the UK (84 per cent) are among homosexual or bisexual men – with the exception of Scotland where the largest proportion of AIDS cases by mid-1987 was among intravenous drug users. Heterosexual transmission is the most important route in many African countries where equal proportions of men and women have developed AIDS.[44]

HIV virus has been isolated from other body fluids, including saliva, tears and breast milk, but there is no good evidence that infection can be transmitted through these fluids,[45] although transmission through breast milk may occur.[46]

Most information we have so far on the relationship between sexual activity and HIV infection comes from research among homosexual men. It shows that multiple sexual partners, and receptive anal intercourse are independent risk factors for HIV infection.[47,48] Bleeding during or after intercourse, and any sexual contact involving semen, blood or excretions of infected partners were associated with a high risk of becoming HIV positive.[49]

More recent evidence shows that the HIV virus can also be transmitted heterosexually both from men to women and women to men,[50] and that multiple partners[51] and sex with prostitutes is associated with a high risk of becoming HIV positive in some African countries[52,53] and parts of the USA and Europe.[54] Research on the sexual partners of AIDS sufferers, and of haemophiliacs who are HIV positive, suggests that the virus may be more readily transmitted from women to men than from men to women.[55]

Transmission through transfusion of blood and blood products

Transfusions of blood and blood products were the second most important source of HIV infection in the UK until screening of all blood donors and heat treatment of blood products were introduced in 1985. Those most affected were haemophiliacs who formed the second largest group (5.5 per cent) of AIDS cases in September 1987. Research in British haemophilia centres shows that in 1986, 44 per cent of people with haemophilia A and up to 60 per cent of severe haemophiliacs (who need multiple transfusions) were HIV positive by 1986.[56]

Transmission through injecting intravenous drugs

Those who inject intravenous drugs are at high risk of developing AIDS even though they form only a small proportion (about one per cent in 1987) of the total number of AIDS cases throughout the UK. Evidence from the USA where intravenous drug users accounted for nearly one in five AIDS cases in 1986, suggests that the potential of this route of viral transmission has been hitherto underestimated.[57] The virus is easily, and often rapidly, spread among intravenous drug users, and those most at risk of becoming HIV positive are those who share injecting equipment[58] and those who inject frequently or who go to 'shooting galleries'.[59] Although evidence is scanty, the injection of intravenous drugs may be a more efficient way of transmitting the virus[60] than sexual intercourse, and this is evidenced in the very short period over which groups of drug users who are known for sharing 'works' have become HIV positive.[61-63] European intravenous drug users with AIDS are much younger than other AIDS sufferers: three quarters are under 30,[64] and by September 1986 over 50 per cent of intravenous drug users in one Edinburgh general practice were HIV positive.[65] This uniquely high rate in Edinburgh probably explains why a much higher proportion of AIDS cases in Scotland are among drug users.

HIV infection can also be transmitted from a pregnant woman to her infant either during pregnancy, birth or shortly after.[66] All 12 cases of HIV positive infants documented by September 1987 were born to women who used intravenous drugs. The risk of an HIV positive woman transmitting the virus is high, probably about 30–50 per cent, but more research is needed to clarify continuing uncertainties.

Predicting the future size of the AIDS epidemic

Attempts to make predictions have resulted in widely differing estimates for the number of people likely to become HIV positive and to develop AIDS.[67] For such predictions to be useful we need to know more about the sexual behaviour of the population at risk; about changes in sexual behaviour over time; about the relationship between HIV infection and eventual disease outcome; and how long it takes from infection with HIV to the development of AIDS.[68] Extrapolations from past UK· and American data, or even from models which make assumptions about these largely unknown aspects of HIV infection, can lead to an unhelpfully alarmist view of possible future trends.

While there is no accurate way of predicting the future impact of the AIDS epidemic, we can make a number of general observations about trends in the UK so far and their implications for the future. First, we know that the number of reported cases of AIDS continues to increase exponentially, with the number of cases doubling every ten or eleven months. While the proportion of homosexual men attending STD clinics who are HIV positive has increased from under four per cent in 1982[69] to just over 25 per cent by 1986, these levels are much lower than in the USA where up to 60 per cent of homosexual men (in selected samples) are now HIV positive.[70] Evidence from the UK, USA and elsewhere suggests that there have been two waves in the AIDS epidemic so far. Infection of the homosexual male community took place first and HIV infection probably spread rapidly among a minority of highly sexually active men with multiple sexual partners.[71] The second wave occurred much later among intravenous drug users (the first case of AIDS associated with intravenous drug use was reported in 1984) and has spread very rapidly among certain regionally distinct groups of users. In Scotland, for example, the proportion of HIV positive drug users reported as 1.5 per cent in 1983 had risen to 38 per cent in an Edinburgh hospital group of drug users by 1985, and to over 50 per cent in a general practice population by 1986.[72]

Evidence from the small number of AIDS cases who do not belong to the major risk groups, together with the almost negligible

66

numbers of blood donors who are HIV positive, suggests that spread to the heterosexual population (aside from drug users) has been minimal – so far. The two main sources of spread to the heterosexual population are likely to be through bisexual men and intravenous drug users.[73] The likely contribution from each source requires better knowledge of the distribution of bisexuality in the population, and a more detailed understanding of the likelihood of sexual relationships between heterosexual drug users and non-users. While it has been agreed that the intravenous wave of the AIDS epidemic will be the most important means by which AIDS spreads to the heterosexual population,[74] it is possible that sexual and social insularity may provide a barrier to the spread of sexually transmitted HIV infection from the very young and deprived group of HIV positive drug users to the more heterogeneous general population who do not use drugs.[75]

6 Road accidents

No one should be free to harm others.

JOHN STUART MILL

Introduction Although we have already indicated in Chapter 2 that the UK's good international record for death rates among young people is mainly due to lower death rates from road traffic accidents, there is still a great deal of scope remaining for prevention. Accidents (road traffic accidents in particular) and poisonings remain the third most important source of life-years lost under the age of 85. This chapter considers the pattern and impact of road injuries on society. It examines those potentially avoidable factors which influence road injuries, and assesses trends in road deaths and casualties among different road users over the last decade. We consider the implications for policy in Chapter 7.

The impact of the problem In 1985 nearly 5,200 people died and 71,000 were seriously injured on the roads in Great Britain. Although road deaths represent only one per cent of all deaths, the majority of victims were young – 39 per cent were under 25. Road accidents were the single most important cause of death in 5–24 year olds in 1985, and represented over two-thirds of all deaths in this age group (see Table 12). Moreover the children of manual workers are at much higher risk of being killed in road accidents than the children of non-manual workers.

Because young people are a major risk group, the cost of road accidents to society is high – estimated at over £2,800 million in 1985 (see Table 13). Although it is impossible to give the true cost of road

Table 12 Death on the roads in Britain (1985)

Age	Number of road deaths (registered)	Road deaths as percentage of all accidental deaths	Percentage of all deaths (in each age group)
0–4	97	24	1
5–9	162	69	24
10–14	241	65	27
15–19	823	80	38
20–24	830	76	31
25–34	675	61	13
65+	1,348	19	<1
ALL	5,583	39	1

Source: Department of Transport. Road accidents in Great Britain 1985. London, HMSO, 1986.

68

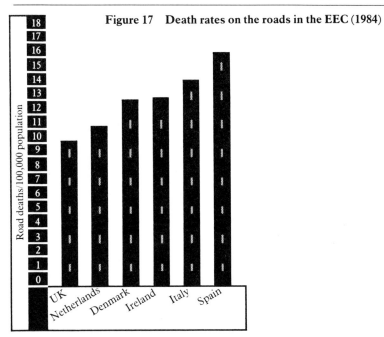

Figure 17   Death rates on the roads in the EEC (1984)

Source: Department of Transport. Road accidents in Great Britain 1985. London, HMSO, 1986.

accidents to society, or to compare them directly with the estimated costs of other public health problems, road accidents still rank high among other pressing challenges to public health, such as tobacco and alcohol. In 1983, 105,000 years of life were lost due to road traffic accidents in England and Wales, compared, for example, with 54,000 from lung cancer and 215,000 from coronary heart disease.

Comparison with other European countries In spite of these avoidable costs, the UK's safety record is among the best in the world – at least for car users. In 1984 the UK had the lowest overall death rates from road accidents in the EEC (see Figure 17) and in world terms was only just bettered by Sweden, Norway

Table 13   The social cost of road accidents in Great Britain (1985)

1	To industry (lost output)	£800m
2	To the NHS (ambulance and hospital treatment)	£140m
3	Damage to property/vehicles	£1,000m
4	Police/insurance/administrative costs	£150m
5	Pain/grief and suffering	£630m
	TOTAL	£2,820m

Source: Department of Transport. Road accidents in Great Britain 1985. London, HMSO, 1986.

and Japan. These figures may not be strictly comparable because deaths are determined by the volume and pattern of use of motorised traffic, which vary widely from country to country. Nevertheless, the UK still compares well – in overall terms – with countries like Japan and the Netherlands whose patterns of roads in built-up areas and levels of car ownership are similar to the UK. Within the UK, the lowest road death rates in 1984 were in Wales (8.8 per 100,000) and the highest in Northern Ireland (12 per 100,000).

Accidents or avoidable injuries? We tend to think of accidents as unavoidable events. But detailed research into their patterns and causes suggests that 'accident' may be an inappropriate word to describe a clear set of potentially avoidable events which result in injury. Every road casualty results from the interaction of the road user, the vehicles involved, the environment, and transport policy. While human error is clearly a factor in nearly all cases, the Transport Road Research Laboratory (TRRL) – the Department of Transport's research arm – has estimated that environmental factors are involved in 28 per cent of cases and vehicular factors in 8.5 per cent.[1,2]

The road environment While increasing vehicle ownership is related to a rising death toll on the roads throughout the world, deaths per vehicle tend to fall again once a certain level of car ownership has been reached.[3] This may reflect increasing levels of development accompanied by higher density, slower-moving traffic and the gradual implementation of road safety measures. Most (77 per cent) road deaths occur in built-up areas, although the highest *risk* of death is in non-built-up areas. Road casualties are twice as likely to occur at night as during the day.[4] Locally based accident investigations show that accident 'blackspot' areas tend to have poor road surfaces, poor traffic control or poor road design. Child casualties are most likely to occur very close to home.

The road user While the largest *number* of deaths are among car occupants, followed closely by pedestrians, the *risk* of being involved in a fatal or serious accident is lowest in trains, buses and coaches. Motorcyclists, followed by cyclists are most at risk. Although this is in part due to the fact that motor cyclists and pedal cyclists tend to be much younger and more inexperienced than other road users, casualty rates for motor cyclists and pedal cyclists are still much higher than those for car drivers of the same age.[5] Moreover, motorcycle accidents are different from cycling accidents. First, motorbike accidents are essentially a problem among young men: in 1985, 87 per cent involved young men, of which the largest proportion (28 per cent) was among 20–24 years old. And second, motorcyclists are more likely than cyclists to be involved in accidents which kill others. Pedestrians are the third largest at-risk group, with most casualties occurring at both extremes of the age spectrum.

Drinking and driving The TRRL has estimated that in 1984, 1,500 deaths – about 25 per cent of all road fatalities – were alcohol-associated. The percentage rises to about 60 per cent at night. Young men of 20–24 were the most likely to be convicted of drinking and driving offences in 1985, and the highest conviction rates are in the summer – not at Christmas.

Evidence for the involvement of alcohol in road deaths and injuries is convincing, and is based on an important controlled study which showed that, compared with someone who is sober, a driver with blood alcohol levels of 80 mg/100 ml (or 80 mg per cent which is the UK legal limit) is twice as likely to be involved in an accident. At 150 mg per cent the risk increases to ten-fold, and at 200 mg to twenty-fold.[6] The findings of this study form the basis of our current

Figure 18   Trends in road deaths in Great Britain (1950–1985)

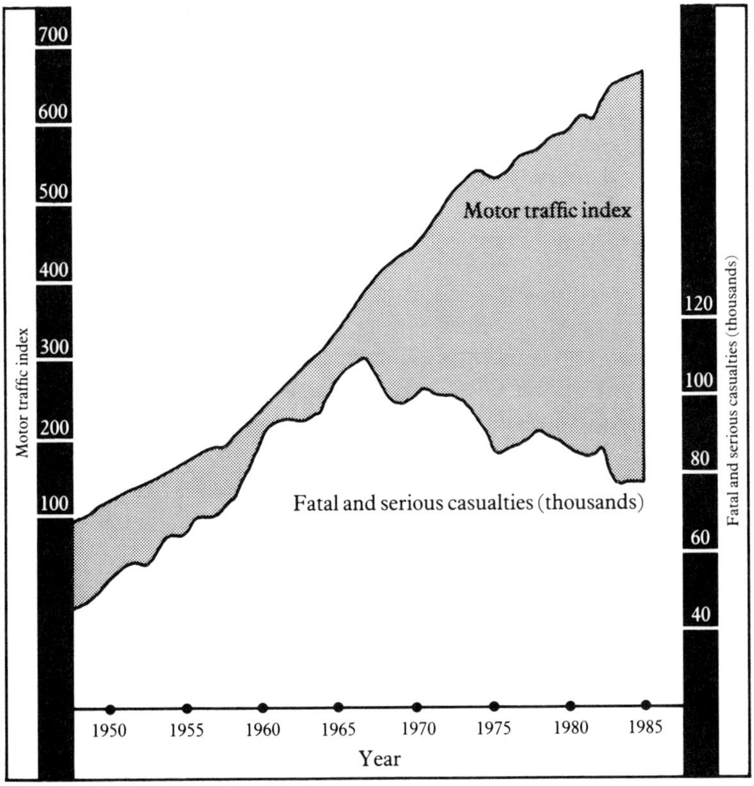

Source: Transport Road and Research Laboratory, 1986.

drink and driving legislation. More recent research from TRRL shows that the risk is much higher for young, inexperienced, drivers (and drinkers) and rises steeply at 30 mg per cent.[7,8]

Figure 19 Fatal and serious road casualties by type of road user (1972–1985)

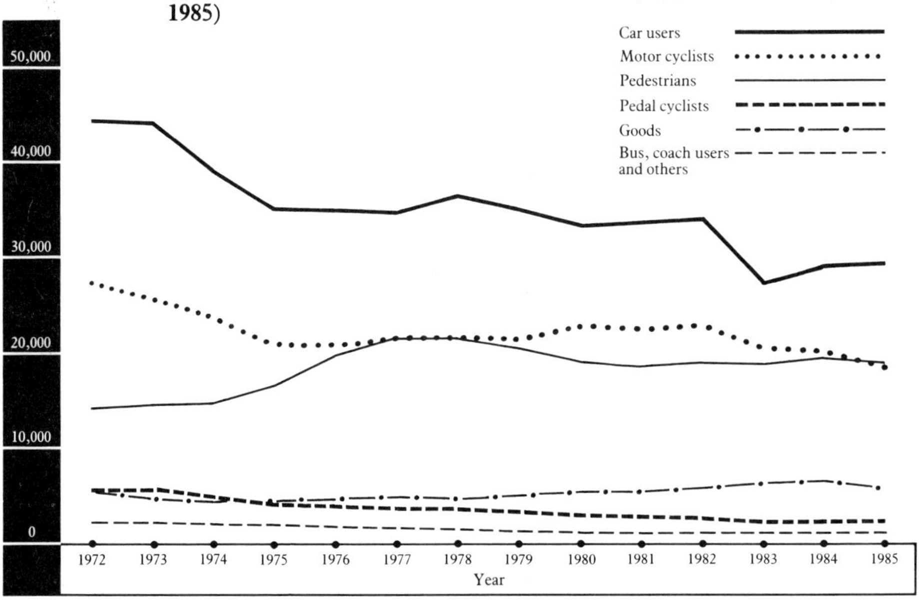

Source: Department of Transport. Road accidents in Great Britain 1985. London, HMSO, 1986.

The vehicles Vehicle size and design is important in accidents. First, two wheeled vehicles are more vulnerable than cars – the structure of which absorbs some of the impact in an accident. Two wheeled vehicles are less visible. Back seat car (and light van) passengers and pedestrians are now relatively more vulnerable than front seat passengers who are required by law to wear a seat belt. Although the commonest injury in all road users is head injury, motorcyclists are now less likely to be admitted to hospital with head injury than other road users.[9] This is most likely to be due to almost full compliance with the law which requires riders of two wheeled motor vehicles to wear crash helmets.

In 1983 the maximum possible speed of new cars bought by the average motorist was 50 per cent in excess of the maximum speed limit.[10] The evidence linking excessive speed to higher accident risk is supported by good evidence.[11,12] The TRRL estimates that high speed directly accounts for 10–20 per cent of accidents. A major review on road safety summarising more than 30 separate studies on the effect of speed limits on road accident rates showed, with a few exceptions, that raising the speed limit increased the number and

72

Figure 20   Recent trends in seat belt wearing rates among front seat occupants of cars and light vans (Great Britain)

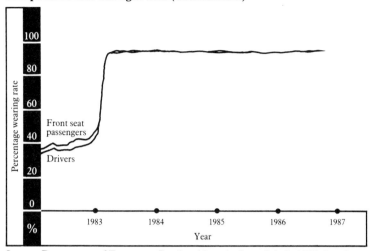

Source: Department of Transport. Road accidents in Great Britain 1985. London, HMSO, 1986.

severity of casualties, and lowering it resulted in a reduction in casualties.[13]

The 1983 TRRL speed survey showed that:

- 40 per cent of cars and up to 90 per cent of coaches and HGVs exceeded the speed limit on motorways;
- 50 per cent of vehicles in residential areas exceeded the limit.

Although opinion polls show that the public do not think that the speed limit should be increased, as many as two-thirds of young male car drivers claimed to drive regularly at over 70 mph.[14] In 1983 the risk of being found guilty of speeding was estimated at less than once in a lifetime.[15]

Trends in road safety

1985 saw the lowest number of people killed on the roads in Great Britain for three decades. The number of fatal and serious casualties has continued to fall since the mid-1960s, and fell by a further nine per cent between 1975 and 1985 – despite a 39 per cent increase in the volume of traffic (see Figure 18).

But there have been few major reductions in total *casualties* within most sub-groups of road user, except pedestrians, where total casualties fell by 11 per cent between 1975–85. Casualties among cyclists rose by 29 per cent compared with a 21 per cent increase in cycle traffic, although the number of fatalities rose by only three per cent. Two wheeled motor vehicle traffic (mainly motorcycles) rose by 55 per cent over the decade, but total casualties showed no increase.

73

Figure 19 shows that the most striking fall among those killed or seriously injured in the last decade occurred in car users following the legislation which made the use of seat belts mandatory in the front seats of cars and light vans in 1981. The evidence for its effectiveness is strong, and we review it in Chapter 7. Regular monitoring of seat belt use by the Department of Transport shows that compliance increased from an average of 37 per cent before the legislation to 95 per cent afterwards (see Figure 20) and that immediate reductions occurred in fatal and serious casualties of about 25 per cent for drivers and 30 per cent for front seat passengers.[16] As might be expected, the legislation had no effect on rear seat passengers or on other road users.

7 Promoting a healthy lifestyle

One should eat to live, not live to eat.

MOLIERE

Introduction   In Chapters 3–6 we analysed trends in the major causes of premature death, and the part played in each by what has become known as our 'lifestyle'. 'Lifestyle' is a useful but much misunderstood term. It is sometimes seen as a set of individually determined behaviours – such as smoking, excessive drinking, and a lack of exercise – which cause ill health. The implication is that *individuals* have sole responsibility for their health, and that society has no part to play. This is a narrow view for two reasons. First, there are many aspects of our lifestyle which are conducive to *health* rather than to disease, and we consider some of these in later chapters. Second, it would run counter to the evidence to assume that people's patterns of smoking, drinking, eating and sexual activity are determined by individual choices that are unaffected by social, economic or legislative factors.

In this chapter we examine the evidence for the effectiveness of both environmental and individually oriented measures in the promotion of a healthier lifestyle. Because most diseases are due to many causes, and individual risk factors contribute to a wide range of diseases, we now move away from individual diseases and concentrate instead on those specific determinants of health and disease which we have so far identified as being capable of contributing to health. We start with strategies for reducing cigarette consumption. We then consider diet, alcohol misuse, road use, and finally sexual and reproductive practices. In Part II of the report we consider the promotion of physical activity, the maintenance of social support networks (Chapter 9) and illicit drug misuse (Chapter 13).

Strategies for prevention   Two broad strategies for the prevention of disease and promotion of health have been identified.

- **The population strategy** This involves measures applied throughout the community, and is akin to the major, public health initiatives of the nineteenth century such as the building of sewers. Today, it might involve mass measures such as increases in tobacco and alcohol taxation, or seatbelt legislation.
- **The high risk approach** This involves identifying and intervening *only* among those sections of the community who are perceived to be at risk of developing a disease or a health problem. This might mean offering heavy drinkers a programme for cutting down, or

treating those with high blood pressure or high blood cholesterol levels.

The relative merits of each of these approaches have generated considerable debate – especially in the field of dietary change to reduce coronary heart disease.[1-3] In practice, the two approaches are not mutually exclusive, but interdependent,[4] for the more successful the population approach is in reducing a problem, the fewer the remaining high risk individuals who need to be identified and treated or supported.

The 'high risk' approach is complementary to the 'population approach', and each has its advantages and disadvantages. Although the health benefits of the 'population approach' are likely to be greater overall than those of the 'high risk' approach, the population-wide measures usually offer small and sometimes imperceptible benefits for the individual. This phenomenon has been termed the 'prevention paradox'.[5] The 'high risk' approach, on the other hand, offers bigger, obvious benefits for the individuals selected for it (such as the treatment of high blood pressure), and could be seen as less wasteful than the population approach which must be applied across the whole community. The 'high risk' approach also offers individuals a choice to opt in or out of an intervention at any stage, whereas population-based measures such as the mandatory use of seat belts or fiscal measures to discourage consumption of harmful products, have bigger implications for individual freedom. This highlights the need for the widest possible debate on all public health measures before their implementation.

Table 14 Public support for measures to control cigarette smoking

	Percentage agreeing (strongly or slightly)		
	All (N = 1563)	*Smokers* (N = 612)	*Non-smokers* (N = 951)
Those 'for a ban on cigarette advertising'	55	47	59
'The government should spend more money to encourage people to stop smoking'	67	60	73
'The government should increase the tax on cigarettes'	47	26	64
'Employers should ban smoking at work'	26	32	63
Those for 'a ban on smoking in all public places'	40	25	53

Source: Marsh A, Matheson J. Smoking attitudes and behaviour. Social Survey Division, OPCS. London, HMSO, 1983.

Figure 21   Consumer expenditure on cigarettes in relation to changes in the real price of cigarettes (1970–1982)

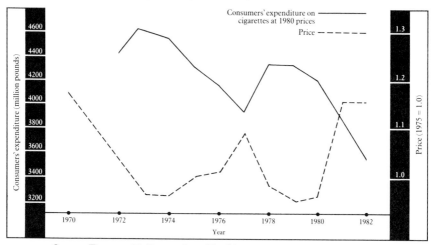

Source: Townsend J. Economic and health consequences of reduced smoking. In: Williams A (ed). Health and economics. London, Macmillan, 1987.

Tobacco The ultimate public health objective for cigarette smoking can be seen as the elimination of all but occasional cigarette smoking. This puts cigarettes in a totally different category from other aspects of lifestyle such as alcohol, diet, and road use where the aim would be to promote healthy, safe and enjoyable patterns of use or consumption. A five-part strategy for the reduction of cigarette consumption forms the basis of recommendations made on successive occasions by WHO,[6,7] two UK government reports[8,9] and the Royal College of Physicians.[10-12] It comprises the following measures:

- regular increases in the real price of tobacco;
- a legislative ban on all forms of tobacco advertising or promotion;
- the creation of a non-smoking norm in public places;
- adequately funded public and professional education and information programmes;
- health warnings on all cigarette packs (and promotional material until a ban takes place).

These measures are also suported by the BMA, the royal medical colleges and the Royal College of Nursing. A majority of the public supports more control on cigarette advertising, and nearly half supports increases in cigarette taxation (see Table 14).

Reducing the demand for cigarettes: taxation There is now a large body of research on the factors affecting the commencement, maintenance and cessation of smoking. There is a close correspondence between the price of tobacco and cigarette consumption levels. Increases in the real price of cigarettes are

77

usually followed by decreases in consumption[13] (see Figure 21).

Economic analyses suggest that increases in cigarette taxation are an effective, if blunt, means of reducing cigarette consumption: for every one per cent increase in the price of cigarettes there is approximately a 0.5 per cent decrease in cigarette consumption per head.[14,15] Children starting to smoke, however, appear to be more sensitive to price changes than adults.[16] Research based on data for the mid-1970s suggested that a policy of major tax increases (a 56 per cent increase in the 1972–3 price of cigarettes), education and control of cigarette advertising might achieve as much as a 40 per cent reduction in cigarette consumption.[17] Fears that increases in cigarette taxation would result in a loss of tax revenue, that price rises would discriminate heavily against the manual classes and would contribute to unemployment, are not supported by research. First, cigarette consumption is relatively insensitive to price changes, which means that price rises only reduce consumption by a small amount and tend to *increase* rather than decrease government revenue from cigarettes[18] (see Figure 22). Second, recent analyses suggest that people in social classes IV and V may be *more* responsive than those in social classes I and II to price increases, and that the *lack* of adequate price increases over the last two decades may have contributed to social class inequalities in smoking rates.[19] A recent analysis of tobacco pricing policy in Finland[20] came to the following important conclusions:

- increases in tobacco prices are effective in reducing consumption, but those which occurred in Finland between 1960–84 were not big enough;
- pricing policy cannot operate in isolation from other aspects of tobacco control policy such as education.

Finally, a detailed, independent analysis of the effects of prevention policy on employment in the tobacco industry concluded that the numbers directly employed by the industry are usually exaggerated. In 1985 there were 20,000 directly employed in the tobacco industry, and the development of new technology within these industries has had a much bigger impact on the numbers employed than prevention policy, although recent tax increases in cigarettes have speeded up the contraction.[21]

Smoking: education and information   It has proved difficult to disentangle the impact of education on smoking trends from that of taxation or other measures, as they are mutually reinforcing. In recent years, the build-up of regular anti-smoking campaigns in the mass media and elsewhere have had a more sustained effect which was evident before the early 1980s when the real price of cigarettes began to increase. It seems probable that

78

Figure 22   Tobacco tax revenue and the real price of cigarettes (1970–1982)

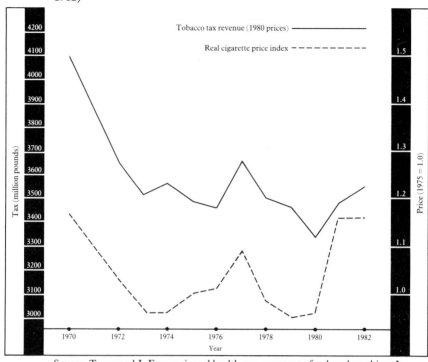

Source: Townsend J. Economic and health consequences of reduced smoking. In: Williams A (ed). Health and economics. London, Macmillan, 1987.

the steadily increasing volume of high quality editorial coverage of smoking and health in the mass media[22,23] is likely to have had a reinforcing role.

The importance of supplementing national measures with action tailored for individuals has been well-documented. General practitioners[24-26] and workplace schemes[27,28] have both been shown to be effective in helping people to stop smoking.

Early efforts to demonstrate behaviour change through anti-smoking programmes at schools were disappointing but some later randomised controlled trials showed that programmes such as My Body were able to significantly delay the decision to start smoking.[29,30] The ability of this and other smoking and health programmes to exert a beneficial long-term effect on smoking behaviour reflect the importance of operating in a 'healthy' social climate.

Smoking: advertising and promotion Economic analyses of the impact of cigarette advertising on consumption are fraught with methodological difficulties. The tobacco industry spends at least £100 million each year promoting smoking. Industry-funded research has concluded that cigarette advertising does not increase total consumption, but merely affects brand preference.[31] An independent review of studies in the field showed that the findings are limited by incomplete information on expenditure on advertising and sponsorship, by varying assumptions about the impact of diverse kinds of advertising, and by an inability to select out the potentially greater impact that advertising is likely to have on children.[32] Nevertheless, of the two independent studies conducted, both found advertising to increase total consumption.[33,34] No study has so far shown that a ban on cigarette promotion would reduce consumption, because most bans are partial and research has not taken this or other factors into account.[35,36]

None of these studies has taken into account the effect of cigarette advertising on the general image of smoking, and its ability to outweigh the government's smoking and health message. The social climate is crucial in reinforcing the idea among children that smoking is still a socially acceptable practice.[37] There is a growing body of research which shows that children are more vulnerable to cigarette advertising than adults, that they are more likely to smoke those brands which are most heavily advertised, and that brand-switching is an important part of the process of becoming a new smoker.[38,39] Moreover, there is now strong evidence from Norway – which introduced a comprehensive legislative package to reduce smoking in 1975 – that the ban on cigarette promotion together with other measures has had a much bigger effect in reducing smoking among teenagers than in adults.[40]

Smoking: what progress has been made? It is now a generation since the RCP published its first report on the dangers of smoking. The British response to repeated calls for action since then has slowly gathered momentum. There are probably more local initiatives throughout the country to reduce smoking than in almost any other public health field. Yet there are no nationally agreed objectives for smoking and health, and government action has been piecemeal.

Under continuing pressure from the royal medical colleges and organisations such as ASH (Action on Smoking and Health) and the former HEC, SHEG and the BMA, significant policy changes have occurred in three areas over the last decade:

- cigarette taxation;
- public education and information;
- advertising and promotion.

The tax on cigarettes has been increased nearly every year since 1974, although there was no increase in the 1987 pre-election budget. The real price of cigarettes rose by 30 per cent between 1980 and 1985. Despite this, cigarettes are still over 20 per cent cheaper in real terms than they were in 1948.[41]

There has been a modest increase in the budgets for anti-smoking education from £0.5 million in the mid-1970s to about £3.5 million in 1985–86. Even though more money was spent by the former HEC and SHEG on education against smoking than on any single other issue, the total amount is still small compared with the promotional resources of the tobacco industry. Baseline information on smoking trends and attitudes is better than in most other public health fields, although not all of it is published. The regular publication of tar, nicotine, and more recently carbon monoxide yields of cigarettes, has provided the tobacco companies with an extra incentive to reduce further the tar yields of cigarettes.

Progress on the control of cigarette promotion has been poor. The 1965 legislative ban on TV advertising is frequently circumvented, and in 1984 there were more than 300 hours of tobacco-sponsored sport on TV. Cigarette advertising in the press, and cigarette sponsorship, have been subject to a series of voluntary agreements between the government and the tobacco industry that are regularly flouted. The latest agreement in 1986 did, however, introduce six new health warnings, and imposed a ban on all cigarette advertising in cinemas. There is a partial ban on cigarette advertising in some, but not all women's magazines read by teenagers, but the latest agreement on tobacco sponsorship falls short of the voluntary code imposed recently by the BBC and Independent Television on all tobacco-sponsored sport.

The main response by the tobacco industry over the last decade has been to make signs available to tobacco retailers reminding them that it is illegal to sell cigarettes to children under 16. The law is still regularly broken.

Despite small budgets, the former HEC and SHEG have maintained a series of smoking and health initiatives at many levels ranging from mass media campaigns to long-term school programmes, community education projects such as Look After Yourself (see Chapter 9), and the regionally based Project Smokefree which is a five-year community-wide campaign in Manchester. The former HEC and ASH, together with 11 other organisations, including the DHSS and the cancer and heart disease research charities, organise an annual National No-Smoking Day which has had widespread publicity as well as supporting an estimated six per cent of the population in attempts to stop smoking.[42] The publication in 1983 of the SHECC (Scottish Health Education Coordinating Committee) expert report[43] on smoking followed by a report from ASH in Scotland giving a breakdown of smoking-related disease by parliamentary and local authority constituencies significantly renewed concern about the need for further action on smoking.[44] The exercise was repeated for England and Wales in 1986 and published jointly by the former HEC and BMA in a report *The Big Kill*.[45]

Although it is beyond the scope of this report to give a comprehensive account of the breadth and number of local initiatives on smoking, major changes have taken place in health authorities and in primary care. The publication by ASH of *Smoking Prevention – A Health Promotion Guide for the NHS*, together with the work of the growing number of health education officers, prompted many authorities to develop smoking and health policies. A survey of regional health authorities (RHAs) commissioned for this project in late 1985 showed that smoking and health was an explicit part of the strategic plans of all but two English RHAs.[46] A survey by the former HEC of all district health authorities (DHAs) in the same year showed that 40–75 per cent had developed, or were implementing, their own smoking control policies.[47] This was the case in nearly all Scottish Health Boards.[48] An ASH survey of local authorities showed that by 1985 four out of five had followed suit;[49] in Scotland every single local authority had taken some action to restrict smoking.[50] One of the most striking examples of joint health board/local authority cooperation has been the establishment of Glasgow 2000, a community-wide project which aims to make Glasgow a smoke-free city by the year 2000.

Following the Royal College of General Practitioners' (RCGP) initiative on the prevention of arterial disease,[51] advice and monitoring of patients' smoking is becoming usual practice in some primary care settings.

Promoting dietary change

In Chapter 3 we summarised the international scientific consensus on the role of diet in coronary heart disease, cancers and a number of other important health problems such as obesity, diabetes and bowel disease. Although much research remains to be done on the relationship between diet and various cancers, there is a striking consistency in the evidence concerning the *kind* of diet that would be conducive to health and would prevent a wide variety of diseases. We also summarised the quantitative dietary guidelines recommended by NACNE for the reduction of total energy derived from fats and saturated fats, an increase in fibre intake, and a decrease in sugar and salt intakes in the UK (see Chapter 3).

Are such goals achievable, and if so, how can they be achieved? There is already evidence that dietary habits have changed towards the NACNE goals over the last decade (see Chapter 3), and that during the last war, when a national nutrition policy was in being, aspects of our diet approached the NACNE goals.[52]

In 1982 a WHO expert group identified the need for a comprehensive strategy involving a combination of the population and high risk approaches to heart disease prevention together with effective treatment.[53] Two subsequent WHO reports in 1984 developed more detailed plans for implementing the 1982 recommendations,[54,55] and have been endorsed in the main by other more recent expert reports.[56–59] Central to their recommendations were the following components:

- government should develop a national nutrition policy and should establish a mechanism for interdepartmental liaison;
- food and agricultural policies should be reviewed and brought into line with national nutritional goals;
- nutritional labelling of foods;
- locally coordinated, community-based prevention programmes;
- community and professional education.

The COMA report *Diet and Cardiovascular Disease* commissioned by the DHSS was the first major UK report to recommend how dietary change might be brought about to reduce heart disease. Its recommendations focussed largely on public and professional education, but it identified other components of the strategy, including legislation to make the nutritional labelling of fats mandatory, and an examination of ways of influencing the Common Agricultural Policy in the interests of nutrition and health.[60]

The most detailed implementation plans so far arose out of a conference organised by the Coronary Prevention Group, known as the Canterbury Conference, which was sponsored by 17 health organisations.[61] It agreed a carefully worked out plan for agencies ranging from EEC, government and health education to primary health care and the media. Many of its recommendations have since been endorsed by the BMA[62] and have become part of health authority health promotion programmes.

Effective strategies for diet

There is a large body of agricultural, economic and market research on factors affecting food consumption patterns. Much of it concerns products that are irrelevant to health. Little effort has been specifically directed towards assessing how food policy might be oriented in the interests of health. Our own conclusions are necessarily based on limited information from educational and community intervention studies, and the findings of nutritionally motivated market research. Five broad strategies for implementation of the NACNE goals have been identified:[63]

- *education and information* through schools, the community and product labelling;
- *pricing* to assist in the switch from harmful to healthy foods;
- *substitution* of harmful, hidden or additional products such as salt

or sugar;
- *provision* of more healthy foods in catering establishments;
- *regulation* by good nutritional surveillance and control of the composition of goods and food advertising.

Diet: education and information

We have already summarised the evidence (see Chapter 3) which shows that dietary advice forms an essential part of successful community intervention in the prevention of coronary heart disease. The Oxford Heart Disease and Stroke Prevention Project has shown that it is feasible, using nurse practitioners, both to monitor dietary practices and to give dietary advice. Preliminary results suggest that the employment of a nurse 'facilitator' on a district-wide basis can significantly increase a practice's ability to record information on smoking and blood pressure as well as diet[64,65] but has not yet evaluated its effect on health outcomes.

Recent market research into consumer attitudes and behaviour in relation to food and health give us a better picture of the kind of nutritional labelling that would be most informative, but a survey commissioned by the British Nutrition Foundation in 1981–2 suggested that having appropriate knowledge and attitudes to diet does not necessarily lead to healthy buying patterns.[66] This is likely to be because food prices, advertising, personal and cultural preferences are also influential.

A joint survey conducted for the Consumers' Association, Ministry of Agriculture, Fisheries and Foods (MAFF) and the National Consumer Council in 1985,[67] whose results were developed into a rational strategy by CPG,[68] came to some important conclusions about what consumers understand about nutrition, what information they wanted through labelling, and how best it might be put across:

- Although people claimed to be eating more healthily, less than 30 per cent were classed as 'nutritionally aware' or knowledgeable about which aspects of diet should be changed in the interests of health.
- Over 90 per cent thought that it was important to show nutritional information on foods, 80 per cent said there should be information on fats, sugar and salt, and 70 per cent on fibre.
- Of the two preferred formats for nutritional labelling, people were most likely to recall nutritional information accurately from labels which gave simple, qualitative information using the 'traffic lights' or 'high', 'medium' and 'low' approach rather than detailed quantitive information.

Diet: prices, substitution and regulation

Evidence we review in Chapter 8 suggests that price and variable availability of foods influences food consumption patterns among the least well-off. The way in which a food pricing policy might be used to support healthy consumer choices has not been seriously explored. The full impact of UK and EEC policy on the price of foods, and their impact on eating patterns await analysis. There is scope for reducing the salt and sugar content of processed foods. The role of food advertising – 40 per cent of which is for confectionery – in influencing consumer choices needs to be examined. Pressure on consumers – especially women – to cut down on starchy foods because they may be seen to be 'fattening' is misleading, and runs counter to the recommendations of the NACNE report.

Diet: the achievements of a decade

As in the case of tobacco, much has been achieved through local initiatives. The health aspects of national food policy appear to be restricted to marginal issues such as the control of additives and contaminants, rather than the development of an overall nutrition policy. There is no clear ministerial responsibility for nutrition which is currently divided between MAFF and DHSS. The legislation on nutritional labelling recommended by the COMA report in 1984, has not yet taken place. A new EEC directive on nutritional guidelines is expected to lead to further delays. Current MAFF suggestions for labelling cover only fats, although there is a clear need to advise the public on the dietary fibre, sugar and salt content of foods as well. The format currently being considered is not of the 'traffic lights' kind which consumers have found most helpful, but that preferred by the food manufacturers, and which consumers have found difficult to understand.[69] There have been no attempts to review the use of agricultural and manufacturing techniques from a health perspective.

The government's contradictory attitudes to public education on diet and health over the last decade are well documented.[70] In 1987 the Joint Advisory Committee on Nutrition Education (JACNE), which compiled *Eating for Health* was disbanded. DHSS and HEC's successor, the Health Education Authority (HEA) launched a new Healthy Lifestyles campaign in Spring 1987 – a component of which is the promotion of a healthier diet. Known as Look After Your Heart, the £2.5 million campaign aims to add to existing efforts to reduce heart disease and cites the WHO target for the year 2000 of reducing heart disease by 15 per cent among those under 65. While this effort falls short of a national strategy, new efforts are to be made to liaise with the NHS, industry, community organisations, schools and the mass media.

Most analyses of the decade point to the importance of the publication of the NACNE report by the HEC in 1983 in reinforcing the renewed interest in diet. Its impact of food and health policy within the NHS has been especially marked. In 1981 there were only three DHAs in England and Wales with food and health policies. By

1984, after publication of the NACNE report, 22 per cent had policies and a further 38 per cent were formulating them.[71] Preliminary results from the most recent survey of the whole of the UK showed that 90 per cent of DHAs and health boards either have a food and health policy or are developing one.[72] These welcome changes are beginning to extend to schools and local authority premises. A survey of 151 employers in 1985, however, showed that only 27 per cent provided health-orientated choices on canteen menus.[73]

A further important, but inadequately researched, spin-off from the publication of the NACNE report has been the growth of media coverage of diet and health. The BBC in particular has a record of food and health coverage that pre-dates the NACNE report. But its coverage increased after the report's publication and included the launch of its own 'food and health campaign', and two major documentary series. This was followed by a further series on healthy cooking. It is not possible to gauge the extent to which the promotion of healthy eating has become part of primary care, and the effect of the call for action from the RCGP[74] has not been formally assessed. But a Welsh community survey in 1985 gives us some idea of the extent to which GPs advise their patients on aspects of lifestyle. Advice about diet is still low on their list of priorities.[75] Despite this, some innovative projects are under way which use the ordinary consultation as a means of 'opportunistically' advising patients about diet and other risk factors for heart disease and stroke.

Although the UK has been slower to develop community-wide initiatives than have the USA and Scandinavia, a review of UK-wide initiatives in the field of heart disease prevention in 1986 was able to identify six major regional initiatives which contained a dietary component,[76] including Heartbeat Wales, a five-year project established in 1985 and aimed at involving the whole Welsh community in the reduction of heart disease. Funded by the former Health Education Council, the Welsh Office and local industry, it is the largest project of its kind in Europe, and has stimulated the DHSS in England and Northern Ireland as well as the Scottish Office to launch their own initiatives. Heartbeat Wales, with its quantified goals and targets, offers a model that, given local commitment and funds, could be adopted in any other part of the country.[77]

Another recent development has been the growing interest within some retail sectors of the food industry in developing healthier products. Some have adopted more informative nutritional labelling systems than those currently proposed by the government, together with a wider range of higher fibre, lower fat products – some of which are now advertised on television. The former HEC successfully negotiated an agreement with the Federation of Bakers whereby it agreed gradually to reduce the salt content of bread in exchange for being able to use HEC's logo in its promotion.

Alcohol: minimising the harm

Alcohol, unlike cigarette smoking, presents a complex public health challenge: how to minimise the harm without jeopardising the benefits. Based on the evidence we assessed in Chapter 5, it is clear that the objective for alcohol is *not* to prevent people from starting to drink, but to reduce average levels of consumption *throughout the community*. The WHO[78] has recommended three main methods of achieving these aims:

- fiscal measures to maintain the price of alcohol above that of inflation;
- controls on the availability of alcohol through licensing restrictions;
- public and professional education.

In the UK, these approaches have received broad support from the government's former Central Policy Review Staff, the Royal College of Psychiatrists, the RCP, the RCGP, the BMA, the SHECC and the Health Education Advisory Committee for Wales (HEACW).[79-86] The Royal College of Psychiatrists has set a modest aim for the nation: to halt the current rise in alcohol consumption with the aim of a gradual reduction in the longer term. This, it suggests, can be achieved by a concerted strategy including interdepartmental government coordination, increases in alcohol tax, closer monitoring of licensing and advertising, improved education, training and treatment services as well as increased roadside breath-testing. The RCGP report emphasised the role of the GP in detecting and supporting patients in their efforts to cut down on drinking. The College of Psychiatrists' views have further been translated into quantitive terms by Action on Alcohol Abuse (AAA),[87] but the most detailed implementation strategy so far comes from the SHECC and the HEACW reports which have laid out clear plans for action by a wide range of agencies from government and the NHS to local authorities, industry and trades unions, the media, voluntary organisations, and the courts.

Factors governing the demand for alcohol

Factors governing alcohol consumption fall into two groups: those affecting demand and those affecting availability. Among the most obvious and most complex are national, cultural and religious traditions. It is likely that the social and cultural features of the local area might also influence consumption patterns, although a recent OPCS study of two English regions which differ widely in levels of consumption and alcohol-related harm, failed to show any locality-specific factor.[88]

Price of alcohol   In the UK, and in many other affluent countries, the best-documented influence on per capita consumption is consumer purchasing power. Alcohol consumption increases with rising prosperity (as in the 1960s), and falls during economic recession – as evidenced in the UK between 1979 and 1982 when unemployment rose sharply. The real price of alcohol (in terms of disposable income) is also a key determinant of per capita consumption.[89,90]

The price of alcohol has halved relative to disposable income, and consumption doubled, in the two decades from 1960 (see Figure 23). In 1964 it took a manual worker six hours of work to earn the price of a bottle of whisky. Increases in disposable income over the next two decades meant that it took one-third of this time to earn the price of an equivalent bottle in 1984. As a reduction in disposable income is clearly undesirable, the best documented means of reducing alcohol-related damage would be to increase the real price of alcohol beyond that of inflation. Scottish research has shown that the real increase in the price of beer, which occurred in the March 1981 budget, resulted in a significant decrease in per capita consumption in a study representative of the community (although 20 per cent of this decline was attributable to unemployment).[91] The research also showed that reductions in consumption occurred among heavy *and* moderate drinkers as well as lighter drinkers.

From the behaviour of the alcohol market, economists have attempted to predict the sensitivity (or elasticity) of consumption to price and income changes. Although findings vary, it is generally agreed that elasticity varies with different kinds of alcohol and that beer consumption is less sensitive than that of wine or spirits.[92] The Central Statistical Office estimates that one per cent increase in the real price of alcohol will reduce per capita consumption of spirits by an estimated 1.6 per cent, but of beer by only 0.2 per cent.

Although independent economic analyses have not been able to show whether alcohol advertising increases total consumption, it would be naive to assume that the £180 million spent annually on the promotion of alcohol has no cumulative effect at all. The alcohol industry currently spends nearly 200 times as much in promoting drinking as is spent on health education to advocate sensible drinking. The alcohol industry argues that advertising informs the consumer, yet in practice there is little information relevant to health on its products, and none at all in its advertisements. We need to know more about the role alcohol promotion plays in reinforcing a social climate that encourages heavy drinking and whether the images presented undermine the consumer's ability to make healthy

Figure 23   Alcohol consumption and its relationship to price and disposable income

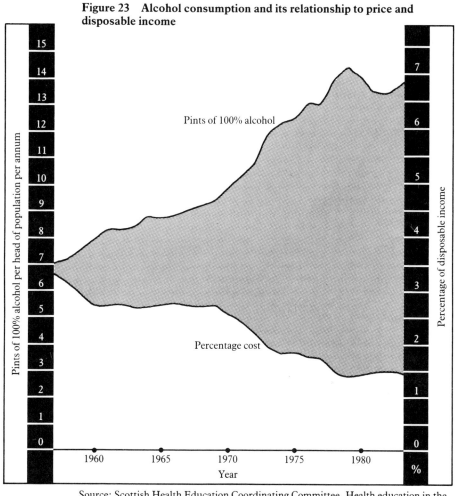

Source: Scottish Health Education Coordinating Committee. Health education in the prevention of alcohol-related disease. Edinburgh, SHEEC, 1985.

choices. Moreover, the relative contribution that glamorised TV images of drinking might make is unknown. A detailed analysis of the portrayal of alcohol on TV showed that seven out of ten fictional characters were portrayed drinking. The dangers of drinking were rarely emphasised, and alcohol was mostly portrayed as a glamorous social lubricant.[93]

Education about alcohol   Beliefs in the ability of isolated public education campaigns to change drinking patterns have been shown to be unrealistic. The most effective educational strategies are those which are linked to legislation, and preferably to a comprehensive national strategy to reduce alcohol consumption.[94] Alcohol education continues to

89

receive a low priority in policy and resource terms in the UK. There is a need for a sustained national effort to educate the community about the sensible use of alcohol. A national survey conducted by the former HEC in 1985[95] showed that the public is ill-informed about alcohol: a majority thought it only harmed those who were 'dependent', and most did not understand that one standard unit of beer was no different from one unit of whisky or wine.

The need for better education for doctors is emphasised in research which shows uncertainty among GPs about what constitutes safe drinking.[96,97] Evaluations of SHEG and HEC's former campaigns in Scotland and north east England over the last decade confirm that mass media initiatives increased awareness of the problem, but the response was short-lived and had no demonstrable effect on behaviour.[98] The north east campaign resulted in a serious oversaturation of the alcohol treatment services.[99] We await the results of a more recent HEC initiative *Understanding Alcohol* in south west England,[100] which aims to progress through local cooperation and long-term planning rather than exclusive use of the mass media.

The best researched educational initiatives so far have been directed at the minority of people who are dependent on alcohol. Alcohol consumption can be reduced in about 60 per cent of clients, and one session of simple counselling may be as effective as longer term outpatient treatment programmes.[101] With the exception of seriously dependent drinkers, total abstinence is neither a necessary nor appropriate goal for the majority who are able to limit themselves to sensible long-term drinking.[102] A randomised trial showed that community-based day centre facilities were more effective in reducing alcohol consumption than both hospital and outpatient treatment.[103]

Preliminary research by SHEG into two further approaches designed to reach problem drinkers has been promising. Evaluation of a self help manual,[104] *So You Want to Cut Down Your Drinking*, and a kit for use by GPs known as DRAMS (Drinking Reasonably with Moderate Self Control) suggest that they could form a useful part of an overall programme.[105]

The availability of alcohol

The availability of alcohol is largely governed by controls on the number and type of outlets selling alcohol, their hours of licensing, together with a minimum legal age for drinking, which is 18 throughout the UK. Relaxation of the licensing laws in the 1960s led to a massive proliferation in the number of outlets which sold alcohol. In 1983 there were 180,000 – representing a 40 per cent increase since 1973. While these increases were accompanied by increases in per capita consumption (see page 62), the specific effects of licensing laws on consumption patterns are difficult to interpret.

Experience worldwide suggests that dramatic relaxation (which occurred in Finland in 1969) or reduction in the number of outlets and/or licensing hours (which occurred in the UK in 1915) is followed by correspondingly dramatic increases (or decreases) in alcohol consumption (and damage). Against a background of many other influential socioeconomic factors it is much harder to assess the impact of minor changes in licensing, such as the small extension in licensing hours which occurred in Scotland in 1976. Although there has been no adequately controlled research on the impact of the Scottish changes on per capita alcohol consumption, overall trends in alcohol-related damage have been broadly similar for men and women in both Scotland and England and Wales[106] (where licensing remains unchanged). There is no evidence either from Scotland, or elsewhere in the world, that relaxation of licensing laws can confer any benefit to health. Indeed, recent evidence from the USA suggests the opposite may be true.[107]

Drinking among young people

A reduction in the short-term, often fatal, consequences of alcohol misuse among the young, may be achieved not so much by reducing total consumption as by changes in the environments which promote inappropriate drinking. There is clearly potential for joint initiatives between the police and publicans to enforce the existing licensing laws governing under-age drinking. A joint educational and enforcement initiative between police and publicans in Devonshire demonstrated a significant reduction (nearly 30 per cent) in alcohol-related convictions over the period (and area) that the policy operated.[108] In the light of research which shows that the clustering of pubs in inner cities may contribute to alcohol-related crime among under 21s,[109] there is further scope for responsible use of licensing, together with efficient public transport services, in preventing alcohol-related damage among young people.

While the pub is a fundamental part of social life in both urban and rural communities, alcohol need not be seen as the only way to ensure social cohesion. The provision of a wider variety of cheap non-alcoholic drinks (which at present are often overpriced), together with a range of snacks, may relieve some of the traditional pressure on pub-goers to drink alcohol exclusively.

Alcohol: Progress in the UK

Compared with the centrally coordinated strategy (see Chapter 12) for the prevention of illicit drug use, there has been little government action on alcohol.[110] It has been largely confined to a preliminary statement in 1981[111] and sporadic initiatives on drinking and driving (see Chapter 6). Alcohol taxation, which raises over £6,000 million annually in government revenue, is not used to control consumption, and government funding for public education on

91

alcohol has contracted rather than expanded in real terms. The total alcohol education budget for SHEG and HEC in 1985 was about £400,000 – 15 times less than that spent on mass media campaigns against illicit drugs. Limited funds have permitted only infrequent public education and information campaigns on alcohol.

The alcohol misuse field has been characterised by too many ineffective agencies with overlapping functions. A DHSS committee which reviewed their functions in England and Wales in 1982 recommended that existing agencies be amalgamated into one national agency for help and support services, that HEC and SHEG deal with public education, and that a new, independent, campaigning agency be established.[112] In the event, there are still several agencies in the field – including Alcohol Concern, the Institute for Alcohol Studies and AAA – with overlapping roles. Alcohol Concern receives government funds, but is not supposed to criticise government. By contrast, AAA, set up by the royal medical colleges with a purely campaigning function, receives no government support.

The potential for promoting sensible alcohol policies at a local level is extensive[113] but has been slow to develop, especially in primary care.[114] A review of action by health education units in England and Wales suggests that alcohol is given priority by a minority, with up to 17 per cent having designated a health education officer with specific responsibility for alcohol as well as a form of community alcohol control team.[115] Progress in Scotland has been in many sectors. In the two years following the SHECC report on alcohol, a series of conferences and seminars had been organised for multidisciplinary audiences involving health boards, local authorities as well as contacts with GPs, local councillors, trades unions and the judiciary.

Alcohol: progress in other countries

While culture and history make it difficult to translate experience from other countries directly to the UK, the relaxation of previous controls on alcohol and the increase in consumption that took place between the mid-1950s and mid-1970s was a world-wide phenomenon which has led, in the last decade, to more effective action being taken in countries other than the UK. There have been extensive health education programmes in France together with some pressure on the wine industry to convert vineyards to other crops. Alcohol consumption fell by 17 per cent between 1977 and 1984. In the USA, constituent states have been compelled by federal government to raise the legal minimum age for drinking to curb drunken driving by teenagers. In the USSR, extensive fiscal, licensing and production restrictions introduced in 1986 are said to have reduced per capita consumption by 38 per cent. A multi-faceted programme in Sweden which included fiscal and educational measures together with a ban on alcohol advertising, a reduction in the alcohol content of beer, and restrictions on licensing hours, was associated with a 17 per cent fall in per capita consumption between 1977 and 1982, together with nearly a 30 per cent reduction in death rates from cirrhosis of the liver.[116] The UK government, by contrast, has taken little action, and supports further relaxation in the licensing laws in England. Moreover the Chancellor did not increase the excise duty on any alcoholic beverage in either 1986 or 1987, allowing the real price of alcohol to continue falling.

Road use The promotion of safe road use, and the prevention of unnecessary deaths on the roads, is not always seen as a 'lifestyle' issue. But the cars we drive, the way we learn to use the road and the influence transport policy has on us forms part of our 'lifestyle' and can adversely affect our health, as do cigarettes, diet and alcohol. In Chapter 6 we examined the major determinants of road safety and the progress made in reducing the death toll on the roads over the last decade. Here we assess those policies which have contributed, or could contribute, towards further improvements.

Seat belts – lifesaving or risk compensation? We have already shown in Chapter 6 how seat belt use increased following the legislation and was followed by a dramatic fall in deaths to front seat car (and light van) occupants. It has been argued that while the legislation has saved the lives of front seat car occupants, it may have encouraged more dangerous driving – known as 'risk compensation' – and resulted in increases in casualties among other road users.[117] Although there is good reason to believe that 'risk compensation' does indeed occur when drivers have *direct feedback*, such as in the case of improved brakes or tyres, nearly all the available evidence suggests that it does not take place among seat belt users.[118,119] First, there is no clear upward trend in casualties among other road users such as pedestrians or cyclists. Indeed, between 1984 and 1985 they fell three per cent and 13 per cent respectively. Second, observational studies show, if anything, that people who wear seat belts – voluntarily or compulsorily – are inclined to take fewer rather than greater risks on the road.[120] Third, a major DHSS case-control study in 15 hospitals throughout the UK showed that the legislation resulted in a 25 per cent reduction in casualties and a 20 per cent reduction in hospital admissions in the year following the seat belt legislation.[121]

Motorcyclists The 1981 Transport Act imposed new regulations on motorcyclists, limiting provisional licences to two years and requiring a more stringent, two-part driving test. The maximum allowable engine size for learners was also reduced from 250 cc to 125 cc. Although overall casualty rates for motorcyclists remained static, the number of 17-19 year old motorcyclists who became involved in accidents fell by 36 per cent between 1982 and 1985.

Local road safety measures

The reorganisation of local authorities in 1974 saw the transfer of responsibility for road safety in residential areas to local authorities, most of which have since developed accident investigation and prevention teams. Their road safety officers are now responsible for the educational aspects of road safety. Although national figures cannot reflect local initiatives, individual authorities have demonstrated substantial reductions in casualties at local accident black-spots.[122] Low cost measures such as the redesign of junctions, improvements in lights and reduced speed limits were implemented by the former GLC at 1,500 sites, and resulted in an estimated saving of 3,000 accidents per year.[123]

Drinking and driving

The 1967 Road Safety Act introduced the 'breathalyser' and made it illegal to drive a motor vehicle with a blood alcohol level over 80 mg per cent (milligrams per 100 millilitres). In the first year when public awareness and publicity surrounding the Act was high, casualties fell by 11 per cent and road deaths by 15 per cent.[124] The Department of Transport has estimated that the legislation saved 5,000 lives and prevented 200,000 road casualties in its first seven years of operation. But convictions for drunken driving rose in the mid-1970s, and by 1980 they were ten times the 1967 levels in England and Wales, and twice the 1967 levels in Scotland.[125] Although part of this rise may be attributable to increased police enforcement, there is no good evidence that this has occurred – except sporadically. The rise in drunken driving offences led the government to set up the Blennerhassett committee which concluded in 1976 that it was not so much that the Act was ineffective, but that it was not being properly enforced.[126] Its recommendations formed the basis for part of the 1981 Transport Act designed to improve enforcement of the 1967 Act and included the introduction of evidential breath testing at the roadside.

Although it is too soon to be certain, preliminary analysis by the Department of Transport claims that evidential breath testing, together with more national publicity, has resulted in a reduction in road casualties in non-built up areas. Early returns from coroners for 1985 have shown 23 per cent of cases were over the legal blood alcohol limit – the lowest proportion for a decade.[127]

Education and training in road safety

The Department of Transport spent £1.7 million on promoting road safety in 1985 – about 0.04 per cent of total transport spending in England. Public education initiatives have been fragmented with isolated campaigns directed at individual road user groups. The

Department of Transport acknowledges the difficulty of evaluating the effect of an educational initiative in isolation from other measures, but a controlled experiment on a drink and driving publicity initiative during Christmas 1982 was not able to demonstrate any significant effect.[128]

There is debate over the effect of education and training programmes for young people. While there is evidence that teaching primary school children the Green Cross Code has resulted in a reduction in childhood casualties, this effect is not sustainable.[129] Similarly, the National Cycling Proficiency Scheme has been demonstrated to improve cycling performance, but has had no demonstrable effect on casualties.[130] Of greater concern is the observation that those who are trained in motorcycle proficiency are *more* likely to be involved in accidents than those who are not.[131]

Maximising road safety – could we do better? The TRRL has estimated that if existing practices are pursued, accidents could be reduced by one-sixth in the ten years between 1982–92. If new, effective, measures were introduced, accidents could be reduced by an estimated one-third.[132]

The environment Effective road safety policies require better interdepartmental coordination at national and local levels.[133] Road safety and better planned amenities – especially for pedestrians – are an integral part of transport policy in the Netherlands and Japan whose safety record for pedestrians is much better than in the UK.[134]

As trains and buses offer the demonstrably safest means of travel, more effort might usefully be directed towards ensuring that public transport is not allowed to decline any further. There is some evidence that the operation of the cheaper fares systems by the GLC and the price freeze in south Yorkshire, resulted in an increased use of public transport in those areas – at a time of declining national use – and an associated reduction in road casualties.[135] But government's plans for transport in 1987–88 involve further reductions in subsidies for British Rail, and the promotion of continued deregulation of the bus services.

Although over 60 per cent of households own cars, the principle of controls on access and speed in the interests of pedestrian safety is widely accepted. TRRL analysis has shown that the deliberate provision of separate cycleways leading to major amenities, together with a pedestrian-centred policy like the Dutch *woonerven* (where pedestrians have greater rights than motorised transport) would result in better road safety records among both pedestrians and cyclists in the UK.[136]

The vehicles While car design has improved greatly, much remains to be achieved. Research has shown that design measures such as a reinforced passenger box, rear seat belts, speed governors, and modification of seat belts and the steering column might further minimise passenger – and in some cases pedestrian – injuries.[137,138]

The road users Most technical or environmental measures need educational reinforcement to promote maximal effectiveness. The small budget and the current isolation of national and local education and training initiatives from those with experience in the production and use of educational materials is illogical. This is especially true of the lack of integration of the drink and driving initiatives into the former HEC's overall alcohol education programme. In addition to education, the most effective way of reducing the alcohol-associated injury on the roads is to increase the probability of detection of alcohol-related offences. This has been achieved in Australia through the introduction of frequent or 'random' breath testing in New South Wales which has been shown to be both effective and acceptable to the public.[139,140]

The consequences of what might be perceived as increased police interference in personal liberty might be overcome if the police were to adopt an educational rather than authoritarian approach. In New South Wales, police spend half an hour of each shift engaged in random breath testing. Random breath testing was recommended by the former government Think Tank, the Central Policy Review Staff,[141] the Department of Transport's Blennerhassett committee,[142] the BMA,[143] and the Royal College of Psychiatrists.[144] In 1982, the New South Wales government further reduced the legal alcohol limit from 80 to 20 mg per cent for 'novice drivers' – that is, those with a full driving licence less than one year old. Preliminary results suggest that this has been effective in reducing road accidents among young people.[145]

Sexual and reproductive practices The tendency to consider the prevention of one disease in isolation from others has hitherto prevented us from seeing the strands of evidence which might unify rather than isolate policies on the prevention of cervical cancer and sexually transmitted disease with those concerning the prevention of the spread of AIDS. We return to this discussion in Chapter 13, where we look further at sexuality and its relationship to family planning. Such an approach might also minimise the waste of scarce resources, as well as highlight the opportunities for *primary* as well as secondary *prevention* of diseases such as cervical cancer.

Primary prevention of sexually transmitted diseases

Education is not the only available means for the prevention of the spread of AIDS. The national strategy for limiting the spread of AIDS already involves a combination of educational and public health measures aimed at the screening of blood and blood products and limiting intravenous drug use and needle-sharing (see Chapter 13). There are two broad approaches which are likely to have an impact on sexually transmitted disease: a reduction in the number of sexual partners and the promotion of what is now known as 'safer sex' – that is, the use of barrier methods of contraception together with the avoidance of sexual practices which involve the exchange of infected body fluids. The value of these approaches will depend on their effectiveness as well as their feasibility, and on the ethics of advocating the required changes. From the evidence so far, we know that changes in sexual behaviour would need to be very substantial in order to influence disease trends. Celibacy is probably not a feasible option but reduction in the number of sexual partners and increased use of barrier methods of contraception are realistic objectives.

Research in the field of sexual behaviour is difficult to conduct and there are still very few studies of the effectiveness of barrier contraception in the prevention of AIDS. Laboratory experiments have shown that the virus does not leak through the major, commercially available, condoms[146] and that the virus is inactivated by spermicides containing nonoxynol-9.[147] Condom use is associated with a lower risk of cervical pre-cancer[148] and of other STDs that are caused by viruses (for example, genital herpes) and bacteria (for example, gonorrhoea).[149]

Some small studies among prostitutes and the sexual partners of AIDS sufferers suggest that condom use reduces the risk of becoming HIV positive,[150] but the dangers of condom use for anal intercourse are likely to be considerable as condom brands currently available have been known to burst and the risk of infection is high in those who practise it.[151] There is little information on the effect of other barrier methods of contraception, although one study has shown that the risk of cervical cancer among diaphragm users is 25 per cent of that among women who use other forms of contraception – even when sexual behaviour is taken into account.[152]

It has been argued that it may not be possible to achieve major changes in patterns of contraceptive use, especially now that the pill is the predominant form of contraception among young heterosexuals. However, methods of contraception have changed relatively quickly over the last two decades, and condoms were the most popular form of contraception until the early 1970s when the pill took over (see Chapter 13). Weighed against this is considerable evidence that condoms are disliked.[153,154] Moreover, the incentive to use condoms to avoid pregnancy is not relevant for homosexual men, and diaphragms have never been used by more than a minority of sexually active women. Recent research has suggested that future mass media and other educational initiatives should concentrate on generating a positive, caring image for condoms rather than on focussing on creating anxiety about AIDS.[155] Such efforts have already been made in New Zealand and Australia where condoms have been promoted as 'parachutes' and 'lifesavers'.

Evidence is also gradually accumulating that a reduction in risky sexual practices, as well as in the number of sexual partners, is an achievable goal among homosexual men. Prospective studies in the US[156,157] have shown that a reduction in transmission of the virus is associated with reductions in the number of sexual partners, in anal intercourse, and in condom use. British studies among homosexual men attending STD clinics have shown that the rate of rise of HIV infection in this group has slowed down since 1984, and that this has also been associated with a significant fall in diagnosis rates for gonorrhoea.[158] These changes have been much less impressive among heterosexual men so far.[159,160] What we do not yet know is whether changes in sexual practices are feasible among those who may not perceive themselves to be at risk, and who practise serial monogamy. In the USA, where the epidemic is three years further advanced than in the UK, many have attributed the slowing down in the exponential growth of the epidemic to changes in sexual behaviour. But this conclusion may be premature, as it could equally be explained by the dynamics of HIV infection.[161]

Secondary prevention: screening for cervical cancer
Screening to detect pre-cancerous stages of the disease is a method of proven value in reducing the incidence and mortality from cervical cancer, as well as of avoiding the trauma of radical surgery. Population screening programmes – when efficiently organised – have been shown to reduce both the incidence and mortality for cervical cancer. The incidence of invasive cancer has fallen by up to 50 per cent in all the Scandinavian countries with organised screening programmes.[162] Although it is more than 25 years since the cervical screening programme was introduced in the UK, it has so far failed to reduce the incidence and mortality from cervical cancer in a substantial way.[163-165] There were three million cervical cancer smears performed in 1980, representing an increase of only 19 per cent between 1972 and 1980. In parts of the country such as Aberdeen and Dundee, where the screening system is efficiently organised and gives reasonable population cover, the incidence of the disease has fallen substantially.[166,167]

National results are disappointing, largely because the screening programme has been organised in a haphazard way, with fragmented responsibility for its implementation. There are no national estimates for the proportion of women who are screened in each age group; the national, computerised call-recall system has only recently been established, and it is operational in a minority of health districts. We know from individual studies that over half of the smears are taken from women under 35, and that 80 per cent of women who have invasive cervical cancer have never had a smear. We also know that women are poorly informed about the purpose and value of cervical screening.[168]

Although GPs are paid to perform smears only on women over 35 years of age every five years, the evidence suggests that this has had little effect on the distribution of screening, which remains substantially concentrated on younger women. Some of the continuing fall in incidence and mortality that occurred in women aged 35–54 during the 1970s is probably attributable to screening. It has been estimated that in the 15 years prior to 1978, screening may have prevented up to 25 per cent of potentially invasive disease.[169]

Effective screening programmes have the following identifiable features in common.[170-175]

- They are organised with the explicit aim of reducing mortality from cervical cancer, and the aim is to cover *the whole adult female population*.
- There is a computerised call-recall system based on population registers, and women are followed up until they attend.
- One person has overall responsibility for coordination and liaison with the local service.
- Adequate resources are available for taking, examining and reporting on smears efficiently.
- Women have the option of being examined by a woman doctor.
- Women are informed of the value and function of a screening programme.
- There is a built-in monitoring system to assess efficiency and effectiveness.

Some recent research has suggested that there may be a more quickly invasive variant of cervical cancer in young women[176] which may warrant changes in both screening and referral policy. Overall trends however, do not support this view,[177] and it would be premature to change current policy.

Some claim that the cost of cervical screening is higher than can be justified.[178] Their argument is essentially that, at £10 per examination, we spend £30 million per year on screening in the UK, and the most that could be claimed is that it has saved about 100 lives per year. This works out at £300,000 per life saved. Others disagree with this estimated number of lives saved, suggesting that the present screening programme may now be preventing as many as 2,000 cases

Table 15   Estimated potential effects of different screening policies for women aged 20–64, in England and Wales, assuming 100% acceptance of screening

Screening policy	Number of cancers per annum	Number of cancers prevented	Number of smears per annum*	Cost of smears per annum
No screening	4,600			
Present 'opportunistic' system	2,700	1,900	3,400,000	£34,000,000
5-yearly ALL women aged 20–64	700	3,900	3,400,000	£34,000,000
3-yearly ALL women aged 20–64	400	4,200	5,500,000	£55,000,000
Annually ALL women aged 20–64	300	4,300	16,500,000	£165,000,000

*The estimates of number of smears allow for the fact that about 20 per cent of the workload is in non-routine repeat tests on women who have had a previous abnormality.
Source: Smith A, and Chamberlain J. Managing cervical screening. In: Institute of Health Service Management. Information Technology in Health Care. London, Kluwer Publications Ltd, 1987.

of invasive cancer per annum,[179] perhaps half of which would lead to death if not diagnosed until they were invasive.

If present resources were more effectively managed it is probable that the number of cancers prevented and number of lives saved would be substantially greater. Table 15 illustrates the potential effect of five-yearly, three-yearly or annual screening in England and Wales if 100 per cent of women were screened at the stated intervals and not more often. This suggests that our current resources are sufficient to prevent 2,000 more cases each year, perhaps saving 1,000 more lives, than we are achieving with the present opportunistic system.[180] What most escalates the cost of each case prevented and each life saved is the inefficient distribution of screening.

Thus the most immediate priority is to improve the distribution of present screening resources by the methods outlined earlier. Whether or not there should be a change from a five-yearly policy to a three-yearly policy is principally an economic issue. Table 15 shows that such a change would, if fully implemented, prevent an additional 300 cases per year (150 lives saved) at an additional cost of 2,200,000 smears, or somewhat over £22,000,000, giving a marginal value of nearly £75,000 per extra case prevented or £150,000 per extra life saved. Because these figures are based on the target of 100 per cent acceptance of the recommended screening policy through-out life, they can really only be used to illustrate the marginal cost-utility of changing the screening interval. Health authorities who have decided to put more money into cervical screening should consider using it more effectively in measures to increase acceptance rather than shortening the screening interval.

Sexually transmitted disease: progress in the UK

No attempt has yet been made to develop a coherent strategy that links the prevention of sexually transmitted disease with sex education and family planning policy. Nevertheless, substantial progress has been made both at national and local levels to link strategies to reduce the spread of AIDS with those aimed at minimising the use of intravenous drugs (see Chapter 13). In the UK, most action in the field was initially undertaken by voluntary agencies such as the Terrence Higgins Trust, and later by the College of Health and organisations such as Body Positive. The UK government has responded to the need to develop a population-wide approach to AIDS. Public health measures such as screening of all blood donors and the heat treatment of clotting factor concentrates were implemented quickly. Other measures such as syringe ex-change schemes (see Chapter 13) have been introduced experimen-tally, although no attempt has yet been made to make condoms more freely available outside family planning clinics, some STD clinics and some drug dependency and information centres.

In 1986, the government established an interministerial cabinet sub-committee to coordinate national action on AIDS. In the same year, the first national press information campaign was launched. In November 1986, £20 million was allocated to develop mass media educational initiatives on TV and radio as well as a leaflet entitled *AIDS: Don't Die of Ignorance* which was sent to every household. Collaboration with TV culminated in a TV AIDS Week in which all television channels participated. Since then, £14.5 million has been given to the MRC to support research into the development of a vaccine together with £3 million to WHO to support international efforts to combat AIDS. In late 1986, the DHSS established a National Advisory (telephone) Service on AIDS to support BBC radio initiatives and has increased its support to voluntary agencies in the field as well as establishing a new AIDS Trust in 1987, whose aim is to coordinate national and local action. The Health Education Authority has taken over the management of the government's public education campaign, and is piloting a teaching pack on AIDS for use in schools.

Monitoring of knowledge, attitudes and practices related to AIDS between February 1986 and 1987 showed a high awareness of the government's AIDS campaign and a high level of knowledge about

AIDS. There was also evidence, in four waves of market research during the period, that homosexual men, but not heterosexuals, engaged in risky sexual practices less frequently and had reduced the number of their sexual partners.[181] This trend had already begun before the government campaign, and credit must thus also be given to other educational initiatives, both by the media and by voluntary agencies and health professionals at STD clinics. Other research in STD clinics showed that successive phases of the government campaign resulted in waves of anxiety and major increases in attendance rates and requests for HIV counselling and screening.[182,183] While counselling and voluntary HIV testing is an essential part of the STD clinic service, little account has yet been taken of whether it is helpful to generate 'panic' testing and whether sufficient resources have been allocated to STD clinics to deal with the increased workload. Other qualitative research based on SHEG's work in Scotland has demonstrated the need to re-emphasise the dangers of transmission to heterosexuals and to correct misconceptions about the transmission of HIV.[184]

It is beyond the scope of this report to describe in detail the many local initiatives that have been taken by both statutory and voluntary agencies. Nevertheless, we have been concerned about the relative imbalance of resources devoted by government to mass media campaigns at the expense of support that is needed by health education departments for longer term training and educational activities. Attention has also been drawn to this in the Social Services Committee's 1987 report on AIDS.[185] Local authorities have taken a lead in appointing special AIDS prevention officers, and by February 1987, 88 per cent of DHAs had also set up groups to coordinate local AIDS strategies, with nearly half having nominated individual AIDS coordinators.[186]

Limiting AIDS: the future It would be premature to judge the effectiveness of efforts to limit the spread of AIDS, not least because developments in the vaccine and treatment fields, as well as changes in the epidemic itself, may profoundly affect the future impact of HIV disease on society. Current knowledge suggests that the problem of AIDS will persist for at least another half a century. The current challenge is to limit further spread of the virus among intravenous drug users and heterosexuals. We cannot assume that measures which have begun to show results among homosexual men will be equally relevant for other groups, where sexual norms may be very different, and among groups such as intravenous drug users who may prove more difficult to reach. Heterosexuals may perceive themselves to be more at risk if the message is widened to include the prevention of other sexually transmitted diseases.

Breast cancer – reducing the death toll We have already seen in Chapter 4 that breast cancer may be related to reproductive experience and that there is a possible, but as yet incompletely substantiated, association with obesity and a high fat, low fibre diet.

There are few realistic policy options for the primary prevention of breast cancer. It would be inappropriate to attempt to influence reproductive practices, and it is premature to make any recommendations concerning the use of oral contraception. The main policy option for the immediate future rests with early detection and prompt treatment. There is now good international evidence upon which a national mammographic breast screening programme can be based.[187]

- There is no convincing evidence that self examination or screening by clinical examination of the breasts can reduce mortality from breast cancer.
- Screening using an x-ray technique known as mammography can reduce mortality among women aged 50–64 (in some studies up to 74) by one-third or more. A fully implemented UK mammography service would be expected to save 2,000 lives per year among women over 50.
- Screening appears to be acceptable to women, and attendance rates can be maintained at above 60 per cent, although they fall off among women over 65.
- The radiation risk associated with the current techniques of mammography is negligible compared with its benefits, although there are no estimates of its cumulative effects. Mammography is a highly sensitive technique that can accurately detect up to 90 per cent of breast cancers. Recent developments have greatly reduced the proportion of false positives.
- There remain a number of unresolved issues which need further research, such as how often women should be screened, and the psychological impact of screening women.

On the basis of the available evidence a report commissioned by the DHSS (the Forrest report) recommended that a national programme should be gradually established throughout the UK in which women aged 50–64 should be screened every three years, with an eventual possible extension to include older women.[188] The estimated annual cost of such a programme would be £50 million at 1985–86 prices. The Forrest report identified the following essential components of a programme.

- It would require 120 new screening units to be established, each with access to a multidisciplinary team skilled in the diagnosis and management of breast disease. Each unit should serve a population of about 50,000 women covering about two health districts or boards.

- A specific person – probably a community physician – should be designated as responsible for managing the service.
- There should be an up-to-date, preferably computerised, record system which is able to identify, invite and recall all women eligible for screening. This would normally be the FPC register or its Scottish equivalent.
- Every eligible woman should be sent a personal invitation to be screened from her GP.

The government has accepted the recommendations of the Forrest report but had committed only £6 million to support the programme by April 1987. The importance of associated information, education and counselling services was not considered by the Forrest report, and there are currently no obvious plans to develop such services.

8 Promoting equal opportunities for health

> Medicine is a social science, and politics
> nothing but medicine on a grand scale.
> RUDOLPH VIRCHOW

Introduction

In our analysis so far, we have shown that death rates have improved at all ages but that our international position would be much improved by more effective measures to prevent coronary heart disease and cancers. We have also pointed to the continuing social disparities in death rates at every stage in life, and specifically for coronary heart disease and lung cancer. In this chapter we consider inequalities in health across the whole range of disease, their determinants and their trends over the last decade. We consider inequality in health from a number of different standpoints including social class, education, housing tenure and geography, as well as gender and ethnic group. We conclude with an assessment of past policy, and implications of the findings for current policies to promote healthier lifestyles.

Social class and health

Almost all health indicators confirm the association between the prevalence of ill health and poor social and economic circum-

Table 16 Social class differences in death rates among adults in Great Britain (Standardised mortality ratios[1])

Social Class		1959–63[2] Men	Married Women[4]	1970–2[2] Men	Married Women[4]	1979–80 & 1982–83[3] Men	Married Women[4]
I	Professional	76	77	77	82	66	75
II	Intermediate	81	83	81	87	76	83
IIIN	Skilled non-manual	100	103	104	109	106	107
IIIM	Skilled manual						
IV	Semi-skilled	103 } 115	105 } 116	114 } 121	119 } 124	} 129	133
V	Unskilled	143	141	137	135		100
All		100	100	100	100	100	

. SMRs express age-adjusted death rates as a percentage of the average (which = 100) at each date.
. England and Wales, ages 15–64 years.
. Great Britain, age 20–64; 20–59 for married women.
. Married women are classified by their husband's occupations
Sources: OPCS Decennial supplements on occupational mortality. London, HMSO, 1971, 1978, 1986

stances.[1,2] In 1981, the death rate was twice as high in the lowest social classes as in the highest (see Table 16). The expectation of life for a child with parents in social class V is about eight years shorter than for a child whose parents are in social class I.

While there is still an incomplete understanding of this association, recent research has improved the position.

The relative disadvantage of those in the classes comprising the manual workers (classes V, IV and III manual) may be most simply expressed by comparing the actual number of deaths in these classes with the number that would have occurred if they had enjoyed the death rates prevailing among the largely non-manual workers (classes I, II and III non-manual). In 1981:

- men in the manual worker classes had death rates 45 per cent higher than men in the non-manual classes, and women had death rates 43 per cent higher;
- the excess mortality associated with being in the manual worker classes was greater than the total number of deaths from stroke, infectious disease, accidents, lung cancer and other respiratory diseases combined;
- if manual workers had enjoyed the same death rates as non-manual workers there would have been 42,000 fewer deaths during the year in the age-range 16–74;
- if mortality at all ages is also considered, the total excess mortality associated with manual work social classes amounts to the equivalent of a major air crash or shipwreck every day.

What is especially striking is that these socioeconomic differences in mortality experience are not confined to a few diseases in which an excess vulnerability might be associated with specific occupational or social factors. The association between social deprivation and disease is broadly based. Of the 66 'major list' causes of death among men, 62 were more common among social classes IV and V (combined) than among all other men in 1981.[3] Of the 70 major causes of death among women, 64 were more common among women married to men in social classes IV and V.[4]

Trends in health inequalities Social class differences in death rates have widened almost continuously since 1951.[5–8] While overall death rates have fallen over this period (see Chapter 2) the death rates in the non-manual classes have declined more than those in the manual classes (see Table 16). If this increased social class inequality is expressed in terms of the proportion of deaths among men and women that would need to be redistributed in order to equalise death rates, then that proportion has doubled since the second world war.[9]

106

The only evidence of a reduction in health inequalities appears to have been for postneonatal mortality during the 1970s (see Chapter 2). It was associated with a disproportionate reduction in the number of births in the manual classes during that period. Measuring inequality across *all* classes, however, rather than simply comparing extremes, suggests that this improvement has not continued since the late 1970s.

Inequalities in the mortality experience of the social classes has persisted – and probably increased – at a time when general variation in the life-span has actually decreased.[10] This reduced variation in life-span is predominantly attributable to a reduction in the importance of those causes of death that operate especially at younger ages (the infections and accidents), and a consequently greater influence of diseases that characteristically kill in late middle life or in old age. It is the more remarkable that death rates from these diseases continue to show such striking social inequality.

The reliability of the data   Wide social class differences in death rates, and consequently in expectation of life, have been reported since 1921 when social class analysis of mortality was first published by the Registrar General. These statistics, which formed the basis of the Black report on *Inequalities in Health*, published by the DHSS in 1980,[11] have always provided the main (but not the only) evidence of socioeconomic differences in health.

The Black report concluded that the observed disparities in health were real, and had widened continuously among adults since 1951. *The Health Divide*, which reviewed the evidence published since the Black report, came to the same conclusion in 1988.[12] Others have argued that the figures are heavily influenced by the gradual upward movement in the class distribution of the population, and by a particular tendency of the healthiest individuals to upward social mobility.

The question at the centre of this issue is whether people in the lower social classes are less healthy because they are socially deprived and living in poorer circumstances, or whether they have moved into the lower classes because they are less healthy. Recent research suggests that there is a tendency for social mobility to discriminate against the less healthy at both ends of life. Childhood hospitalisation[13] and short stature[14,15] prejudice a person's chances of upward social mobility, and chronic illness later in life limits job choices and opportunities.[16] However, these factors make only minor contributions to the observed class differences in health, and there is no evidence that their influence has increased.[17]

Measures which take account of the changing proportion of the population in different classes show that this process is not responsible for the tendency for social class differences in death rates to widen.[18,19] The possible influence of revisions to the way in which occupations are allocated to the social classes has been examined by restricting the analysis to those occupations which can be consistently identified throughout the time period. The findings do not suggest that this is the source of the apparent widening in mortality differentials.[20]

Inequalities in the experience of illness

Not only are minor ailments more common among the manual classes, there is also evidence that people in manual classes who already have cancers, or heart disease, are less likely to survive.[21] We do not have comprehensive statistics on the occurrence of illness, but interesting data are collected from the General Household Survey which relies on people's own assessments of their health. Although people's assessments of their own health are influenced by varying norms and expectations between classes, reported rates of chronic illness and days of restricted activity in 1983 were twice as high in social class V as in social class I. Differences in the reporting of illnesses which temporarily restricted people's activity were smaller. Surveys of people's perception of their health (as opposed to their sickness) have shown that a sense of wellbeing is also related to social class.[22] While social class differences in height and obesity are small, four times as many people in social class V had no natural teeth, compared with social class I in England and Wales in 1980, and, in 1983, five year olds from manual backgrounds had twice as many decayed teeth as those from professional backgrounds (see Chapter 12).

Newer classifications of deprivation

The observed health gradient is not unique to the Registrar General's social classification. In the largest prospective study of its kind, the Longitudinal Study, analogous gradients can be shown if people are grouped according to whether they own or do not own a car, own or rent their home, or by the amount of education they have had (see Table 17).

These different classifications are not simply different ways of identifying the *same* group of disadvantaged people. If two or more classifications are used simultaneously, even larger differences in death rates are found.[23] Thus, while all men who have access to one or more cars have death rates 15 per cent below the average, those who were also owner-occupiers in 1971–81 had death rates that were 23 per cent below the average.[24]

Because people are allocated to the Registrar General's classes on the basis of their occupation, the classification is more suitable for men of working age than it is for many women, the elderly, the unemployed or the economically inactive (most of whom are women). People who cannot be regarded, for statistical purposes, as attached to a wage earner – and are often the most socially deprived – are left out of the classification. For such groups, classifying by housing tenure, education or income offers an alternative way of assessing health disadvantage.

Table 17 Death rates using various socioeconomic classifications (standardised mortality ratios[1])

	Men (Aged 15–64 at death)	Women (Aged 15–59 at death)
Housing tenure[2]		
Owner occupied	84	83
Privately rented	109	106
Local authority	115	117
Education[3]		
Degree	59	66
Non-degree higher qualification	80	78
A-levels only	91	80
None or not stated	103	102
Access to cars[2]		
One or more cars	85	83
No access to a car	121	135

1 SMRs express age-adjusted mortality as a percentage of the average for deaths in England and Wales 1971–81.
2 Aged 15 years and over in 1971.
3 Aged 18 and over in 1971.
Source: Office of Population Censuses and Surveys. OPCS longitudinal study. Unpublished data provided by Social Statistics Research Unit, City University. Crown copyright reserved.

Gender, class and health inequality

Mortality patterns for women follow generally similar class gradients to those of men when married women are classified according to their husband's occupation. However, two-thirds of married women are now engaged in paid work of their own. The classification may therefore conceal important occupational influences on women's health. There appears to have been an increase in mortality rates from lung cancer and coronary heart disease among women married to manual workers[25] (see Chapters 3 and 4), and it is important to identify any contribution that women's own jobs may make to these trends. This is especially so in the light of evidence that when working women's smoking patterns are analysed by their *own* class, the familiar class gradient disappears and women in social class I have a smoking prevalence similar to that for classes IV and V.[26]

The only major analysis of women's mortality rates in relation to

109

their own individual jobs highlights the need for further research. Cancers of the reproductive system (breast, ovary and uterus) were more common among professional women than among those with manual jobs. Although this may reflect differences in childbearing patterns, the mortality patterns for some textile and ceramic workers and cleaners may be work-related.[27]

Health patterns among women may be compared with those of men – irrespective of class. Women seem to have a health advantage over men because they live longer and have lower death rates than men at every stage in life. On the other hand, women are more likely than men to suffer many kinds of ill health – especially mental ill health[28] (see Chapter 10). They also suffer ill health from sex-specific problems, such as cervical and ovarian cancers which may, in part, explain why young women are heavier users of health services than men. The full explanation, however, is more complex.

While a classification of women by their own occupation would be useful, it would shed no light on that large minority of women (nearly 40 per cent) who fall into the 'economically inactive' group. We have yet to find a satisfactory social classification for women which takes into account both their domestic and paid work. This is likely to be fruitful as we already know that, among women, marital status is not associated with the same patterns of mental ill health as in men.[29]

Health, class and ethnic minorities

There are few studies of the class distribution of health among different ethnic groups in the UK. Studies of immigrants (based on the census classification of people by country of birth) found that only Irish immigrants showed the same social class gradient in mortality as the rest of the population.[30] The absence of a social class mortality gradient among immigrants from Africa, the Caribbean, Europe or the Indian subcontinent, may reflect selection and the insulating effect of their previous culture and environment, and of selection. Evidence from other countries shows that these influences tend to diminish with time, and there is evidence that this is already occurring within the Asian community in the UK. Although overall death rates for first generation immigrants from the Indian subcontinent lacked any clear social class gradient, stillbirths and infant mortality rates for subsequent generations of Asian children studied in Bradford showed a steep gradient.[31]

Geographical inequalities

Socioeconomic differences make an important contribution to the marked geographical differences in death rates found in the UK – especially the higher death rates in the north and in Scotland compared with the south and east of the country (see Table 18). There are climatic, cultural and other natural factors – such as water

Table 18 Social class differences in mortality by region

Social classes	All	I	II	IIIN	IIIM	IV+V
	Standardised Mortality Ratios. Average for Great Britain in 1978–9 and 1982–3 = 100					
Scotland						
M	123	74	90	111	137	157
F	124	83	93	100	130	141
North West						
M	114	70	86	105	120	146
F	113	75	88	97	109	135
North						
M	114	72	83	106	115	152
F	112	65	83	92	103	136
Yorkshire and Humberside						
M	104	75	80	100	105	134
F	102	68	79	84	100	120
Wales						
M	104	68	81	99	101	144
F	105	69	81	87	95	125
West Midlands						
M	102	67	76	93	112	127
F	100	67	79	85	105	113
East Midlands						
M	95	69	75	96	92	122
F	95	70	74	80	93	110
South East						
M	89	61	69	87	97	112
F	90	67	72	84	92	100
South West						
M	87	63	70	85	93	108
F	87	66	71	80	88	96
East Anglia						
M	79	65	65	80	80	93
F	81	61	70	72	79	81

Men 20–64, Women 20–59. Married Women classified by husband's occupation, single women by own occupation; N = Non manual; M = Manual.
Source: Office of Population Censuses and Surveys. Occupational mortality 1979–80 and 1982–3, Series D S No 6. London, HMSO, 1986.

hardness – which may contribute to this geographical pattern, but we know little about how they may exert their effects. The observed regional differences in death rates cannot be accounted for in terms of differences in the social class composition of the regional populations,[32] for regional mortality differentials are still present after adjustment for social class. The socioeconomic differences between regions tend to reflect differences between the circumstances of people in broadly similar occupational class categories, rather than differences in the proportions of people in different classes. In the more prosperous south east, people in *each* occupational category tend to do better than their counterparts elsewhere (see Table 18).

At the other end of the geographical scale, health differences between areas as small as electoral wards do reflect the differences in class composition of residential neighbourhoods. Differences in death rates between electoral wards have been studied in several cities. Findings suggest that 60 to 80 per cent of the variation in death rates is related to socioeconomic circumstances.[33,34]

Inequalities: the contribution of medical treatment

The proportion of deaths in the UK today which are regarded as potentially preventable through good medical treatment is small – about five per cent. While many other diseases are partly treatable, it is generally accepted that medical care has had little impact so far on the overall death rate from some of the most important diseases, such as cancers and heart disease (see Chapters 3 and 4).

Although the data are difficult to interpret, social class differences in the uptake of medical care per episode of illness seem to be small. There are significant differences in the use of *preventive* health services, ranging from child health clinics to cervical screening, although systematic data are not available. While these deficiencies clearly need to be remedied, they are unlikely to affect the death rate from most cancers and heart disease which make the biggest contribution to overall mortality differentials.

The relatively minor influence of medical treatment is confirmed by studies which show that geographical differences in the death rate for all causes combined are more closely related to socioeconomic factors than to differences in medical provision.[35] Variations in the death rate from diseases regarded as 'amenable' to medical care do not reflect differences in the standard of medical services.[36] Although class differences in medically preventable mortality have widened slightly more than differences in mortality not regarded as medically preventable,[37] there is no general relationship between the treatability of a disease and the size of the social class difference in its mortality. Social class inequalities in medical care are therefore not a major explanation of mortality differentials.

112

Hazards at work The contribution made by occupational health hazards to social class differences in death rates is difficult to assess. With the exception of those who work in laboratories, non-manual workers are likely to have much lower rates of exposure to chemical and other physical hazards, and so suffer less from both their known and unknown health effects than manual workers. But the distribution of other risk factors, for instance work-related stress, is unknown. Not only are its various components likely to have different social distributions, but their consequences for health are still uncertain (see Chapter 14).

Only a small proportion of the total mortality resulting from exposure to occupational health hazards is currently identifiable. Even what should be regarded as an occupational risk is hard to define. For instance, if exercise is beneficial to health, should the increasing tendency to sedentary work be regarded as an occupational hazard?

One way of estimating the influence of occupation on mortality is to assume that social class is a good guide to the health risks associated with people's domestic circumstances and way of life, and then to compare the variation in death rates between occupations before and after standardising them for their social class. In a study using 25 occupational categories and six social classes, 80 per cent of the mortality variation seemed to be associated with 'way of life' (that is, with social class), and the rest with occupation.[38] Despite its flaws, this is currently the best guide we have.

Genetic factors and health It has been suggested that innate characteristics of individuals may determine their occupation – and therefore their social class – and that these characteristics may also determine health or the capacity of individuals to protect their own and their children's health. It has further been suggested[39,40] that these characteristics may be multifactorially inherited and that their distribution in each generation is an important determinant of social mobility, and of health, and therefore of an association between health and social class.

Such influences can hardly account for social class mortality gradients that have been reversed in the past few decades – for example, the mortality from hypertension, coronary heart disease, stroke, peptic ulcer and suicide, nor for the steepening class gradient in other causes of death.

In the light of a considerable body of current evidence, we can conclude that material inequalities make an important contribution to continuing inequalities in today's major causes of death, such as heart disease, lung cancer, accidents and suicide. There are clearly other important cultural factors involved, but research in this area is still insufficiently developed for us to draw any reliable conclusions.[41]

Identifying specific risk factors
The available evidence is insufficient to identify more than a few of the risk factors that link specific aspects of socioeconomic disadvantage to health. While we may still lack knowledge of the exact *mechanisms* through which these factors operate, this does not put their contributory role in doubt.

Income and health
Income is clearly associated with health. The evidence is clear that the death rates of old people are affected by changes in the real value of state old age pensions, and also that as occupations move up or down the occupational earnings rankings they show a corresponding and opposite movement in the occupational mortality rate.[42] The implication is that income – perhaps the major determinant of standard of living and of life-style – has a direct effect on health. It is also clear that health is more sensitive to small changes in income at lower than at higher income levels.[43,44]

Unemployment and health
There is strong evidence that the deprivations associated with unemployment are damaging to health.[45] After adjusting for the effects of social class and age, the death rates of unemployed men and their wives are at least 20 per cent higher than expected.[46,47] Unemployment is associated with an estimated 1,500 extra deaths among unemployed men and their wives for each million men unemployed.[48] The two-fold higher death rates from suicide among the unemployed in a given social class, point to the importance of psychosocial factors.[49] The relationship between unemployment and parasuicide (see Chapter 10) and the deterioration and subsequent improvement in mental health following unemployment and re-employment, add weight to the relationship between unemployment and mental ill health.[50] While unemployment undoubtedly damages a person's sense of self-worth, part of the psychosocial impact of unemployment must arise from the material disadvantages it brings.

Lifestyle and socioeconomic disadvantage
The interrelationship of smoking, alcohol consumption, diet, physical activity and socioeconomic disadvantage are far from straightforward. There is a clear social class gradient in the prevalence of smoking, and those in the non-manual classes are more likely to have stopped smoking (see Chapter 4). Smoking is particularly prevalent among the unemployed. There is some evidence that smoking is associated with stress[51,52] and that socioeconomic disadvantage is stressful. However, there is also evidence that stress does not impede smoking cessation.[53]

The relationship between socioeconomic disadvantage and alcohol consumption is more complex. The heaviest drinking is concentrated in the manual classes, but there is heavy drinking in all classes (see Chapter 5).

114

Dietary differences between rich and poor make a major contribution to global inequalities in health. In a relatively affluent country such as the UK, they are most readily detectable among children born to working class parents, who are shorter than children born to professionals. But interest in diet has shifted more recently from simple undernutrition to malnutrition – the consumption of a diet that contains excessive quantities of fats, salt and unrefined sugars – which is known to contribute to coronary heart disease, and a range of other health problems (see Chapters 3 and 4). The National Food Survey shows that those in the lowest income categories eat – in many, but not all, respects – a less healthy diet than those with higher incomes; the poorest groups eat less fresh fruit, green vegetables and wholemeal bread (which is high in fibre), and more white bread and sugar, which contribute to obesity and tooth decay (see Table 19). But there is no equivalent social class gradient in the consumption of fats.

These consumption patterns almost certainly reflect income and cost considerations, as well as differences in culture or education. Research shows that *within* each income group the effect of additional children is to shift the pattern of food consumption nearer to that of poorer families.[54] The nutritional differences between large and small families within each income group are reflected in the tendency for people's height to be related, class for class, to their birth order and family size.[55] Small scale studies[56,57] suggest that

Table 19 Income group differences in food consumption

Food	Ratio of average per capita consumption in high income compared with low income households
Fruit	2.1
Wholemeal and wholewheat bread	1.6
Butter	1.44
Cheese	1.35
Fish	1.25
Vegetables	1.1
Margarine	0.8
Potatoes	0.7
Sugar	0.6

High income denotes households where the earners' average weekly income exceeds £270.
Low income denotes households where the earners' average weekly income is below £83.
Source: Ministry of Agriculture, Fisheries and Foods. Household food consumption and expenditure 1984. London, HMSO, 1986.

those on a low income may not be able to afford the diet recommended by the National Advisory Committee on Nutrition Education (see Chapter 3). Although these findings are based on data from highly selected groups, the lack of availabilty of a healthy range of foods in deprived areas is also an important feature limiting food choices.[58]

People in low income households spend proportionally twice as much of their income on food as those in high income households.[59] There is also evidence of undernutrition among the poor. The diets of many school children leave them below the recommended intake for many nutrients,[60] and seven per cent of old people suffer malnutrition;[61] half of women who are single parents on low incomes cut down on their own food consumption to save money,[62] and 25 per cent of unemployed people do not have enough money for food at the end of the week.[63]

The overall impact of social class differences in nutrition is not yet completely established. But the simultaneous widening of social differences in health and in nutrition during the decade following the end of war-time nutritional policy shows that they are important. Social class differences in total fat consumption remained small during the 1950s, immediately after the end of food rationing, but poorer people ate progressively more sugar while the better off ate increasing quantities of wholemeal bread. This period also saw smoking become more common in the manual classes.[64] The most dramatic change in the distribution of disease was the reversal of the social distribution of heart disease which had previously been more common among non-manual groups.[65]

The importance of diet is also reflected in statistical relationships between nutrition and health which exist across regions as well as classes.[66] White bread, sugar and potatoes are eaten most by working class people and in the north of the country, while wholemeal bread, fresh fruit and green vegetables are eaten more by the non-manual classes, and those in the south. While the class differences in tooth loss are partly a reflection of differences in sugar consumption (see Chapter 12), the social distribution of obesity may also be influenced by differences in physical activity, rather than by the comparatively small differences in total calorie intake between classes. Leisure-time exercise is more common among professionals and high income groups, but some of this difference is offset by differences in physical activity between sedentary and manual occupations, and by the effect that car ownership has on people's walking (see Chapter 9).

Housing and health The differences in death rates among owner occupiers, private and council tenants (see Table 17) reflect the influence of a wide range of socioeconomic factors, rather than of the standard of housing alone. Because people who live in overcrowded or substandard houses usually suffer from many other forms of disadvantage, it is difficult to disentangle the many influences at work. The widespread impression that housing is a direct determinant of health originated in the well known association between insanitary conditions, overcrowding and the high rates of infectious (especially respiratory) diseases in the past. While some modern studies have failed to identify any direct effects, most have found that factors such as overcrowding, structural deficiencies and lack of privacy do make a contribution to poor health.[67-69] The location of housing may also have indirect effects on health. Estates where access to jobs, shops and health services is difficult tend to increase the disadvantage of those who live in them.[70]

Although we are hampered by the lack of research, it is clear that much of the modern contribution which substandard housing makes to ill health arises less from its physical impact than from the social and psychological effects of damp, disrepair, inadequate facilities and cramped living accommodation. Housing is almost certainly an important factor in the large social class differences found in mortality from childhood accidents. The lack of indoor playspace and gardens means that young children are more likely to play unsupervised in the street. Another problem is that of homelessness. In 1985, local authorities received 203,000 housing applications from homeless people and families.[69] The Department of the Environment estimates of 'concealed homelessness' among single people were put at 330,000 in 1981.[70]

Social support and health There is increasing evidence to suggest that close or 'confiding' relationships and social support from friends and relatives may be protective of health[71-73] (see Chapter 9). Evidence from the Whitehall study of civil servants shows that those in the lower grades are less likely than those in administrative grades to have a social contact at home and at work and to see a close confidant daily.[74] It was once widely believed that social ties were closer in some of the stable, urban working class neighbourhoods than in some better-off areas – an impression which was fostered partly by the well known findings of studies like *Family and Kinship in East London*.[75] These close social networks may have been destroyed by the mass clearance of slums but this has not been adequately studied. In addition, social class differences in access to cars and telephones affect people's ability to keep in touch with more distant friends and relations. They are particularly important among elderly people.

The disadvantaged The number of people living in poverty depends on how poverty is defined. While many have argued that it should be higher, DHSS estimates currently use a threshold of 40 per cent above supplementary benefit as a definition. Based on official DHSS data, nearly one in three British adults (16 million people) lived in poverty in 1983 (see Figure 24). This included 85 per cent of the unemployed, nearly two-thirds of pensioners and single parents, and nearly half of families with three or more children. Between 1979–83 – a period for which comparable data are available – the number of people in poverty increased by 42 per cent overall with the biggest increases occurring among the unemployed and married couples with children.

In 1985 there were 3.3 million people officially unemployed. This estimate increases to over 4 million when those not registered are taken into account. At that time, the UK had the fourth highest unemployment rate in the EEC but rates began to fall in 1987. Those now most likely to be unemployed are the under-20s, ethnic minorities and disabled people. The numbers of unemployed

Figure 24   Estimates of people living in poverty in Great Britain (1979–1983)

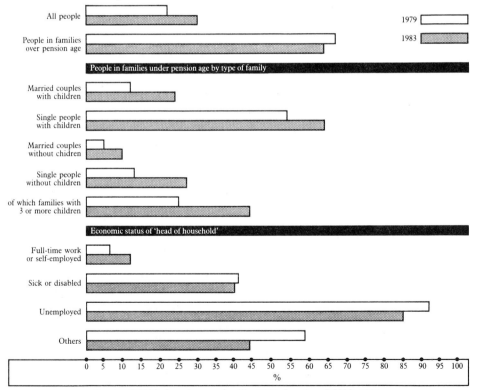

Source: DHSS. Low income families 1983. London, DHSS, 1986.

increased twelve-fold between 1964 and 1985, with the sharpest increases occurring in the late 1970s (see Figure 25).

Figure 25   Trends in unemployment in the United Kingdom (1971–1985)

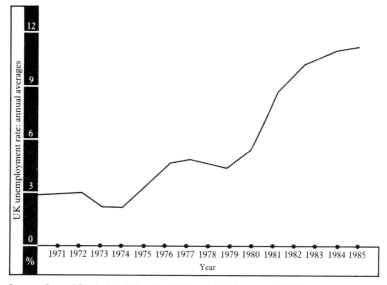

Source: Central Statistical Office. Social Trends 17. London, HMSO, 1987.

Possibilities for the promotion of health and prevention of disease

The reduction of inequalities in health is the first of the WHO's European *Targets for Health for All.*[76] All 33 European states, including the UK, are signatories to this document and have endorsed the aim that by the year 2000 health inequalities should be reduced by 25 per cent. Historically, the major advances in health reflect the fact that changes in social circumstances which are regarded as intrinsically desirable, tend also to be those which favour good health. Thus the kinds of housing, environments, types of employment, leisure activities and items of consumption to which people with greater choice have access, were generally – although not always – beneficial to health. Hence, past improvements in health have appeared more as a by-product of a rising standard of living than as a result of conscious policies to improve health.[77] Our continuing ignorance of the mechanisms through which deprivation operates should not prevent major improvements in health from taking place in the future, any more than it has in the past.

The relationship between deprivation and ill health offers four broad approaches to prevention.

- The economic approach aims to increase wealth and to redistribute resources so as to reduce the deprivation.
- Risk factor reduction aims to sever the link between deprivation

119

and ill health by promoting behaviour change (see Chapter 7).

- The educational approach aims to promote a better educated community – especially among the most disadvantaged.
- The community development approach aims to support and promote self-esteem and autonomous action among the most deprived groups in the community.

Reliance on risk factor reduction alone may inadvertently accentuate disadvantage as health promotion initiatives (for example, smoking) are more rapidly accepted among the more privileged (see Chapter 4). Moreoever, there is a limit to the extent to which risk factors such as smoking, poor diet and physical inactivity can be changed without altering the circumstances in which they arise. In a report on *Health Education in Areas of Multiple Deprivation* from the Scottish Health Education Coordinating Committee (SHECC), the community development approach was strongly advocated, but it was envisaged as part of a wider strategy in which it would be necessary to reduce the deprivation itself.[78] Risk factor reduction, educational initiatives and community development approaches are thus linked with and complementary to economic action.

We believe that efforts to reduce specific risk factors, to promote a better educated community, or to promote community action among disadvantaged groups, are likely to become *more* effective once the burden of socioeconomic disadvantage is reduced. If the greater freedom of the middle classes and their greater command of resources enables them to be more responsive to health information and education, then it is reasonable to suppose that it would benefit health to extend that freedom to other classes. The notion that inequalities in health result from a cultural preference among working class people for a life that is 'short and sweet' is not supported by the evidence.[79] Moreover, a major review of health and happiness showed that happiness and a good quality of life are highly correlated with longevity, as well as good income.[80]

Income policy There are two possible approaches to the reduction of socioeconomic disadvantage: wealth creation and income redistribution. International comparisons of the relationship between income and mortality rates suggest that economic growth (and its associated creation of wealth) is associated with improved mortality rates.[81] But marginal changes in income (that is, income distribution) have also been shown to have a beneficial effect on the least well-off while making little difference to those who are better off.[82–84] Analysis of family incomes in 1983 shows that the incomes of the poorest 20 per cent of families could be doubled by redistributing 17 per cent of the incomes of the richest 20 per cent.[85]

The implication is that wealth creation and income redistribution in favour of the poor are complementary approaches that could substantially improve the population's *overall* mortality rates. International comparisons confirm that there is a close relationship between a nation's income inequality and its average life expectancy.[86,87] This relationship holds in both affluent and poor countries, and is independent of the benefits of economic growth alone.[88]

Analysis of changes in life expectancy earlier this century demonstrate the effects of income redistribution. During the first and second world wars, civilian life expectancy in England and Wales increased two or three times as fast as during the rest of this century. The greatest gains were among the poorest sectors of society.[89] This is probably related to the fact that the wars virtually ended unemployment, were associated with a substantial redistribution of income[90] as well as the development of certain minimum standards – such as food rationing.

Aside from general measures to promote increased wealth and a reduction in material inequalities, we have found few well-researched examples of initiatives which have been able to demonstrate reductions in specific aspects of health inequality. Sweden is often cited as an example of a country which has, through specific socioeconomic policies, narrowed health inequalities in infancy. But the supporting evidence is not clear cut.[91] The reduction in regional differences in death rates in Finland followed a conscious policy of better welfare and health service provision to the deprived.[92] The best evidence comes from measures such as fluoridation and family planning policy, which we review elsewhere in this report. Here, there have been demonstrable reductions in specific aspects of health inequality.

Inequalities: implications for policy

The emerging picture is one which suggests that rather than being an intractable problem the health disadvantage of the working classes might be an area of public health in which major gains can most readily be achieved. Opinion polls have repeatedly shown that a majority of the public see unemployment and health as key areas for government action. Almost half of those polled by MORI in August 1986 also favoured taxation measures, which could achieve a form of income redistribution.

Based on its findings, the Black report recommended what it called a 'comprehensive anti-poverty strategy' with the primary goal of eliminating child poverty. It included the following components.

- A reduction in differences in material standards at work, at home, and in community life.
- Improvement in social security benefits, including child benefit

121

and maternity grants.
- A shift of resources from hospital to community and preventive services within the NHS, including the establishment of a number of 'health development areas' in deprived parts of the country.
- Specific measures to reduce smoking-related deaths and promote road safety.

The government did not accept the major findings of the Black report and its recommendations were rejected on the grounds that they would cost too much to implement.[93] Research has now clarified the contribution of material deprivation to ill health and the findings have been confirmed in *The Health Divide* and in a recent report from the BMA.[94] In 1985, a report from the Archbishop's commission, *Faith in the City*, which assessed aspects of health and community life in inner cities, reiterated many of the findings of the Black report and made a number of recommendations concerning increases in expenditure on housing, the rate support grant, social security benefits and urban renewal projects.[95] The Institute of Fiscal Studies estimated that the proposals of *Faith in the City* would increase the standard income tax rate by 4p in 1985.[96] This compares with the government's estimate in 1979 that implementing the quantifiable Black recommendations might entail an extra 2p on the basic income tax rate, an amount equivalent to the actual reduction in 1988. This estimate did not take into account those recommendations, such as income redistribution, which do not involve any net increase in cost.

In 1988, *The Health Divide* concluded that while much local action had occurred – especially within metropolitan local authorities, by health education departments and primary health care workers – the response by government had been poor.[97] Our own survey of health promotion policy in RHAs however, showed that a commitment to the reduction of inequalities in health was not prominent.[98]

PART II: LIVING BETTER

9 Promoting physical and mental health

> By health I mean the power to live a
> full, adult, living breathing life in close
> contact with what I love – I want to be
> all that I am capable of being.
> KATHERINE MANSFIELD

Introduction While few would deny that reducing the premature death toll from today's major causes of preventable mortality is a key public health priority, there is clearly more to healthy living than survival alone. In this, and the five following chapters, we assess the interactions between physical and mental health, and the potential for preventing ill health as well as promoting well being *during our lives*. In this chapter we assess the effects of different forms of physical activity on health and the quality of life. We then consider the difficulties presented by research on the role of stress in mental and physical health, followed by an assessment of the potential contribution to be made by social support.

Why exercise? Exercise has always been seen to be a good thing for body, soul and nation. While past efforts have been directed at promoting sport among the young and gifted, there has been a renaissance of interest in the value of regular physical activity for the whole community, irrespective of age, ability and state of health. It is based on the belief that regular exercise is not only enjoyable, but makes a major contribution to health and fitness at all ages.

Physical activity is a term for a complex set of activities of which exercise (and sport) form only two sub-categories. Some, but not all, of the components of physical fitness, such as cardiovascular fitness (the ability of the heart to perform effective work) muscular endurance, and strength, flexibility and body composition are now measurable.

Fit for what? Although there are few British data, and much of the evidence relates to middle-aged men, there is a general consensus now in favour of the health benefits of exercise. Much of it has been summarised in a conference report jointly sponsored by the Sports Council, former HEC, and the Medical Research Society in 1983,[1] and in a Sports Council review.[2] Further evidence has accumulated since then,[3] together with a detailed review commissioned by the American government's Centres for Disease Control in 1985.[4] There are still large gaps in the evidence however, and its interpretation is hampered by poorly designed, unrepresentative studies of athletes; nonetheless a number of important conclusions can readily be drawn.

Physical aspects of fitness

The effects of moderate, rhythmic and regular exercise (such as brisk walking, running or swimming with 'overload' for 20–30 minutes about three times each week) have been studied in people up to the age of 70. Such training has a number of demonstrable effects.

- Improved cardiovascular function.
- This results in a better tolerated and sustained work effort, but is *not* necessarily synonymous with a reduction in risk of coronary heart disease (see below).
- Muscle size and strength improve, together with ligament strength. This can result in improved function of muscles which help to maintain posture and thus protect against joint instability and injury, and back pain in pregnancy.
- These benefits can be produced over a three-month period in both men and women of all ages, but are only maintained while the activity(s) is maintained.
- The beneficial effects are more striking in those who are least active (that is, elderly people or those with chronic disease).

Physical activity in old age

Although the maintenance of fitness is beneficial to health at all ages, it is critical in elderly people and can mean the difference between independence and institutionalisation. As people get older there is a steady decline in the capacity to do physical work – maximum oxygen capacity, muscle bulk and strength decrease by about one per cent a year.[5] This decline may eventually result in an elderly person no longer being fit enough to carry heavy shopping or to get up out of a chair without help. Although some of this decline is inevitable (see also Chapter 14), there is now good evidence that about 20 per cent or more is due to disuse, and is thus recoverable at any age.[6] Such an increase in physical fitness might extend the period of independent living in old age by eight or nine years.[7]

If the central goal for health in old age is the promotion of independence and autonomy (see Chapter 14), then the maintenance of stamina, suppleness and strength through physical activity (see Table 20) is an integral part of this process.[8]

Fitness and mental health

It is difficult to interpret some of the research on physical activity and mental health. It is often based on descriptive studies of highly selected groups such as athletes, with few properly controlled studies. Nevertheless the available evidence[9] suggests the following.

126

- The generally held view that exercise makes people 'feel good' is probably true. Population surveys in Canada, and small, randomised controlled trials in children and women have demonstrated that exercise – at least in the short term – results in a significant improvement in measures of self-confidence and self-esteem – both of which are correlated to physical fitness.
- Exercise has an antidepressant effect which has been most reliably demonstrated in the short term among mildly or moderately depressed people in both hospital and community-based populations.
- A number of poorly controlled trials show an association between exercise and a reduction in anxiety.
- Randomised controlled trials have shown that exercise can reduce the immediate physiological response to stress.
- The antidepressant, and possible anti-anxiety effects of exercise are biologically plausible. The epidemiological evidence is supported by some research in brain chemistry which shows that one of the immediate effects of exercise may be an increase in the brain of levels of endorphins – substances whose effects are broadly those of an intrinsic heroin-like substance.

Table 20   Some essential components of fitness in old age

Fitness component	Impact of loss	Activity required to maintain fitness	Effects
STRENGTH	WEAKNESS	Isotonic and isometric exercise not sustained for more than ten seconds per contraction, for example swimming, stair climbing	Improved carrying ability; climbing stairs; getting up out of low chairs; improved mental well being
SUPPLENESS	STIFFNESS	Daily movement of large joints, for example hips and shoulders through full range	Prevention of falls and strains
STAMINA	EASY TIRING/ BREATHLESSNESS	Regular walking, swimming, digging, housework, dancing, about three times a week	Ability to perform a wider daily range of tasks without tiring; improved mental wellbeing

Source: Adapted from Muir Gray J A (ed). Prevention of disease in the elderly. Edinburgh, Churchill Livingstone, 1985.

Exercise and the prevention of disease

Although there are still gaps in the evidence, those who are physically active throughout adult life live longer than those who are sedentary.[10] This conclusion is based on a carefully conducted, if selective, follow-up study of Harvard University graduates whose leisure-time physical activity and its impact on health have been monitored for 16 years. Those who are active (that is, those who expend more than 2000 kcal of energy in leisure-time activities per week – mostly in sports, play and walking) live up to 2.5 years longer than those who are classed as inactive (that is, expend less than 500 kcal of energy per week).

Coronary heart disease

There are now many controlled prospective studies which show that those whose work or leisure involves vigorous, regular exercise, are between one-third and one-half as likely to develop or to die of coronary heart disease as those whose lives are more sedentary.[11-14] The protective effect of exercise persists at all ages, and after other risk factors are taken into account. Although three of the four biggest studies involve men in selected jobs, and there is no corroborative evidence from intervention studies, the evidence is now sufficiently persuasive that vigorous exercise does have an independent, protective action against coronary heart disease.

Physical activity and other conditions

Research on the effects of physical activity on other conditions is less well advanced, but has been best documented for conditions which are themselves risk factors for heart disease, such as high blood pressure, obesity, and diabetes mellitus. This may partly explain the mechanisms through which exercise acts to protect against heart disease (see Chapter 3). Conclusions from the research are as follows.

- The relationship between physical activity and blood pressure (both systolic and diastolic) is inverse: the higher the level of physical activity the lower the blood pressure. Population studies suggest that physically active people have slightly lower diastolic blood pressure. (2–5 mm) and a correspondingly lower systolic pressure than those who are sedentary.
- Physical fitness programmes appear to significantly lower blood pressure, and the effect is most striking among those who already have mild or moderately high blood pressure. Difficulties in measurement and definition of high blood pressure have contributed to the inability to reproduce these findings in fully randomised studies.
- Those who are physically active – especially elderly people – are less likely to be overweight or obese and have been shown to have better control of glucose metabolism. This may result in a reduced risk of the kind of diabetes associated with overweight that is common among older people.

- Physical activity in middle age confers relative protection against those fractures in old age that are caused by thinning bones or osteoporosis (see Chapter 14). While physical activity may help to slow down the bone-thinning process, it probably needs to be life-long and the evidence is not as good as that of the effect of hormone replacement therapy.[15]

The risks of exercise

Different forms of exercise clearly carry specific risks, some of which are well-documented like eye injuries related to squash; muscle, tendon and joint injuries related to running; and specific infections associated with swimming. Many of these are acceptable because they are understood and we know how to avoid them. Current concern, however, is focussed on whether vigorous physical activity of the kind needed to reduce the risk of coronary heart disease might also increase the risk of sudden death (which is almost always due to undiscovered, pre-existing heart disease). Research in this field is inadequate, and we know little about the risks of the most popular kinds of exercise now advocated.[16] While there is good evidence to show that *long-term* moderate and vigorous exercise protects against heart attack and sudden death,[17,18] we have less reliable data on the short-term effects – especially in those unaccustomed to exercise.

The available evidence suggests that the small absolute increase in the short-term risk of sudden death from exercise in adulthood is greatly outweighed by the much larger reduction in the relative risk of heart disease in the long term. As the risk of heart disease in adulthood increases with age, we urgently need to establish more clearly how the short-term risk changes with age, so that the public and health professions can make informed decisions about the risks and benefits of vigorous exercise in middle and older ages.

Who exercises?

Surveys of physical activity vary widely in their findings and the variation is partly due to problems of definition. The two most reliable sources of information in the UK are the General Household Survey (GHS) which covers leisure-time activity in Great Britain, and the Heartbeat Wales community survey which covers work and leisure time activity (see Chapter 7).

GHS data for 1983 show that sport and recreational physical activity is still a minority practice, with about one in three men and only one in five women participating in any activity. Walking remains the most popular activity in all age groups except the youngest, and only 17 per cent of the population participate in any other outdoor activity. Of the ten most popular sports, three (fishing, darts and snooker) involve little physical activity. Participation rates are higher for men than women in every age and socioeconomic group; professional men are three times more likely than women married to unskilled manual workers to be active sports participants. Levels of participation are highest for 16–19 year olds, and there is a steep decline with increasing age (see Figure 26). There is no national monitoring system for physical activity levels among children under 16, but a DES survey of 14–16 year olds in 1983 showed that the 70 per cent participation rates among schoolchildren drop sharply to 57 per cent among school-leavers.[19]

Figure 26 Participation in physical activity by age in Great Britain (1983)

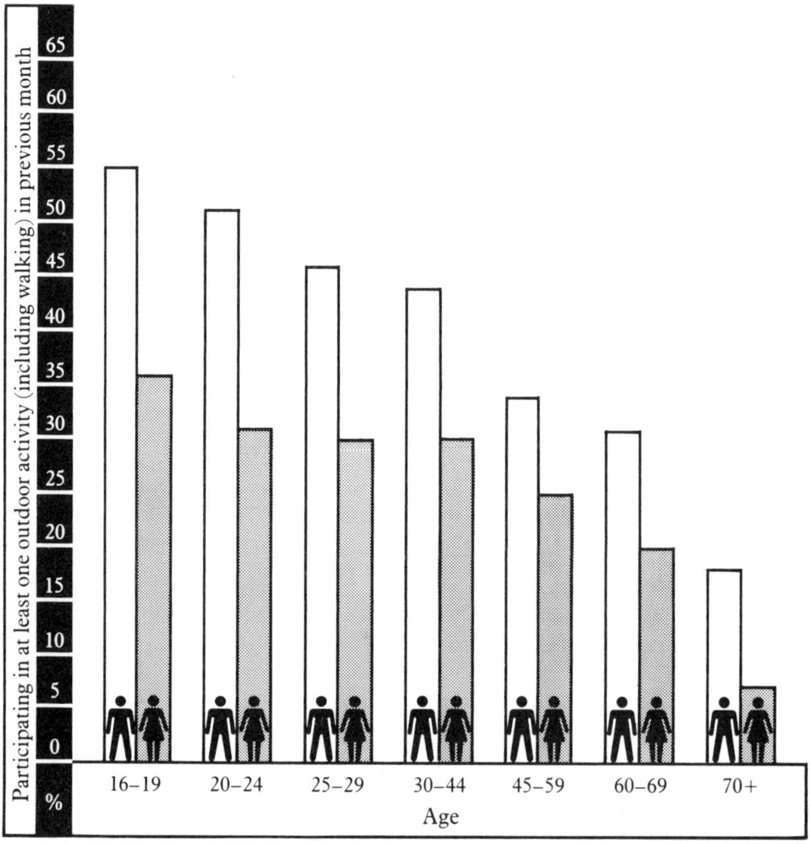

Source: OPCS. General Household Survey 1983. London, HMSO, 1985.

The years 1977–1983 saw a small, but significant, increase in participation rates among both men and women (see Figure 27) in walking, athletics (which includes jogging), swimming and squash. This is in line with the findings of a representative poll commissioned by Fitness Magazine in 1984 which suggested that the proportion of people taking moderate, regular exercise had increased. The age and socioeconomic gradient remained broadly unchanged, but by 1980 men in skilled manual jobs had overtaken

130

professional men in participation rates for indoor sport[20] – although this includes less active sports such as darts and snooker. The Welsh survey in 1985 paints a gloomier picture, although this may reflect lower participation rates in Wales than in other parts of the UK. Based on a composite index of work and leisure activity, it concluded that only one in five men and only two per cent of women were taking sufficiently vigorous exercise to help protect them from heart disease.[21] A national fitness survey, Activity and Health 2000, is in an advanced stage of preparation by the Fitness and Health Advisory Group of the Sports Council and the former HEC.

The determinants of physical activity

Patterns of physical activity are governed by complex factors. The cultural and political climates have been influential in increasing the amount of – often enforced – leisure, and new technology has reduced the amount of physical activity in paid and domestic work. Sex differences in participation in physical activity are heavily influenced by prevailing views of what is regarded as proper behaviour for women and men, and probably explain why women (but not men) use exercise as a means of weight loss.[22]

The available research evidence[23] – nearly all of which is American – offers some important clues as to what prompts people to take exercise.

- Those who are physically active as children are most likely to continue to be so during adulthood.

Figure 27   Trends in participation in sport and physical activities in Great Britain (1977–1983)

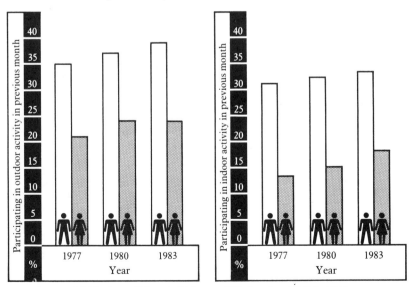

Source: OPCS. General Household Survey 1983. London, HMSO, 1985.

131

- Enjoyment and social contact are more important motives for regular physical activity than health, although a MORI fitness poll in 1984 showed that interest in health and fitness were the second most important reason.
- A positive self-image and confidence in the ability to influence future activity levels.
- There is no evidence, as yet, to suggest that increased knowledge about the effects of exercise on health improves participation.
- Easy access to cheap facilities is an important factor in determining participation.

Physical activity: what has been achieved? The growth of interest in sport pre-dates the current 'fitness movement', and stems from a long-standing concern about the high drop-out rate from sports among school leavers together with a desire to live up to the Council of Europe's 1960s charter, Sport for All. The Sport for All initiative gathered momentum following the creation of a Minister for Sport and, subsequently, the Sports Council, which officially launched the campaign in 1972. The success of the campaign, assessed in a report commissioned by the Sports Council,[24] has been partial.

- Central government funding for sport and specific local authority allocations have helped improve participation in sport.
- Despite small improvements, the Sport for All objective is far from being realised, and inequalities persist.
- Inequalities in the provision of sports facilities have diminished – especially for indoor sport.
- The recent recognition by the Sports Council of the need to reach deprived groups may offer a way forward.
- The shift away from the Sports Council's earlier emphasis on elite sports has been slow, and disproportionately large amounts of the Council's funds are still being spent on elite sport.

The clear strategy and ambitious target-setting exercise embarked upon by the Sports Council has not only permitted effective monitoring, but has helped to stimulate action. In 1965 more than 600 local authorites had no indoor swimming pools and most of the country's 239 sports halls were limited to schools and colleges. In 1972 the Sports Council set national targets to be achieved over the following decade.[25] By 1981 the targets set for swimming pools had been exceeded by nearly 100 per cent and large increases had also occurred in the number of newly built sports centres and golf courses.[26]

Having identified women, school leavers, the over 50s, and low income groups as targets for the future, the Sports Council has begun to use mass media campaigns to reach them, and individual local authorities have made special provision for women and ethnic minority groups. The effect of this shift in policy remains to be seen.

While the Sports Council has helped to promote better provision of facilities, health education, voluntary agencies and local authorities have helped encourage participation. Exercise features as a major component within many of the HEA's nine programmes, including the prevention of heart disease and the promotion of health in old age. The emphasis has been on the use of exercise promotion as a positive rather than negative force for good health in order to link several of the hitherto fragmented but overlapping programmes on health promotion in adulthood. This philosophy is encapsulated in the former HEC's Look After Yourself (LAY) programme which involves the training of tutors who lead adult education courses dealing with exercise, healthy eating, relaxation and a flexible range of other topics, including alcohol and tobacco. This integrated approach to adult education mirrors that now being adopted in schools (see Chapter 12) and preliminary evaluation suggests the results are positive.[27,28] In 1981 there were 187 LAY classes in operation, but by 1986 this had grown to 2,500 involving nearly 100,000 people throughout the country, including public sector employees, as well as 60 per cent of health education units.

Earlier expectations that mass media and high profile promotional events might lead to lasting behaviour change have proved to be unrealistic. Their effect on public attitudes can be significant, however. The SHEG and former HEC's joint sponsorship initiatives with the BBC and the Sports Council in Feeling Great, SHEG's Walk About a Bit campaign, and the former HEC's Sunday Times Fun Run have been important in this respect. One of the most successful promotional initiatives of this kind was the HEC's Great British Fun Run which was a nationally organised round-Britain event with a series of associated local fun runs and health fairs. The evaluation[29] showed that the event achieved a high public awareness, and the commitment and resources given to it have resulted in many health authorities and local councils increasing their own commitment and allocation of resources to the promotion of good health through exercise.

The promotion of innovative forms of exercise in schools has been slow. Evidence suggests that, with notable exception, the commonest kind of exercise at school remains competitive team games which come low on most teenagers' list of sporting preferences.[30] The Teachers' Advisory Council on Drug Education (TACADE), in conjunction with the former HEC, plans to introduce a new approach into secondary schools utilising the LAY philosophy.

While exercise is a well-established part of rehabilitative practice in hospitals, its place within primary care is unclear. The innovative example of the Peckham Experiment in 1935, in which a health centre developed swimming and gymnastic facilities on its premises, has yet to be followed, and may now be inappropriate. A promising initiative by the Sports Council and the Mersey Health Authority has resulted in the creation of a sports development officer who advises individually referred patients about exercise and helps develop local exercise classes, such as LAY courses within primary care.

Physical activity: future policy

Progress over the decade has been substantial, but poorly planned. With the exception of the Sports Council's clear strategy, and the Faculty of Community Medicine's guidelines,[31] there are no national objectives or plans for promoting fitness and health. Federal government in the USA has led the way, and developed a challenging set of targets for the promotion of physical activity. This has more recently been translated into a practical plan for promoting physical activity at different stages in life.[32]

Mental health

Although it is often asserted that mental health is more than simply the absence of mental disorder, theoretical definitions have so far proved difficult to translate into practice. The instruments for measuring mental wellbeing are poor compared with those for mental disorder. There are, however, increasing numbers of validated ways of measuring limited aspects of mental health.

Stress – separating fact from folklore

The complex nature of mental health, has complicated the study of its determinants. While physical health, personality factors and socioeconomic settings (see Chapter 8) are important, the study of stress offers one of the more problematic areas of research. An inadequate understanding of what constitutes stress has led to vague research and findings that are difficult to interpret.

Two fundamental difficulties facing research into stress involve defining what it is, and when it is unhealthy. While we all have a personal understanding and experience of stress, it is hard to translate this into research terms. Stress has been defined by researchers both in terms of environmental stimuli and as responses to such stimuli. This conceptual confusion arises from the need to study the *interrelation* between individuals and their environment as well as from the difficulty of distinguishing between the inevitable stresses of our lives and those which are potentially damaging.

Much of the UK research in this field stems from an important study of the role of life events in depression among women. This showed that major life events involving threat or loss (such as bereavement or unemployment) were most likely to have negative consequences for mental health[33] (see Chapter 10). This has since

134

been supported in other studies.[34-36] Other life events such as the short-term stress of examinations or perhaps loss by theft were not damaging.

The impact of stress on health It has been fashionable to see stress as a major threat to mental and physical health. To what extent is this view sustainable? Research in the 1960s and early 1970s has repeatedly shown an association between stress – in the form of life events – and a wide range of mental and physical health problems.[37-40] However, it is still not clear whether the stress causes ill health or ill health causes stress, or even whether stress is as important as other contributing factors. This is because much of the research has been inadequately designed. In many cases, the data on stress has been retrospectively recollected and other contributing factors have not been taken into account.

These difficulties have still not been entirely overcome, even though there is now evidence that stress – in the form of reliably measurable life events – influences both mental and physical ill health[41] (see also Chapters 3 and 10). There remains no good evidence that stress is associated with cancer in general,[42] or with breast cancer in particular,[43] although it may influence the survival of those with breast cancer. Bereavement has been shown to increase the risk of death from all causes by 40 per cent in the short term.[44] This risk is confined to men, persists for up to ten years, and has been shown to be independent of other major risk factors such as socioeconomic and educational status and cigarette smoking.[45] The effects of adverse life events on the outcome of pregnancy have also been reliably demonstrated (see Chapter 11), as has their role in repeated hospitalisation, and there is evidence of the effect of prolonged marital discord in parents on the health of children.[46] Although statistical pooling of the data[47] suggests that stressful life events make a significant total contribution to mental ill health, individually they account for only a small proportion of reported mental ill health. The scope for prevention is likely to be limited as most of the significant life events are unavoidable. Indeed we know of no intervention studies which have been able to reduce the risk of mental ill health by attempting to reduce the risk of life events.

stress – the role of social support Apart from socioeconomic measures to reduce the stresses associated with low income and unemployment (see Chapter 8), there are few options open to us for relieving stress itself. Many stresses, such as bereavement, divorce or separation from children are an inevitable or common part of life. We thus need to explore ways of reducing the negative consequences of stress. There is now evidence which suggests that good relationships with lovers, relatives and friends are important in the maintenance of good mental health and may help protect against the negative effects of life events.[48,49]

A lack of this kind of social support is associated with depression, anxiety, heavy use of medical services and high blood pressure.[50] Good social support also appears to protect against the negative consequences of stressful life events, including divorce, psychiatric and psychological symptoms, occupational stress and illness in the elderly.[51]

Prospective studies in large, representative communities in the USA have strengthened the evidence that social support confers some protection from depression and depressive symptoms, and appears to exert its most important effect in the presence of environmental stresses. However, well-designed intervention studies are few and far between. There is some evidence – in specific instances – that informal support, such as the provision of lay-women companions to women in labour (see Chapter 11), or to women rearing children with chronic illnesses,[52-54] may improve both mental and physical health outcomes.

The best available evidence linking social support to good health comes from three prospective US community studies.[55-57] These studies must nevertheless be interpreted with caution because objective measures of initial health status and levels of social support were not always used.

Patterns of social support

The most extensive studies of patterns of social support have been in the USA. Although their findings must be translated to the UK with caution, they offer some insight into the scope for intervention studies.

- Women and men have equally large networks, although women's tend to be family-based and men's work-based. Older women tend to have wider social networks than older men.
- Marriage offers a special kind of intimacy and support (although it should be noted that it is also associated with mental ill health in women). Those who are divorced, separated or widowed have the least social support.
- People living in small, rural communities have a wider social network than those living in cities.
- Those who belong to clubs and the church have larger social networks than those who do not.

In the UK, evidence from a large study of male civil servants shows that working class men have less social support than middle class men (see Chapter 8), but the only representative information we have on women comes from the 1985 Welsh Heart Survey.[58] It showed that home-based social support is commoner among younger people and women, whereas social contact outside the home is commonest among young men. There were significant minorities of elderly people with poor social networks, at home and outside the home.

Social support: implications for action
The possible protective effect of social support on mental and physical health requires further research. Well-designed intervention studies are needed which use reliable measures of the quantitative and qualitative aspects of social support. Research on patterns of social support suggest that the scope for health promotion may be limited, because it is the *quality* of support in a marital relationship that is crucial rather than the quantity, and this is not readily amenable to intervention. Nevertheless, those who tend to be socially isolated offer potential opportunities for health promotion, as well as for more research into the support needs of those who care for them (see Chapter 14). The potential for using the temporary social support of counsellors in situations other than bereavement warrants further investigation.

10 Preventing mental ill health

New opinions are always suspected, and
usually opposed, without any other
reason but because they are not already
common.

JOHN LOCKE

Introduction
In the last chapter we focussed on mental and physical health. In this chapter, we examine some of the major forms of mental ill health and the scope for their prevention. We start with a consideration of depression and an assessment of patterns of psychotropic drug prescription. We follow by considering suicide and parasuicide, and schizophrenia. Finally, we consider mental illnesses in children and elderly people.

The size of the problem
More than five million people consult their GP each year because of mental ill health. It is the second most common reason for consultation, accounting for at least 15 per cent of all consultations, and was responsible for the loss of nearly 57 million working days in 1981–82. The DHSS estimated that mental illness and mental handicap cost the NHS £1.5 billion in 1985. About 70 per cent of women and 50 per cent of men will, at some time, consult their GP concerning their mental health. The two commonest problems presented by adults to their GPs are depression and anxiety. Women consult three times more often than men. Although the last decade has seen a pronounced decline in admissions to mental hospitals, there were still 188,000 such admissions in 1983 in England alone. Most were for schizophrenia and depressive illness. The biggest recent increases in admissions were for dementia and for drug and alcohol misuse (see Chapters 5 and 13). Scotland has higher admission rates to mental illness units than England and Wales. This probably reflects the larger number of psychiatric beds and psychiatrists per head of population in Scotland.

Depression and anxiety
Depression and anxiety may be appropriate short-term responses to adverse situations. However, incapacitating forms of depressive illness and anxiety may persist for long periods. Depression is the commonest form of mental ill health in the community today, and is sometimes associated with, but is twice as common as, anxiety alone. Prevalence estimates from representative community studies suggest that about six per cent of men and 12-17 per cent of women suffer from depression – at least half of them long term. The most striking feature of urban surveys among women are the higher levels among

138

working class women, up to one in four of whom suffer from depression.[1] Although comparisons are difficult, the overall rates of depression in rural areas are lower than those in the inner city,[2] and working class women in rural areas do not appear to be at increased risk as they are in inner city areas.

The determinants of depression Although we do not know exactly what causes abnormal depression, it is clear that those at greatest risk are young to middle-aged, working class women. Recent negative 'life events' (see Chapter 9) involving loss are the most clearly identified risk factors for depression[3] but experience of a 'life event' does *not* lead, on its own, to depression.

Early research suggested that there were a number of 'vulnerability factors', which, in the presence of a life event, markedly increase the risk of depression[4] but more recent studies have not confirmed this[5] – except in the case of one kind: the lack of a confiding relationship.[6]

Other individual factors have a role to play in depression. Recent interest has focussed on certain long-standing mental perspectives – known as 'cognitive sets' – which predispose to or protect against depression. More research is needed to elucidate their possible contribution to depression. Overall, the research findings so far do not offer any obvious means of preventing depression.

Benzodiazepines Despite the genuinely high prevalence of depression, doctors' responses to their patients' mental health problems are not always appropriate. In 1983, general practitioners issued 23 million prescriptions for benzodiazepines – the main category of psychotropic (psychologically active) medicine prescribed today. Nearly all of these were for sleeping problems, anxiety and related forms of mental distress. Up to half of these were repeat prescriptions. In 1981 this cost the NHS £37.5 million. An international survey in 1981 showed that nearly seven per cent of British adults had used anti-anxiety and tranquillising medicines in the previous year.[7] While the UK had lower usage rates than either the USA or most other European countries, it ranked third highest of 11 countries in long-term use, with about three per cent (about 1.25 million people) having taken them for over a year.[8]

While benzodiazepines do have a clear role in both hospital and general practice, estimates suggest that 15–44 per cent of long-term users – up to 175,000 people[9] – experience withdrawal symptoms when stopping their use[10] and often make considerable use of the NHS when trying to stop taking them. Moreover, they are often inappropriately prescribed both for depression (usually among women) and to those who have no discernible psychiatric illness at all.[11]

Figure 28   Trends in benzodiazepine prescriptions in the UK (1972–1985)

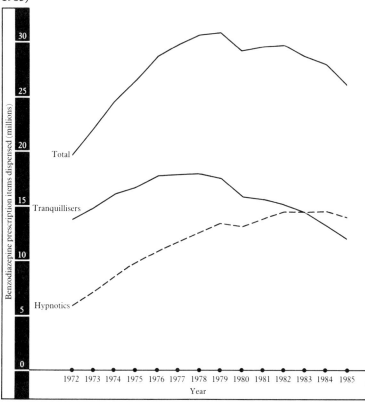

Source: Taylor D. Current usage of benzodiazepines in Britain. In: Freeman H, Rue Yvonne (eds). The benzodiazepines in current practice. Royal Society of Medicine International Congress and Symposium, Series No 114. London, RSM Ltd, 1987.

While the effects of long-term benzodiazepine misuse are not as damaging to health as those of cigarettes, alcohol or some illicit drugs, they demonstrably impair memory and adversely affect driving skills.[12,13] They are associated with a five-fold increase in the risk of road accidents and cause 'hangovers' and confusion among older people. There is a well-established association between taking repeated drug overdoses and the use of psychotropic medicines. In one study of people who deliberately took drug overdoses, over half had been on benzodiazepines, and, of these, one-third had no clearly defined psychiatric illness at all.[14] Moreover, simple counselling in a primary care setting is as effective as benzodiazepine treatment in the treatment of anxiety.[15]

140

Benzodiazepines: trends in the last decade

Benzodiazepines were introduced into the UK in the mid-1960s. Following heavy promotional campaigns, they gradually took over from barbiturates as the new 'remedy' for insomnia and anxiety. Between 1970 and 1980 there was an eight-fold reduction in barbiturate prescriptions. This was associated with concerted action by the medical profession to curb their use following the realisation that they were addictive, and potentially lethal. Recognition of the over-prescribing of benzodiazepines came in the late 1970s. The issue of benzodiazepine prescriptions for anxiety rose to a peak in 1979 and there has since been a 16 per cent fall to 1985. The prescription of benzodiazepine hypnotics (sleeping tablets) rose steadily, however, by 58 per cent between 1972 and 1985 (see Figure 28). Some of the fall in sedative prescriptions can be attributed to the well-orchestrated campaigns by MIND – the National Association for Mental Health – supported by the media. The potential for further reduction – especially in inappropriate long-term use – lies in the education of future doctors and the public.

Suicide and deliberate self-harm

Suicide is an important cause of premature death and parasuicide (deliberate self-harm) is a major cause of suffering. Although we have one of the lowest suicide rates in the affluent world, 4,300 people in England and Wales committed suicide in 1984, and a further 100,000 were admitted to hospital for self-poisoning. Suicide is the third leading cause of death among 15–34 years olds, and parasuicide is the second commonest reason for emergency medical

Table 21   Suicide and parasuicide – a comparison of risk factors

	Suicide	Parasuicide
Age	Rate increases with age Peaks at over 60	Rates highest in young women under 30
Sex	Men more than women	Women : 2.5 times the risk of men
Marital status	Divorced, widowed, single men	Divorced
Social position	Unemployment No social class differences	Unemployment Working class
Precipitating 'life events'	Present	Present
Methods used	Planned Lethal	Unplanned Non-lethal
Previous psychiatric illness	Depression in two-thirds	No illness in two-thirds

admission – costing the NHS an estimated £15–20 million annually in the mid-1980s.[16]

Although each suicidal act results from a unique combination of social and psychological factors, some important general features emerge from overall patterns of suicide and parasuicide that point to the scope for their prevention. First, suicide and parasuicide differ in many important respects (see Table 21). Most suicides occur in middle age: *rates* are currently highest among men over 60 who are either widowed, divorced or single. Parasuicide, on the other hand, is more likely to occur in divorced young women in the manual classes.[17] However, there are some important similarities between the two. Both suicide and parasuicide are much more common among the unemployed living in areas of multiple deprivation [18] (see Chapter 8) and 40 per cent of those who commit suicide have a history of parasuicide.[19] This has implications for prevention – *if* it is possible to identify those parasuicides at high risk of committing suicide.

Suicide trends and implications for prevention

Suicides reached a peak in 1963 and then fell dramatically until the mid-1970s (see Figure 29). Since then there has been a steady increase among men of working age which closely parallels the increase in unemployment (see Chapter 8). There has been no similar increase among women. Indeed, there was a small (five per cent) fall in rates between 1975 and 1984[20] among women aged 15–34.

Suicide has always been a recognisable feature of most cultures. Despite this, the dramatically changing overall pattern over the last two decades, together with other factors associated with suicidal behaviour, suggest that there is some scope for prevention. First, trends in the UK show that the single most important factor in reducing overall suicide rates since the 1960s has been the elimination of carbon monoxide from domestic gas supplies.[21] The implication is that controlling the availability of methods for committing suicide may further reduce death rates. In addition, suicide is influenced by glamorised reporting of suicides in the media.[22,23] Better public and professional awareness of the need to throw away unused or unwanted medicines from the home, together with restriction and supervision of the availability of painkillers in chemists and supermarkets, may help but are unlikely to have a major impact.

The majority of people who commit suicide have suffered depressive illness and have contacted their GP in the month beforehand.[24] Primary care would seem to have a potential role to play in suicide prevention. Bereavement counselling has been shown to be effective in preventing a deterioration in mental health – especially among older widows and widowers who are at risk of

Figure 29   Trends in suicide by sex in England and Wales (1950–1982)

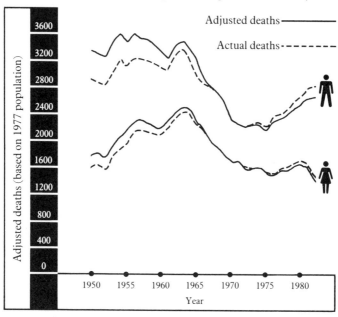

Source: Alderson M R. Suicides 1950–1982. Population Trends 1984, Spring, 35: 11–17.

Figure 30   Trends in self-poisoning (parasuicide) among women in England and Wales (1953–1982)

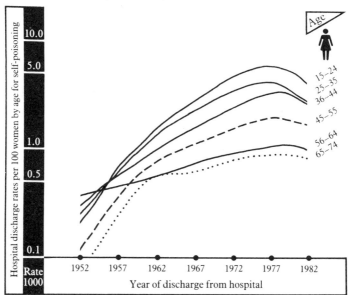

Source: Alderson M R. National trends in self poisoning in women. The Lancet 1985, 27 April: 974–975.

143

suicide.[25] More research is needed to assess the effectiveness of such skills in other age groups. Community-based suicide prevention schemes like the Samaritans' telephone counselling service are beneficial in many ways, but have not been able to demonstrate any beneficial effect on suicide rates.[26] Efforts to screen for those who are at high risk of committing suicide have not yet proved to be feasible on a large scale.[27-29]

Trends in para-suicide and the potential for prevention
In the three decades before 1977 there was a sharp rise in hospital discharge rates for parasuicide among women.[30] But rates in every age group have since fallen (see Figure 30). The more detailed analysis collected by the Edinburgh Poisons Unit, which covers all Edinburgh residents, confirms this trend for women, although the trend for men is not clear.[31] We do not know what underlies these changes in the pattern of parasuicide. Although there is little evidence to go on, the challenges raised in the prevention of parasuicide seem different from those of suicide. In parasuicide we need to prevent what is often an impulsive act. There is no evidence so far that contact with the Samaritans has any impact on the parasuicide rate, and intervention studies aimed at preventing repetitions among those who have already taken an overdose have all had negative results[32-34] – although other beneficial effects were noted. As research shows that minor tranquillisers (mainly benzodiazepines) and non-prescription pain killers are the commonest means used in parasuicide,[35] one of the more obvious approaches to its prevention lies in avoiding unnecessary benzodiazepine prescriptions.

Schizophrenia
There are about 150,000 people suffering from schizophrenia in the UK. While numbers are small compared with other types of mental illness, schizophrenia usually starts in early adulthood and imposes a heavy burden of care on families, the community and the NHS. It often requires a lifetime of medical follow-up with intermittent hospital admission. In England alone there were 28,000 admissions for schizophrenia in 1983. About 60–70,000 patients are in day care. The annual health care costs imposed by schizophrenia were estimated at over £200 million in 1978.[36]

We do not know what causes schizophrenia, but twin and adoption studies show that there is a strong genetic component to the disease. Biochemical evidence of abnormalities in chemical messengers in the brain may ultimately lead to a better understanding of its cause. We know little, however, about the role of specific environmental factors in schizophrenia, especially as its incidence – with one or two exceptions – is similar in widely differing cultures. Although disharmony within families and social deprivation are

144

associated with schizophrenia, evidence so far suggests that family members who are excessively critical or emotionally over-involved with those who develop schizophrenia, are more likely to affect the *course* rather than the *onset* of schizophrenia.[37] On the basis of current knowledge, we can do little to prevent the onset of schizophrenia, but the scope for minimising the disability it causes is much larger.[38]

Mental ill health and handicap in children

The scope for the prevention of mental ill health in children is broad and has been outlined in a major report from the WHO in 1977[39] and more recently in a report from the RCGP.[40] We assess in other chapters many of the specific measures which can demonstrably contribute to the prevention of childhood mental handicap and psychiatric disorder. Some of the most exciting possibilities for prevention are in the field of mental handicap. The most important measures to prevent mental ill health in childhood include the following.

- The reduction of unwanted and unplanned pregnancies through the provision of family planning and abortion services (see Chapter 13).
- Antenatal screening and the offer of termination of pregnancy for the prevention of Down's syndrome and spina bifida. Newer techniques of gene mapping and sampling offer major opportunities in the near future for the prevention of genetic diseases (see Chapter 11).
- Avoidance of smoking and heavy drinking during pregnancy to prevent retardation of fetal growth and development (see Chapters 4, 5, 11).
- Prevention of premature births and of brain damage during delivery (see Chapter 11).
- Screening after birth for phenylketonuria and congenital hypothyroidism to prevent impaired intellectual development (see Chapter 11).
- Immunisation against rubella and measles (see Chapter 12).

More controversial has been the evidence concerning the effect of low levels of environmental lead on intellectual development. Although a DHSS expert group, and a subsequent review of the field,[41,42] concluded that the evidence linking lead to intellectual impairment fell short of proof, public concern, together with a major campaign in the UK, has led to a 60 per cent reduction of lead levels in petrol. We believe that there is persuasive evidence linking environmental lead and intellectual impairment in children and that, since the reduction of atmospheric lead was both feasible and potentially desirable, there was sufficient justification for action.

More recently, concern has been expressed about the role of tartrazine (an artificial food colouring) in childhood hyperactivity. The evidence implicating tartrazine is weak, largely based on individual instances of behaviour disturbance. Hyperactivity is unlikely to be due to tartrazine alone.[43] A consensus development conference on the issue held by the National Institute for Health in 1982 concluded that more research was needed before any action should be considered. Concern about tartrazine should not be seen in isolation, and there is a need to look at the effects of a wide range of other food additives and constituents.

Child abuse The emotional, physical and sexual abuse of children has only recently been recognised as a major problem. Despite recent publicity and justifiable concern, there is little evidence to suggest that the incidence of physical child abuse is rising. While NSPCC child abuse registers have recorded a 42 per cent increase in recorded cases of child abuse between 1985 and 1986[44] much of this is likely to be due to increased recognition and recording of a previously hidden problem.

A more reliable survey based on all cases of child abuse resulting in physical injury in South Glamorgan between 1970–81 has shown a *fall* in severe injury with a steep rise in milder injuries since 1973.[45] The most likely explanation for these trends is that the concept of the 'battered child' did not reach official consciousness until the late 1960s, and since then the increase in reporting represents formal recognition of what was already happening. The decrease in severity of recorded injury, and earlier professional intervention, may be a positive reflection of that increased recognition. Similarly, increased awareness of the sexual abuse of children has led to a rise in the number of cases reported to paediatric departments.[46,47] The victims are usually girls under 10, and the perpetrators are usually men – commonly fathers and stepfathers living in the family home.[48,49]

Although we know that children most at risk of physical abuse tend to come from multiply deprived families, where young parents often live in over-crowded conditions, sexual abuse can occur in any social group. We do not at present know how to prevent either kind of abuse.

Public and political concern about recent individual cases of physical abuse has led to more clearly defined ways of managing and following up children after admission into hospital. A full inquiry into ways of minimising the damage to 'at risk' children resulted from an individual case in 1986. The inquiry recommended changes in training and coordination of a wide range of professional activities, translated by the DHSS into a set of guidelines for future inter-agency cooperation. We await the provision of guidelines on

146

sexual abuse. Social measures may be expected to make a positive contribution to the prevention of physical abuse, together with early identification of parents at risk, although this has yet to be demonstrated. The provision of emotional support and, occasionally, emergency substitute child care may be life-saving in an emergency.[50] Where biological parents are unable to look after their children themselves, long-term fostering and, preferably, adoption is the best means of preventing later emotional disorders in childhood.[51]

Emotional and behaviour disturbances in children
Emotional disorders affect about five per cent of children. Overprotective parents, families with severe marital problems, or ambivalence about a pregnancy are associated risk factors.[52] Overprotectiveness may result from past experience of miscarriage, or from a combination of a physically handicapped child and an anxious parental personality. Early recognition of the problem together with child-centred counselling may be helpful. Sensitive hospitalisation policies which allow frequent parental visiting may reduce a subsequent overprotective reaction.[53]

Conduct disorders ('delinquency') in older children and teenagers include aggressive behaviour, truancy and stealing. In the last two decades there has been a trebling of the deliquency rate among 14–17 year old boys. Although delinquency is still about five times as common in boys as girls, this ratio has been falling.[54] There is now clear evidence that conduct disorders, as well as other emotional disorders in adolescents, are twice as common in inner city as in rural areas.[55,56] A major study comparing inner London with the Isle of Wight[57] came to the following conclusions,

- The two-fold difference in prevalence is real and not due to ethnic differences or the drifting of the mentally ill into the inner city.
- While poverty and low socioeconomic status play a part in the higher inner city rates, they explain only a small part of the differences.
- Differences in patterns of disorders among parents were the same as among children.
- Inner city problems were most likely to be chronic, starting early in childhood.

A number of different research approaches have shed further light on those aspects of inner cities that may predispose children (and their parents) to mental ill health.

- The higher inner city rates are not simply due to high population density or urbanisation, and city living on its own is not a sufficient explanation.[58,59]

- Rates vary widely within the inner city. Children living above the fifth floor in housing estates have higher levels than those living on lower floors.[60]
- Research shows clearly (see Chapter 12) that the school itself has an independent, influential role in truancy and scholastic performance.
- Psychosocial adversity in the family has a key role, and those families with high adversity rates in *either* inner London or the Isle of Wight were equally at risk of having children with psychiatric disorder.[61] It is likely, therefore, that the main adverse effect is indirectly exerted on children through direct adverse effects on parents.

Although there is little supporting evidence as yet, the following areas have been identified for potential public health action:

- improved building design with more security and privacy;[62]
- better supervision and planning, together with control of alcohol at football matches;
- improved leisure facilities – delinquency rates are highest in cities with fewest leisure provisions;[63]
- improved school organisation (see Chapter 12).

Older people The prevention of mental ill health in an expanding population of older people is one of today's biggest public health challenges. Although the majority of over 65s are neither mentally nor physically ill (see Chapter 14), both depression and dementia are important problems. Fifteen per cent of over 75s (and 20 per cent of the over 85s) suffer from dementia. In 1983, 18,000 people in England were admitted to hospital with dementia, but by far the largest burden of responsibility falls on the community, either through surviving relatives, neighbours and friends, or on health and social services; more than five times as many demented people live in their own homes as in institutions. Inadequate data makes it difficult to estimate the total cost of dementia to the NHS, but in 1977 £138 million was spent on the care of the demented in psychiatric units and residential homes.[64]

Dementia Although the age-specific prevalence of dementia has remained unchanged, continuing expansion of the elderly population, especially among those over 75 and 85, has meant that the crude prevalence of dementia has risen very quickly and is likely to continue to do so for at least another 20 years (see Figure 31).

The outlook for the prevention of dementia is limited at present, but not wholly bleak. Dementia is of two major kinds: the Alzheimer type (in which there is a gradual degeneration of brain tissue) and

148

Figure 31   Women residents in Scottish mental illness hospitals and units: percentage distribution by age in 1963 and 1981

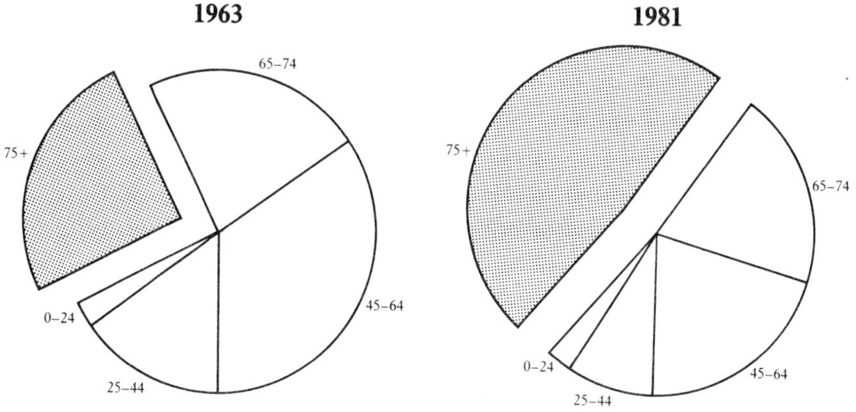

Source: Scottish Information Services Division, unpublished.

multi-infarct dementia (which is caused by a series of small strokes which gradually reduce active brain substance). Although there is little we can do at present to prevent the Alzheimer type, enough is now known about its biochemistry to offer scope for research into its prevention in the near future. The multi-infarct kind of dementia accounts for up to 30 per cent of all dementia,[65] and high blood pressure is a risk factor. A reduction in blood pressure in middle age will therefore not only reduce the risk of coronary heart disease and stroke, but may also reduce the incidence of dementia – although this has yet to be demonstrated.

While we do not yet know how to prevent dementia, knowledge of those who are at risk may help prevent some of its consequences. In an average general practice where one in ten people over 65 will be demented, as many as 80 per cent may be unknown to their GPs.[66] There is still untested scope for developing a system of regular, outside support for the demented living at home which may minimise the distress of dementia both to older people themselves and to those who care for them. This could also offer an opportunity for reviewing unnecessary drug prescriptions – expecially benzodiazepines which can lead to an incorrect diagnosis of dementia. Support through respite care for those who bear the brunt of looking after elderly relatives with dementia may not merely be humane, it may also avoid depression among carers themselves (see Chapter 14).

Depression in old age   Dementia is not the only major psychological problem in old age. Indeed, more than three times as many people over 65 suffer from depression. Representative community surveys suggest that about 17 per cent of people over 65 are depressed – about the same

149

prevalence as among younger women. Again, the rates are twice as high for older women (23 per cent) as for men (12 per cent).[67]

Three major sets of factors are important features associated with depression in old age: deteriorating brain function; physical disease; and psycholocial factors. The last two offer most potential for prevention. As people get older they are more likely to become physically ill. As many as 60 per cent of depressed elderly people also have significant accompanying physical illness.[68] If this can be shown to be a cause of depression, then it offers scope for prevention. Because 'life events' involving loss and bereavement are important factors in depression, the elderly are clearly vulnerable, although they show less severe bereavement reactions than people in other age groups. Bereavement counselling by both professionals and trained lay people can be of value,[69,70] especially as 30 per cent of people over 65 live alone and may not be able to express their grief to anyone else. These findings need to be translated into better preventive practice in primary care since one large study showed that as many as two-thirds of elderly widows were not visited by their GP in the six months following a bereavement.[71]

11 A healthy maternity

It is the customary fate of new truths to
begin as heresies and end as
superstitions.

THOMAS HENRY HUXLEY

Introduction
In the last two chapters we assessed the potential for promoting physical and mental health and for preventing illness throughout the age spectrum. In this and the next three chapters we consider the potential for promoting specific aspects of health at different stages in the life cycle. We begin with maternity and move on, in the following chapters, to childhood, adolescence, adulthood and old age. We do not attempt to be comprehensive, but rather to use each stage of the lifecycle as an opportunity to focus on several key areas which offer potential for the prevention of disease and promotion of health. In this chapter we start with an assessment of changes in the experience and outcome of pregnancy over the last decade, and the contribution made by the maternity services.

Recent trends and today's challenges
Carrying and giving birth to a wanted child remains one of the most significant and rewarding events in the lives of women and men. It is also a safer experience today than ever before for both mother and child. Death of the mother during, or as a result of, childbirth is now rare and only eight women in every 100,000 died as a result of childbirth in England and Wales in 1984. As we have seen in Chapter 2, mortality around birth and in early infancy continues to decline – especially perinatal mortality.

The limited scope for further reduction in perinatal deaths has led to a broadening of the objectives of the maternity and allied services. Official policy reflected in the two reports from the House of Commons Social Services Committee on perinatal and neonatal mortality known as the Short reports;[1,2] the government's reply to the first[3] and the subsequent guidelines issued by DHSS's Maternity Services Advisory Committee,[4-6] now endorse these wider goals which might be summarised as follows:

- to reduce perinatal and neonatal mortality rates;
- to eliminate disparities in these death rates between different sections of the community;
- to minimise impairment, disability and handicap;
- to promote the social and emotional wellbeing of parents and children.

The reduction of the social disparity in perinatal mortality rates between non-manual and manual social classes (see Chapter 8) remains a challenge. In 1984, babies born to the manual classes (IV and V combined) were nearly 160 per cent more likely to die in the perinatal period than those born to professional classes (I and II). The relative disparity has remained unchanged over the last decade (see Figure 32). Analysis by ethnic origin reveals that the highest death rates of all were among the babies of women of Pakistani origin whose perinatal death rates were nearly 18/1000 births in 1985, compared with 9.5 among babies born to women of UK origin.

Figure 32 Trends in perinatal mortality rates by social class for England and Wales (1975–1984)

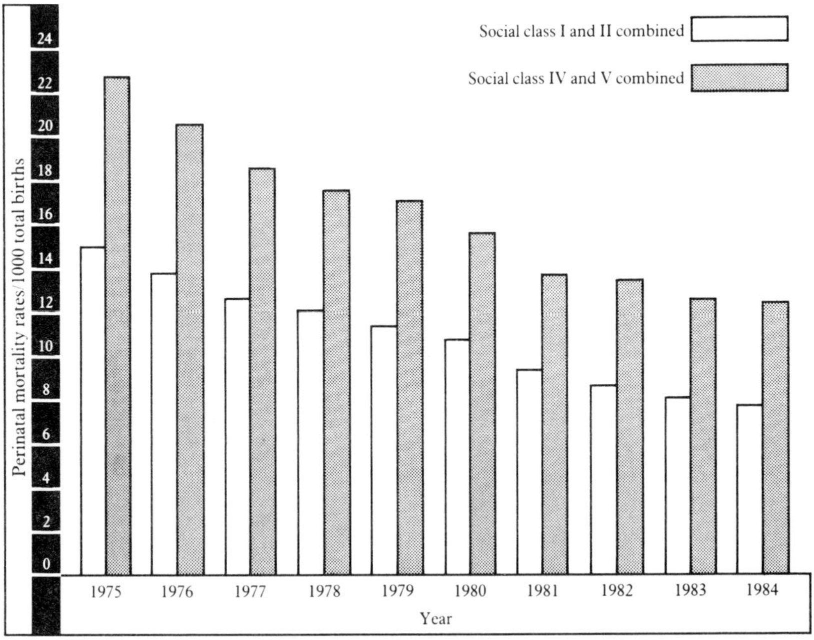

Source: Whitehead M. The health divide: inequalities in health in the 1980s. London, Health Education Council, 1987.

The Scottish Perinatal Mortality Survey, which has conducted a confidential inquiry into every perinatal death since 1977, shows that low birthweight and congenital malformations are the most important determinants of perinatal death.[7,8] Although perinatal mortality rates are sometimes used as indicators of the quality of the maternity services, low birthweight is more closely associated with poverty than with medical care. Poverty is further associated with higher maternal smoking rates which are also associated with low birthweight. It has been argued that in comparing the perinatal mortality in different countries, adjustments should be made for differences in the birth prevalence of low birthweight and congenital abnormalities. When these adjustments were made to statistics for 1978, the adjusted perinatal mortality rates for the UK compared favourably with those of Scandinavia and other parts of Europe, where crude perinatal mortality rates have always been much lower.

Although this suggests that our treatment services cope very well with low birthweight babies, it strongly suggests the need to concentrate on *preventing* low birthweight and congenital abnormality which explain much of the UK's poor international record. In 1984, 5.3 per cent of babies born to fathers in social class I in England and Wales weighed less than 2,500 gm (the usually accepted threshold for babies in social class V). Perinatal death rates among babies weighing less than 2,500 gm were 92.6 per 1,000 in 1984, compared with 2.8 per 1,000 for normal birthweight babies (3,000–3,500 gm). Two-thirds of low birthweight babies are born to working class mothers and despite improvements in the survival of babies in all birthweight categories the total proportion of low birthweight babies has remained unchanged at seven per cent over the last three decades. Although this figure is lower than for the USA and parts of Eastern Europe, the proportion of low birthweight babies in Sweden and Finland is less than five per cent.

In Chapter 8 we assessed the contribution made by material deprivation to health in general. Although its contribution in perinatal mortality is important, we do not know how big it is.[9] Congenital abnormality continues to account for one in five of all perinatal deaths. Death rates vary markedly throughout the UK and the rest of the world. This is largely a reflection of the varying incidence of low birthweight and central nervous system malformations which manifest either in their fatal form (anencephaly) or in a related, seriously disabling form (spina bifida).

Childhood disability and handicap There is no reliable information on the current extent of childhood disability, and still less on handicap. The most reliable estimates suggest that in 1978 five to six per cent of children suffered from moderate or severe physical or intellectual impairment. Of these, 1,000 cases in England and Wales were thought to be associated with perinatal factors and, therefore, potentially preventable through maternity care.[10] Even less identifiable are the estimated two per cent of the population who suffer mild intellectual impairment (with an IQ between 50–70) which is concentrated among low birthweight babies from working class families.[11]

Sudden infant death syndrome (SIDS)

It has been suggested that there is considerable scope for the reduction of mortality due to SIDS or 'cot deaths'. As we have shown in Chapter 2, SIDS now represents a major cause of death in the first four months of life. Wide variation in reporting has led to difficulty in interpreting the data, but respiratory disease is the most commonly associated factor. There is no associated cause in up to 48 per cent of cases.[12] While we are far from clear about the causes of SIDS, one intervention study in Sheffield suggests that about 15 per cent of these deaths may be preventable by the use of a scoring system to detect high risk babies at birth, together with extra health visiting support during the first 20 weeks of life.[13] If such a scheme were implemented on a national basis it would cost an estimated £5–7 million at 1986 prices. Claims that such a programme is cost-effective[14] are probably premature, for the Sheffield findings need confirmation elsewhere.[15]

Social features of childbearing

Surveys of women's experiences of pregnancy and childbirth, based on selected samples, suggest that while many women find childbirth an enjoyable experience,[16] hospital and antenatal care is characterised by long waiting times, poorly organised and dreary surroundings, and impersonal care.[17]

A review of innovations in antenatal care,[18] together with more recent surveys of users in 1981 and 1983,[19] suggest that there has been a conscious effort by some authorities to provide more flexible and supportive services. The availability of good health education material like the former HEC's *Pregnancy Book* and SHEG's *Book of the Child*, as well as information on antenatal care in a number of other languages, has increased, but there is little evidence that the antenatal clinic is being used as an opportunity for the exchange of information and advice. Most maternity units now allow fathers to attend and assist in the birth and more mothers are now given their babies to hold immediately after birth.[20] Mothers are also given support with breast feeding, largely by health visitors, midwives and counsellors. Two national surveys of breast feeding reflect this new emphasis: in 1980, 42 per cent of women in England and Wales were still breast feeding at six weeks compared with 24 per cent in 1975

Table 22 Trends in breast feeding in England and Wales and Scotland (in brackets)

	Attempting breast feeding at birth (%)	Still feeding at six weeks (%)	Introducing solids at 3 months (%)
1975	51	24	85
1980	67 (50)	42 (32)	55 (62)

Source: Martin J, Monk J. Infant feeding 1980, London, OPCS, 1982.

(see Table 22).

There are still wide regional and social class disparities in breast feeding, the proportion being highest (76 per cent) in south east England and lowest in Scotland (50 per cent). Older, professional woman are more likely to breast feed than younger, working class women.[21]

How have the maternity services changed? Virtually all women receive some form of maternity care, although the women suffering most social deprivation – especially Bengali women – are least likely to attend early or be adequately informed of maternity services.[22,23] Efforts to change this position by a DHSS-funded Asian Link Worker Scheme are slowly being implemented. The most striking change occurring over the last decade has been increased medical intervention at all stages of pregnancy, childbirth and the neonatal period. There was a profound shift of responsibility

Figure 33   Trends in the place of delivery 1960–1980 (England and Wales)

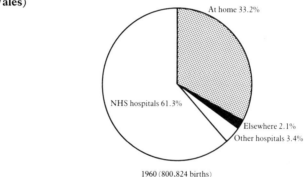

1960 (800,824 births)

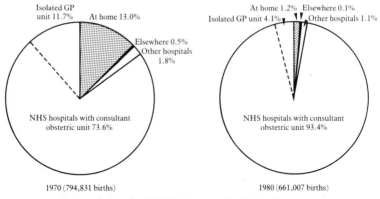

Source: MacFarlane A, Mugford M. Birth counts. Statistics of pregnancy and childbirth. National Perinatal Epidemiology Unit (in collaboration with OPCS). London, HMSO, 1984.

155

for antenatal care from the midwife and the GP to the hospital consultant in the 1970s. In the 1970 British Births Survey, only 22 per cent of women were seen exclusively in a hospital unit, whereas in a study of the whole of Aberdeen in 1979 this proportion had increased to 71 per cent.[24] While Aberdeen may be atypical, the figures do reflect a genuine increase that took place over this period. Although there are no national data, there has been some shift back to shared GP/midwife/consultant care since then, with some consultants – notably in Scotland and inner London – holding antenatal clinics in the community.

Although there are no national estimates, more and more pregnant women are undergoing antenatal investigation, with an estimated 80 per cent now having a routine ultrasound scan at 16–18 weeks of pregnancy.[25] Screening services for the detection of Down's syndrome are patchy, with poor overall uptake, but screening for neural tube defects is now available in every health authority. Counselling provision – especially in the genetic field – had developed in about 20 centres by 1983.

In 1983, 99 per cent of babies in Great Britain were born in hospital. This is the culmination of a trend away from home and GP

Figure 34   Trends in obstetric intervention in England and Wales (1955–1978)

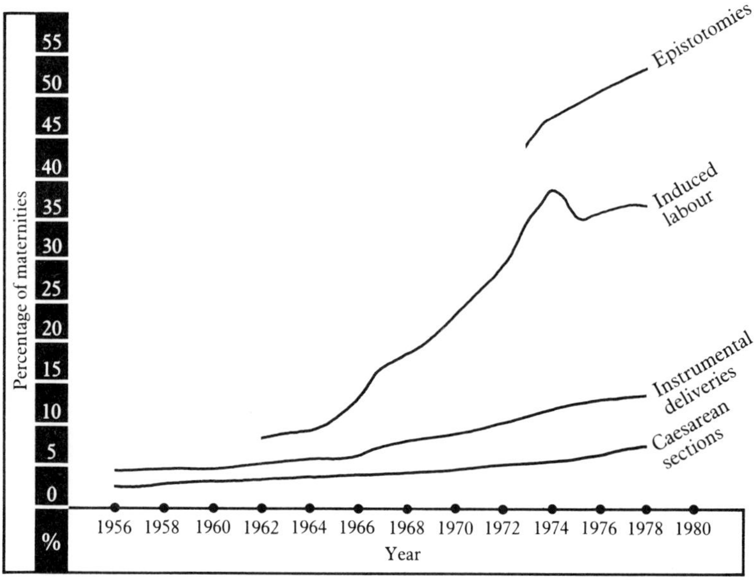

Source: MacFarlane A, Mugford M. Birth counts. Statistics of pregnancy and childbirth. National Perinatal Epidemiology Unit (in collaboration with OPCS). London, HMSO, 1984.

unit deliveries which has taken place over the last two decades (see Figure 33). A shift in government policy has led to the closure of many isolated GP maternity units with a relative concentration of deliveries in larger, consultant units. There has been a concomitant increase in intervention in labour (see Figure 34) with large increases in the proportion of women having episiotomies – a procedure whereby the skin around the opening of the vulva is cut, ostensibly to prevent serious tears when the baby is born. The artificial induction of labour increased to a peak in 1974, then fell and remained at about 35 per cent until 1980. It has since fallen to about 18 per cent. The caesarean section rate doubled in England and Wales from 4.3 per cent of deliveries in 1970 to 10 per cent in 1983. The picture is similar in Scotland with an increase in caesarean section rates from 8.5 per cent in 1975 to 12.5 per cent in 1983.

Following a series of recommendations from the Short report, the British Paediatric Association and the Royal College of Obstetricians and Gynaecologists, there has been an increase in the provision and use of special and intensive care baby units. By 1977 as many as 20 per cent of newborns were nursed in special care baby units, but since 1983 this proportion had fallen to 11 per cent because the criteria for admission have been revised.[26]

The rationale for the changes

Antenatal care The Short reports have reiterated their belief that antenatal care, and early attendance in particular, is effective in reducing perinatal mortality. Although there is an inverse relationship between perinatal mortality and frequency of attendance at antenatal clinics,[27,28] the effect of early attendance on perinatal mortality has never been properly tested. Moreover, the observed association may be explained by the fact that women who book early at antenatal clinics are more likely to come from professional backgrounds and thus to have a lower risk of perinatal death – irrespective of whether they attend early or not.

Antenatal care is a complex mixture of interventions that would make a randomised control trial impracticable, and probably unacceptable. However, recent research offers a more realistic picture of what we can expect from it. A study of all pregnant women in Aberdeen in 1975 showed that many of the problems arising in pregnancy are unpredictable, and that antenatal visits up to the 32nd week of pregnancy (excluding screening for genetic and chromosomal disease which was not assessed in the study) are diagnostically relatively unproductive. The study concluded that antenatal visits for low risk women could be reduced and blood pressure screening tests more efficiently and comfortably performed by the midwife at home or in primary care.[29]

157

Psychosocial interventions The widely held belief in the value of the prevention of anxiety and provision of a socially supportive environment during pregnancy and labour is increasingly borne out by the evidence. Not only can stressful experiences for the mother adversely affect events from conception to birth[30] but intervention consciously designed to support women can positively affect the outcome of pregnancy.[31]

A statistical pooling analysis of 29 registered randomised controlled trials up to 1985[32] of some form of social support (all non-clinical interventions involving information, health education, counselling and changes in the organisation or environment of care were defined as 'social support') showed that it had the following significant, beneficial effects:

- a reduction in the amount of drugs used for pain relief in labour (this was mostly as a result of antenatal education/preparation classes);

Table 23   The main antenatal and neonatal screening tests of proven effectiveness

Problem	Approx prevalence/ 1000 births	Levels of implementation in the NHS
DISORDERS AFFECTING THE FETUS		
1 Anencephaly ⎫ Neural tube defects	20	Probably variable
2 Spina bifida ⎭ (NTDs)	20	
3 Down's syndrome	15	Partial and variable
4 Rhesus disease	70	Full
5 Thalassemia major	5	Experimental
6 Haemophilia	0.4	?
ANTENATAL DISORDERS AFFECTING THE MOTHER		
1 Eclampsia	20	Probably good
2 Iron deficiency	10–3000	Full
3 Rubella	3	Full
4 Sickle cell anaemia	1	Probably full
5 Congenital syphilis	2	Full
DISORDERS AFFECTING THE NEWBORN		
1 Congenital dislocation of the hip	10	Probably good
2 Congenital hypothyoidism (underactive thyroid)	2	Full
3 Phenylketonuria (genetic defect in protein metabolism)	1	Full

Source: Adapted from Wald N (ed). Antenatal and Neonatal Screening. Oxford, Oxford University Press, 1984.

- a reduction in the risk of prolonged labour;
- a reduced risk of instrumental delivery, maternal anxiety and postnatal depression.

Although the pooling exercise did not demonstrate a significant effect on the proportion of low birthweight deliveries *overall*, a significant beneficial effect was detectable in one of the trials among women in the highest risk categories. Although this may be an isolated finding, it offers a possible way of reducing the incidence of low birthweight babies among working class women[33] who are under more stress than other women.[34] This approach has produced promising results in the field of smoking in pregnancy, where working class women have higher rates than professional women (see Chapters 4 and 8). Randomised trials suggest that *supportive*, rather than didactic, advice given about smoking during pregnancy is more effective.[35] We await the results of other trials of social support offered by midwives or their aides to women in high risk groups.

Antenatal and neonatal screening Screening of the parents and fetus for risk of abnormality during pregnancy (antenatal screening) and after birth (neonatal screening) is one of the best researched areas of maternity care. It has been estimated[36] that if antenatal and neonatal screening tests (and treatment) of proven value (see Table 23) are effectively implemented:

- perinatal mortality in the UK could be reduced by 20 per cent;
- 11–13 per cent of severe childhood disability (mental and physical) could be prevented.

Table 23 summarises the main cost-effective antenatal and neonatal screening tests which are currently available. Screening for neural tube defects (NTDs) – that is, spina bifida and anencephaly – and Downs' syndrome, currently offer the most important means of reducing the birth prevalence of congenital abnormality.

While there is no firm evidence yet to justify the routine use of ultrasound to screen all pregnant women, it has beneficial outcomes in specific instances, such as the confirmation of the diagnosis of neural tube defects and genetic diseases linked to the sex chromosome (for example, haemophilia) where ultrasound diagnosis of the baby's sex is now very accurate.[37,38] It has been argued that because ultrasound has been shown to be a relatively safe test all women should be tested. Others suggest that women feel reassured following a normal ultrasound scan, although the findings of existing studies are mixed.[39] A fully controlled trial of ultrasound is needed to answer many of these and other remaining questions.

Neural tube defects (NTDs) Eighty-four per cent of babies who survive with open spina bifida (the kind of NTD detectable by antenatal screening) are severely disabled.[40] The risk of NTDs increases for women who have had a previously affected child, but the major determinants lie in the environment and are thus potentially preventable. There is marked geographical variation in these conditions in the UK, with Wales, Northern Ireland and Scotland having the highest rates, together with the north and western parts of England. Preliminary studies suggest that multi-vitamins – especially folic acid found in leafy vegetables – may be protective. We await the results of a major MRC trial of vitamin supplementation.

The detection of a high level of a protein known as alphafetopro-tein (AFP) in the mother's blood between 16 and 18 weeks of pregnancy is an effective screening test for NTDs. If backed up with a further test – amniocentesis, which shows high levels of AFP in the fluid surrounding the fetus – about three-quarters of open spina bifida and nearly all anencephaly can be detected. Further investigation with an ultrasound scan can increase the detection rate of spina bifida to 91 per cent.[41] At 1980 prices, the total cost of the screening process, including scanning and amniocentesis, was £6.50 per woman screened. Assuming a detection rate of at least 75 per cent, the benefit to cost ratio was estimated at 8:5.[42] In other words, for every £5 spent on screening, £8 will be saved by preventing NTDs.

Between 1976 and 1985 the notified birth prevalence of congenital malformations of the central nervous system (mostly NTDs) fell by two-thirds; spina bifida by 63 per cent, and anencephaly by 92 per cent (see Figure 35). Only about one-third of the decline can be directly attributed to screening (together with termination) – as was confirmed by associated terminations occurring mainly after screening was implemented on a national scale. The rest is unexplained, but may be due to environmental factors such as dietary change.

Down's syndrome Ninety-five per cent of cases of Down's syndrome result from a non-heritable abnormality in the 21st chromosome which is accurately detectable by amniocentesis. Down's syndrome is the commonest cause of institutionalisation for mental handicap, and among children of school age 30 per cent of those with learning difficulties suffer from Down's syndrome. The risk of giving birth to a baby with Down's syndrome increases with the mother's age and rises to one in 250 between the ages of 35 and 39, and one in 45 over the age of 45. Economic studies show that the benefits of screening for Down's syndrome outweigh the costs if it is used in women aged 35 and over – the age when the risk of having a Down's baby exceeds that of abortion due to amniocentesis (up to 1 in 100).[43]

Although the evidence supporting screening for Down's syndrome at 35 and over is good, the 1980 Short report recommended

160

that only women over 40 should be offered amniocentesis. Despite inadequate information about policy and practice, the available evidence suggests that screening is offered in a patchy fashion to women at ages which vary from health authority to health authority. In 1978, 14 per cent of women aged 35–39 and only 41 per cent of over 40s had amniocentesis in the UK.[44] More recent evidence from individual health authorities suggests that uptake had increased only to 49 per cent in women over 38 by 1980.[45] We urgently need to know whether this poor progress is due to a lack of availability of screening services around the country and their poor organisation, or whether women are inadequately informed or counselled about it or have ethical objections to it.

The lack of an overall downward trend in the notification of Down's syndrome (see Figure 35) reflects only in part the patchy implementation of screening policy. While older women still have the highest risk of having a baby with Down's syndrome the largest *numbers* (about 80 per cent) of affected women are now in the younger age groups. These trends have important implications for other public health policy areas (see Chapter 7) – especially on diet or alcohol and even AIDS – where measures designed *only* to reach high risk sectors of the community will leave the problem largely unresolved.[46]

However the future offers a potentially cost-effective means of

Figure 35   Notification of congenital malformations in England and Wales (1964–1980)

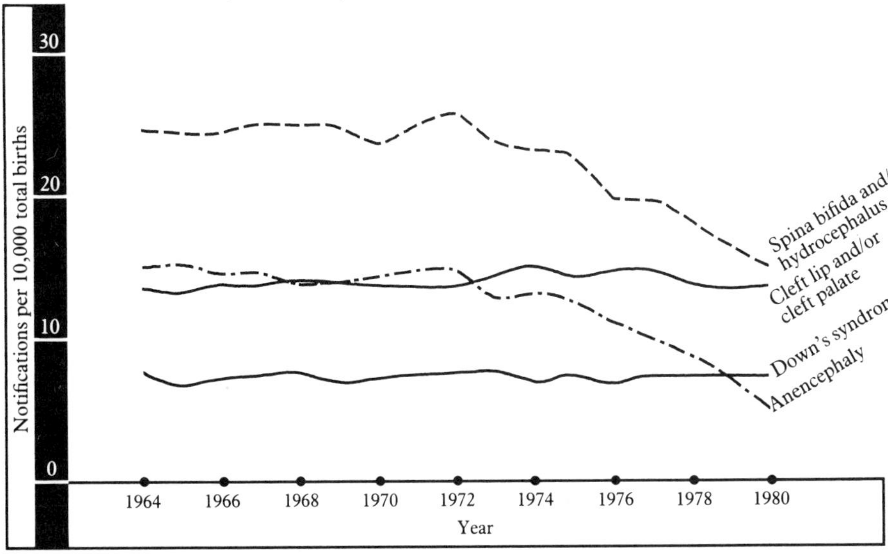

Source: MacFarlane A, Mugford M. Birth counts. Statistics of pregnancy and childbirth. National Perinatal Epidemiology Unit (in collaboration with OPCS). London, HMSO, 1984.

161

extending screening for Down's syndrome to younger women. For there is now good evidence that Down's syndrome is related to abnormally *low* levels of AFP in the mother's blood which can be detected by the screening test already used for NTDs.[47,48] Preliminary research in one health authority suggests that a policy which combines amniocentesis in older women with AFP screening for under 35s could detect 40 per cent of all Down's syndrome babies – a five-fold improvement on the current position.[49] These conclusions are now supported by the early findings of a multi-centre trial in the USA.[50]

Innovations in screening for genetic disease The development of methods for mapping faulty genes, and even, ultimately, for replacing them (through developments in recombinant DNA techniques) offers scope for the future prevention of genetic disease. This scope is limited, however, to the detection of defects in single genes, which account for only a small proportion of all genetic disease. The gene responsible for cystic fibrosis – the commonest disabling genetic disease in the UK – has recently been identified and much progress has been and could be made in the prevention of genetic diseases such as thalassemia major and sickle cell disease which are caused by single gene defects in the haemoglobin molecule and represent a major worldwide challenge.

The most promising recent development in the screening field has been chorionic villous sampling (CVS) – a technique in which a small sample of fetal tissue can be removed for genetic and chromosomal analysis. Its main potential advantage is that it is performed much earlier in pregnancy (8–11 weeks) than amniocentesis (16–18 weeks), and may offer an effective means of earlier detection. CVS, when used in conjunction with an information and counselling service, has been shown to reduce the birthrate for thalassemia major by 60 per cent in the Cypriot community and by 20 per cent among Asians of East African origin in the UK.[51] While the service was regarded as acceptable to these two communities, it was not by women of Pakistani origin who now give birth to more babies with thalassemia than other ethnic groups in the UK.

CVS,[52] along with developments in gene-mapping and potential 'gene therapy', may offer a cost effective means of preventing increasing numbers of genetic diseases such as sickle cell disease and fragile X syndrome – a cause of mental handicap in males second only to Down's syndrome. The successful implementation of CVS depends not only on trials of its effectiveness but on full discussion of its ethical implications with those most likely to be affected. This is why the unique involvement of user groups in the MRC trial of CVS is of considerable importance.

Intervening during labour The use of many previously untested

162

obstetric interventions has recently been called into question. Research has shown that practices such as shaving the pubic area, giving enemas and the use of gowns, masks and sterilising procedures in normal deliveries are unnecessary. The belief that episiotomy is better than no intervention at all is unfounded.[53] A major randomised controlled trial of fetal monitoring in labour, compared with traditional intermittent monitoring with a fetal stethoscope, showed that if used with monitoring of pH (acidity levels) in the baby's blood it was better able to detect fetal distress in high risk, prolonged labours. It was also able to reduce convulsions significantly in the newborn by more than 50 per cent. The study has not been followed up for long enough yet to detect whether this policy has any effect on subsequent disability. Conclusions so far suggest that such monitoring should be restricted to women in high risk categories only.[54,55]

Recent debate has been about the increasing use of caesarean sections and the move away from home and GP unit deliveries to hospital birth. While it is clear that caesarean sections can be life-saving for the baby in certain situations, there is disagreement on the exact indications for the operation and this is reflected in the wide variations in the proportion of caesarean deliveries throughout the UK. Concern stems from the desire to minimise unnecessary intervention during childbirth[56] and to avoid the small, but significant, extra risk that caesarean section imposes on the mother. Increases in what is often unjustified medical intervention in labour account for more than half of the rise in caesarean sections over the last decade.[57] There is thus scope for reducing unnecessary caesareans by the more judicious use of techniques such as fetal monitoring.[58]

The 1980 Short report recommended a shift away from home and GP unit births to hospital births for all mothers. This conclusion was based on data for home-versus-hospital births in 1975 which seemed to suggest that perinatal mortality rates were higher at home than in hospital.[59] But detailed analysis of the data, together with more recent findings from the Cardiff Births Survey, has shown that these conclusions were unfounded. When home deliveries are analysed by *intended* place of delivery it is clear that they fall into two distinct groups: intended or planned home deliveries which are safe, and unplanned deliveries in which illness and death rates among the newborn were higher than for planned deliveries.[60] Analysis of all home births in England and Wales in 1979 showed that when births were analysed by *intended* place of delivery rather than by where they happened to occur, perinatal mortality rates for intended home deliveries were substantially *lower* than in consultant units.[61]

More recently, research from New Zealand, where nearly one

third of births take place in small GP units, has shown that for babies weighing over 1500 gm perinatal mortality rates were significantly lower in GP units than in larger, consultant units. Only babies weighing less than 1500 gm benefited significantly from delivery in a consultant unit.[62] While these findings should give us cause to review our own policies, there are problems of comparability presented by this and other research from abroad.[63]

Intensive care of the newborn A detailed consideration of neonatal intensive care is beyond the scope of this report, but its rapid growth raises some important ethical issues. While the provision of effective neonatal intensive care has contributed to the improved survival of very low birthweight babies,[64] there is growing concern that this may lead to a rapid increase in the prevalence of seriously disabled children.[65] For the risk of impairment – especially cerebral palsy (spastic children) – rises as birthweight falls. This is already apparent in Sweden where the incidence of cerebral palsy has been rising since the 1960s.[66] Although there are no comparable national UK data, results of research into the births of all children born in one region showed no increased prevalence of disabled children at the age of three – despite a concomitant fall in perinatal mortality in recent years.[67] This study was not large enough to settle this important issue. A number of questions require wide public discussion: for instance, does the salvage of increasingly small babies result in a greater burden of disability in the community and, if so, are we prepared to accept *and* act on the consequences?

12 Promoting child health

Love is like the measles; we all have to
go through it.

JEROME K JEROME

Introduction The health of children is an important indicator of the nation's overall health and childhood is a time when opportunities for maximising health potential are likely to be great. It is disappointing, therefore, that there is little reliable national information (apart from that on mortality) on health, disease and disability in childhood, and still less on the possible relationship between child health and adult health.

From the limited data so far available it is clear that health in childhood can be shaped by influences acting long before birth and childhood itself. Children born to manual workers are less likely to survive infancy and early childhood, and those brought up in deprived, inner city areas are more at risk of conduct and other emotional disorders (see Chapter 10). Children's physical and mental health can be significantly affected by their parents' family planning practices (see Chapter 13) as well as by events which may take place during pregnancy and around birth (see Chapter 11). In this chapter we assess opportunities for promoting health during childhood itself. We focus on the general contributions made by the family and the school, and assess the value of specific contributions made by the health service. We then consider two specific areas in more detail: immunisation and dental health.

Parents – an important resource The health of children and their parents is inextricably linked. The impact of parents' health and behaviour on that of their children is well-documented in some respects, and we know that parents who smoke or drink heavily are more likely to produce children who do likewise. We also know that postnatal depression, family disharmony, parental neglect, and, of course, abuse, can have profound effects on children's wellbeing and development (see Chapter 10). But we have neglected in both research and policy terms the impact that children can have on their parents' wellbeing. A commitment to promote health in childhood must therefore also involve a consideration of factors which promote or compromise the health of parents who are primarily dedicated to the healthy development of their children.

There is now evidence that bringing up a mentally handicapped child takes a toll of the mental health of the child's parents –

especially its mother.[1] But rearing healthy children can have adverse effects on the mental health of their mothers – especially working class women (see Chapter 10). A small but important study of the impact of caring for pre-school children on the health of mothers in 102 families has shown that most mothers bear the brunt of all childcare and spend 70 per cent of their 15 hour working day with their children. This leaves little time for relaxation and is associated with symptoms of emotional upset in most mothers.[2]

This study also highlighted the positive contribution that parents make to their children's emotional and physical development. Eighty per cent of the mother's activities recorded in a diary were deemed to be oriented towards their children's nutrition and health. This reinforces other research into more specific aspects of child health which show that parents deal with 90 per cent of childhood illnesses themselves and that parental participation in the use of preventive services such as child health clinics can improve both their effectiveness and efficiency.

An important recent social change has been the increasing proportion of women in paid employment. This is likely to have major implications for child health and development. Projections for 1986 suggest that over two-thirds of women of working age are in paid work and that this figure will rise among young women.[3] The available evidence suggests that women have neither abandoned their traditional child rearing responsibilities nor transferred more of that responsibility to their partners.[4]

Nursery provision State and workplace nurseries can offer an acceptable solution for the increasing numbers of families where both parents are in paid employment. State provision of such facilities is virtually non-existent in the UK – except for children from multiply deprived families. This position reflects a long standing British concern about the potential adverse effects that separation from the mother may have on the young child, together with possible adverse effects of nursery care itself.

In the postwar period it was widely believed that children between the ages of six months and three years could suffer what became known as 'maternal deprivation' resulting in permanent emotional damage if separated from their mother.[5] More recent research has shown this view to be poorly founded as it was based on observations of unrepresentative samples of institutionalised children who had been emotionally deprived for other reasons.[6] The available evidence today[7] shows that separation of a child from its mother is not harmful in itself and that emotional disturbances in children are more likely to originate from family discord. While attachment relationships are important in the promotion of good child develop-

166

ment, a child's attachment to its mother is not a unique, irreplaceable relationship. There is no evidence that day care in nurseries is damaging to children and *high quality* care confers some social advantages on attenders. The relative effects of different forms of day care (including childminding) are at present the subject of a major study.

ent progress in legislation

Family policy is poorly developed in the UK, and while we have kept pace with other European countries in equal pay and opportunities legislation we compare poorly in employment protection, parental leave and nursery care provisions. Although the 1980 Employment Protection Act goes some way towards protecting the mental and physical health of both mother and child in the first six months of the child's life, a survey of the EEC in 1985 showed that the UK was the only country which pays less than 75 per cent of previous earnings during maternity leave and requires a woman to have been employed continuously for two years to be eligible for leave.[8] Moreover, the UK is one of only three EEC countries which make no statutory provision for parental leave following maternity leave.

ducation for health

While we have documented throughout this report the impact of specific health education initiatives on children's health and behaviour, there has been little emphasis so far on the role of education *in general* in promoting healthy development among children. It is widely agreed that pre-school education – either through play groups or nursery school – has a favourable effect on children's emotional and intellectual development. It is therefore encouraging that attendance at nursery school in England has increased over the last decade from 28 per cent of under fives in 1975 to 43 per cent in 1985.

The most detailed research on the direct impact of schooling has been conducted on children of secondary school age. There is now compelling evidence that, after taking other major factors into account, some schools have protective effect on scholastic achievement, attendance rates and even delinquency rates.[9] In a major controlled study of 12 schools in inner London, the following factors were significantly associated with successful achievement at school and low delinquency rates:

- a good mix of intellectually able and less able pupils;
- the use of rewards and praise;
- an attractive school environment;
- encouragement for children to participate in the running of the school together with firm leadership and participation by the teaching staff;

167

- teachers' attitudes and behaviour.

These findings[10] add to the debate about how schools might be organised in the interests of promoting the social and emotional development of children.

Growing recognition of the potential of the school as a medium for promoting health has resulted in a marked move away from one-off, topic-based health education teaching towards integration of health education throughout the curriculum.[11] The importance of encouraging pupils of all ages to participate actively in their own learning about health is now recognised. The impetus for this change came from a number of joint initiatives between the Schools Council and the former HEC which resulted in the development of programmes such as All About Me for 5–8 year olds and Think Well for 9–13 year olds. They have gained wide acceptance and have been implemented in one form or another throughout the UK. The Schools Council programmes are founded on three main principles which are now official policy at DES.[12]

- The success of the educational approach depends on fulfilling social and emotionally defined outcomes as well as medical objectives.
- The programmes need to be integrated right across the curriculum.
- Learning in general, and health-related behaviour in particular, are enhanced by methods geared towards promoting a child's self confidence and decision-making skills.

Careful evaluation in 120 schools showed that many of the objectives are achievable when measured in terms of teacher/pupil acceptability and the development of self-esteem, although changes in health-related behaviour such as smoking and diet were difficult to detect.[13]

Parallel approaches designed for older secondary school students have been developed since the mid-1970s. These are based on research into small group work to help promote the development of 'life skills'. Such approaches, now to be found in operation within social education curricula, are deliberately designed to help students develop a positive self-image to foster the idea that they can take charge of their own lives and relationships.

While specific issues such as smoking, drug-taking and sexually transmitted disease arise in discussion, they are *not* the central theme of this approach and are discussed in the context in which they arise. The aim is to allow the students, ultimately, to make informed *choices* about health-related behaviours. Evaluation of this approach has shown increases in confidence and self-awareness among students and that it is widely accepted by teachers throughout the country.[14–16]

Child health
surveillance
Modern ideas about child health surveillance stem from the need to see child health in terms which are broader than the prevention of disease alone. This is clearly reflected in a recent policy statement from the Health Visitors' Association (HVA)[17] which is consistent with WHO objectives for child health.[18] The HVA has identified four essential components of surveillance: screening tests (procedures designed to detect specific disorders); health promotion support (advice on all aspects of child health including immunisation); developmental screening (examining the child to detect any deviation from the normal range of development); and developmental assessment (assessment of abnormal findings identified by screening).[19]

Screening tests for hypothyroidism (an underactive thyroid) and phenylketonuria (a genetic disorder of metabolism) in the newborn have been shown to be effective (see Chapter 11). But other potentially effective tests for problems such as undescended testes, congenital dislocation of the hip, and hearing and visual impairment, have been inadequately evaluated.[20] Although the WHO has concluded that screening tests for hearing and visual impairment are of proven efficacy,[21] we still do not have information on when or how often children should be screened or who is best qualified to perform such tests.[22] While there is evidence that systematic screening policies in a primary care setting are able to detect a number of childhood disorders, false-positive and negative diagnosis rates are high[23,24] and there have been no intervention trials to demonstrate that screening has a beneficial impact on health.[25]

Despite the absence of systematic data, a considerable body of information has accumulated from three postwar prospective studies of child health and development. In the case of visual and hearing impairment, where there are effective interventions for preventing disability, these studies point to some of the prerequisites for establishing an effective screening programme.[26,27] Visual and hearing impairment are common problems in childhood. About four per cent of children aged 5–7 have moderate visual impairment, and six per cent of 7 year olds have significant hearing deficits. Untreated visual impairments such as squint can result in permanent damage and subsequent reading difficulty. Children with untreated hearing impairment are more likely to be educationally and psychosocially handicapped than normal children at age seven.[28] Screening at repeated intervals is essential, because one normal result may be followed by the detection of subsequent abnormalities – especially in the case of visual impairments such as myopia (short-sightedness) which is not usually apparent before the age of seven.

Health promotion support The potential impact of support and advice on health in childhood is a neglected area of research.

Although we know that health visitors and GPs are important and valued sources of advice and support for parents of pre-school children, we do not know whether this advice beneficially affects health outcomes. Information on some health-related trends in childhood is now sufficiently detailed to prompt intervention studies on the effect of advice from health professionals in these areas. We know, for example, that although the average height of children continued to increase between 1972 and 1980, there is still scope for improvement as children from less well-off families remain shorter than children from well-to-do families.[29]

Developmental screening and assessment Developmental screening was introduced in the UK more than 25 years ago. Yet there is still no good information on which tests are valid, effective and reliable; when it is best to do them; and how much emphasis should be placed on their results.[30,31] While it has a potential role to play in reassuring parents about their childrens' development, one of its main difficulties is that there are no *fixed* points in a child's development which offer *clear-cut* distinctions between normal and abnormal development. This raises a number of problems concerning the value of screening tests.[32] Delay in achieving developmental milestones is a poor predictor of subsequent abnormality and most children who start walking or talking late turn out to be normal. The assumption that delayed development in early years is critical and leaves irreversible damage is unfounded, for development is a dynamic process and children can learn new skills throughout childhood. While education and early stimulation of children from deprived backgrounds can result in developmental benefits, these may be temporary unless parents also play an active role. Although there is some evidence that early intervention can reduce speech, language and behaviour problems,[33] there is little firm overall evidence that it has any lasting effect.

Little thought has been given to the potential anxiety that developmental screening could create among parents and their children, and still less to the possible misdirection of effort from advice and support towards time-consuming, untested observations which parents are mostly well-equipped to do themselves.[34]

Implications for policy A series of major reports on child health, led by the government's 1976 report *Fit for the Future*,[35] (known as the Court report) at once reflect and attempt to overcome the uncertainties in the field of child health surveillance. The Court report, and its sequels from the National Children's Bureau in 1987, the BMA, British Paediatric Association (BPA), HVA, RCGP, and Faculty of Community Medicine,[36–40] have identified two further important barriers to improving child health services:

- a lack of national commitment to the development of an integrated child health service;
- the inability of the diverse professional groups involved to reach agreement on responsibilities within the field.

Although differing professional perceptions and allegiances have led to a variety of recommendations on exactly what tests to perform, at what stages, and by whom, there is broad agreement about several essential elements within strategies laid out so far.

- Child health services should be integrated within primary health care and child health surveillance should be the joint responsibility of parents, health visitors and GPs. There will be a continuing need for clinical medical officers – especially in inner city areas.[41]
- Immunisation, screening for hearing and visual impairment, and for undescended testes and congenital dislocation of the hip, form legitimate components of a surveillance programme.
- While the validity and reliability of developmental screening remains in question, there should be an agreed means of assessing a child's development throughout the pre-school and school years. It may be best to adopt an 'anticipatory care' approach in which opportunities for advising and reassuring parents about aspects of child development are created within the ordinary consultation process.
- There should be clear agreement about professionals' responsibilities for different aspects of child health surveillance. This is currently the subject of an interdisciplinary Joint Surveillance Working Party established by the HVA with the BPA, the BMA and the RCGP.
- There should be a reliable national and regional monitoring service, and this is slowly being built up through the Child Health Computing System.

Immunisation – a challenge to the child health services

Immunisation remains one of the best documented ways of protecting health and is a central feature of all child health care programmes. There is also evidence that the benefit-to-cost ratio of immunisation programmes is favourable. Economic analysis of the successful US measles and rubella programmes in 1981 suggests that the costs imposed by these diseases were 15 and 11 times greater than the costs of the respective immunisation programmes.[42] We must, however, be cautious in translating these findings to the UK.[43] While we must await a full analysis of the UK position, preliminary results suggest that the benefits of the UK programme outweigh the costs.[44]

Figure 36 Trends in immunisation uptake in England and Wales, and Scotland (1974–1985)

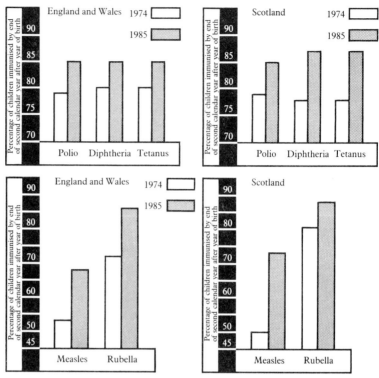

Rubella immunisation applies to girls immunised by the end of their 14th year after birth.
Rubella immunisation in Scotland excludes Greater Glasgow and Lothian Health Boards for which comparable figures are not available. Figures for 1981-85 record girls immunised by 30 June of 14th year after birth.
Comparisons for rubella immunisation are only available from 1978 onwards.

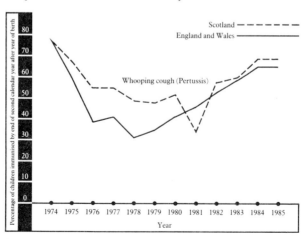

Source: Comparative data for England and Scotland prepared by Scottish Health Service, Information and Statistics Division.

Goals for immunisation policy

WHO aims to eliminate measles, polio, tetanus in the newborn, diphtheria and congenital rubella by the year 2000. In support of this goal they have set a target of 90 per cent immunisation uptake rates for each of these diseases to be achieved for all European children under two by 1990.[45] While such immunisation targets might be achievable, the total eradication of these diseases may not be possible.[46] However, more realistic goals have been set for the USA for major reductions in these diseases (without elimination) by the year 1990.[47]

The European targets – with the exception of past rubella policy – are all translatable into UK policy. But the DHSS has only so far set a firm target for 95 per cent uptake of measles vaccine by 1990, with the aim of total elimination by 1995. Whatever the criteria used, achievements in the UK have, so far, been mixed. Although diphtheria, polio and tetanus have all but disappeared from the mortality and disease statistics, and there is a welcome upward trend in immunisation uptake rates for other diseases (see Figure 36), the UK still falls far short of reaching either national or international targets for rubella, measles and pertussis (whooping cough). This unsatisfactory position was highlighted in two major British reports to Parliament in 1986.[48,49] The UK record is also poor in an international context. Not only does it do worse than the USA and most of eastern, and some of north western, Europe, but it also lags behind an increasing number of third world countries such as Chile, Brazil and the Gambia[50] which have better immunisation uptake rates for measles and pertussis.

National averages hide what can be achieved regionally. Scotland does better than England, and the Borders Health Board had the best immunisation uptake levels in the UK in 1984. In England and Wales the gaps between the best levels achieved in Wessex RHA and the worst in the North Western RHA need further research. Local findings so far suggest that social class disadvantage (see Chapter 8) is only part of the explanation and that varying commitment and organisation of district immunisation programmes play an important role.[51,52]

Measles

Although measles is now rarely fatal in the UK, there are still up to 100,000 reported cases each year and this is likely to be at least a 50 per cent underestimate. Measles is still a serious disease. Up to 10 per cent of children develop complications, including four per cent with chest infections and 0.5 per cent with a rare but serious form of encephalitis (inflammation of brain tissue). Measles itself is at least ten times more likely to cause permanent damage to the nervous system than the measles vaccine, where adverse effects are extremely rare. Since its introduction in 1968, the impact of the measles

173

immunisation programme has been substantial: the annual number of reported cases is now about one-fifth of what it was in the pre-vaccine era (see Figure 37), but in the last decade the number of reported cases has remained between 50–100,000. The biannual epidemic pattern has now been replaced by an annual one. The national immunisation level of 68 per cent in England (73 per cent in Scotland) is still well below the DHSS target of 90 per cent by 1990 (see Figure 36).

Experience from the USA and Scandinavia suggests that the UK record could be better. In the USA, immunisation is a legal precondition for school entry and, in some states, for pre-school entry too. By 1981, 97 per cent of children at school entry had proven evidence of measles immunisation.[53] This, together with a major public education programme, surveillance and active intervention on individually reported cases, has brought the USA close to reaching its own and WHO's targets for the year 2000 (see Figure 37).

Figure 37   Measles in England and Wales, and in the USA: trends in reported cases (1961-1987)

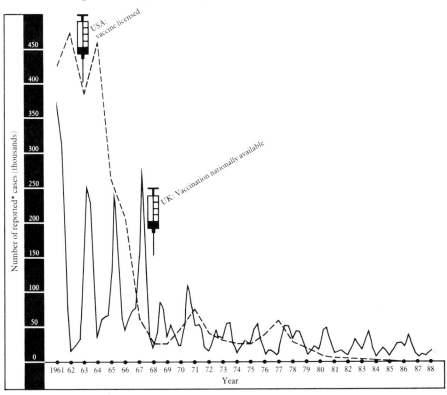

*Cases in England and Wales are reported quarterly
Sources: Centre for Disease Surveillance and Control, 1988.
Centre for Disease Control, Atlanta, USA.

Measles: improving UK performance

Despite sporadic, national health education campaigns, local research in Scotland[54] suggests the barriers are fourfold.

- A third of parents do not see measles as a serious condition.
- More than half had doubts about the vaccine's safety.
- Although eight in ten GPs supported immunisation, only three in ten had an active recall system for children of fifteen months.
- Although health visitors and community physicians were convinced of the value of the vaccine, a minority of GPs thought it was ineffective or dangerous.

The disparity between the American and British programmes has led to a 160-fold higher notified incidence in the UK in 1985.

Rubella

Rubella, or German measles, is a minor childhood illness, but infection during pregnancy can, if contracted in the first three months, lead to congenital rubella syndrome (CRS). Most CRS babies have serious, multiple disabilities including deafness, blindness and mental impairment. Estimates for England and Wales in the pre-vaccine era suggest that 15 per cent of deafness of neurological origin was due to rubella – about 225 cases per year.[55] In 1987 the lifetime health costs of caring for a child with CRS were estimated at £175,000.[56]

CRS is one of the few congenital problems that is, in principle, wholly preventable. The objective of past UK immunisation policy has been to eliminate CRS without attempting to eliminate rubella itself. The method proposed to achieve this was – until recently – the immunisation of all girls aged 10–13. It was introduced in 1970 and backed up in 1976 with screening and immunisation of all non-pregnant women of childbearing age who were not immune (seronegative). In 1983, the DHSS, together with the national health education bodies and the Rubella Council, launched a £2 million educational drive to increase rubella vaccine uptake. Its effects should already be in evidence as the first generation of girls eligible for the vaccine are now well into their childbearing years. Some, but not all, of the signs are encouraging. Vaccine uptake in schoolgirls increased by 17 percentage points to 86 per cent between 1976 and 1985 in England, and to 88 per cent in Scotland (see Figure 36) and surveys of girls and young women show that 90 per cent or more are now immune or seropositive.[57] Evidence from a major study in Manchester has demonstrated that with careful coordination through a responsible nurse it is possible (in a hospital setting) to increase total immunisation uptakes among adult women to 85 per cent. Between 1979 and 1984 the proportion of women who were still seronegative after childbirth was reduced from 6.4 per cent to 2.7 per cent.[58] Yet despite this impressive coverage, CRS has not been eliminated from Manchester.

Evidence for the success of the UK programme must ultimately come from a combined analysis of trends in CRS cases and rubella-associated terminations. Continuous monitoring by the National Congenital Rubella Surveillance Programme between 1971 and 1984 shows that during the worst epidemic of the decade (1978/79) the immunisation programme did not prevent an increase in either the number of cases of CRS or the number of rubella-associated abortions (see Figure 38). During the more moderate epidemic in 1982/83, the number of CRS cases did not rise as much as expected,[59] and the number of rubella-associated terminations fell by 53 per cent between 1982 and 1985.

The US rubella immunisation programme has been quite different from the UK programme so far. In the US, the aim is to *eliminate*

Figure 38   Trends in rubella infection and rubella-associated abortion in England and Wales (1977-1985) and in CRS in the UK (1970-1984)

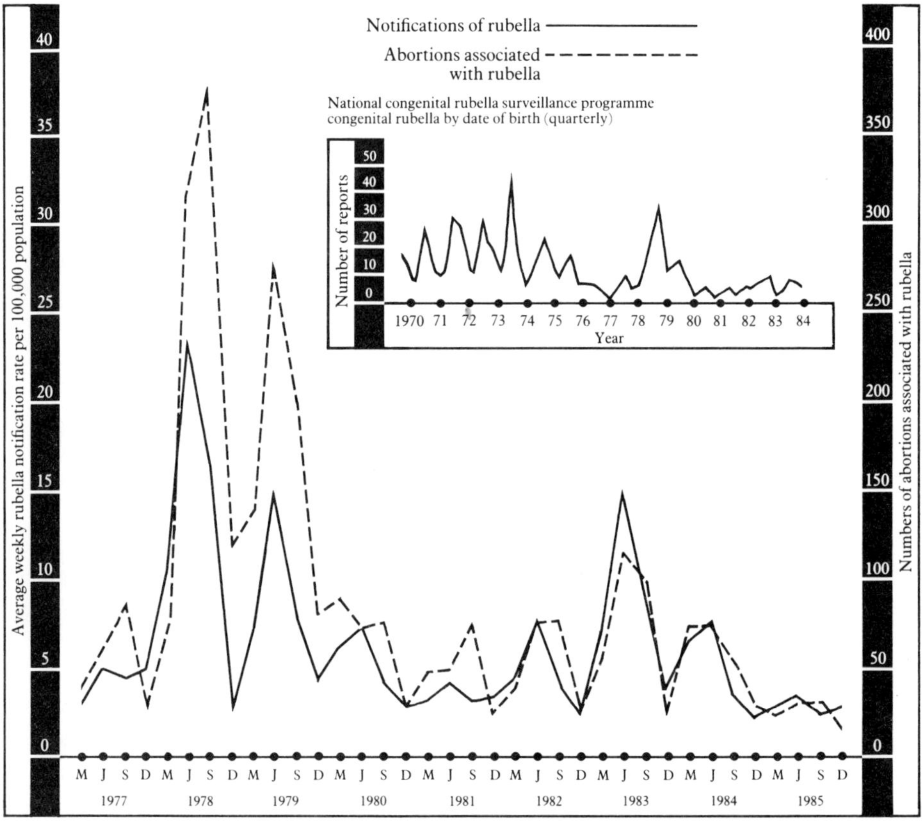

Source: OPCS: Rubella associated terminations of pregnancy. OPCS Monitor, AB 86/5. 9 September 1986.

176

rubella as well as CRS through compulsory immunisation of both boys and girls aged 12–15 months. All the evidence so far suggests that the US approach has had substantial success (see Figure 39), although the number of reported CRS cases may be underestimated by up to 90 per cent[60] and the absence of data on rubella-associated terminations makes it difficult to be certain. The programme is probably cheaper and certainly less complicated to implement than its British counterpart. It also has the advantage of being administered to children as a combined vaccine with measles and mumps. In the light of this and other evidence, the DHSS has announced that from the end of 1988 rubella vaccination policy will change: all children will be given rubella immunisation as part of a new triple vaccine for mumps, measles and rubella (MMR).

Pertussis (whooping cough) Pertussis, like measles, now rarely causes death or permanent damage to children in the UK. Nevertheless it is still a serious disease for infants under six months, 60 per cent of whom need to be

Figure 39 Trends in rubella and CRS in the USA (1966–1981)

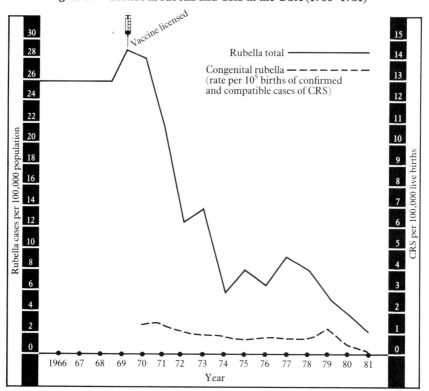

Source: Gruenberg E M (ed). Vaccinating against brain syndromes: the campaign against measles and rubella. Oxford, Oxford University Press, 1986.

admitted to hospital – often to intensive care. Following the introduction of an effective vaccine during the 1950s, immunisation uptake reached 80 per cent and the four-yearly pertussis epidemics were substantially reduced (see Figure 40). There was, however, a resurgence of the disease in the late-1970s. Immunisation uptake rates fell to a very low level of 31 per cent in 1978 following widespread publicity given to the possibility that the vaccine might cause brain damage. The powerful impact of the mass media on parents' decisions is illustrated by the fact that while pertussis immunisation levels fell, levels for diphtheria and tetanus – the other two components of the vaccine – remained steady. There was a new pertussis epidemic in 1977–1979 in which there were over 100,000 cases reported with a death toll of 27.

The National Childhood Encephalopathy Study was set up in 1976 to examine the alleged connection between pertussis vaccine and brain damage. It found that the risk of severe, acute neurological illnesses (those affecting the brain and nervous system) related to pertussis itself was *greater* than that attributable to the vaccine. Although no vaccine can be entirely risk-free, the risk of such illness attributable to whooping cough vaccine is very small: about one in 100,000 doses.[61]

Since then, recent public education campaigns, together with renewed efforts by health professionals to restore parents' confidence in the safety of pertussis immunisation, have begun to be effective. Uptake has more than doubled since 1978, reaching 65 per cent in England and Wales and 69 per cent in Scotland in 1984 (see Figure 36). This still falls short of the peak of 81 per cent reached in 1969 which substantially reduced past epidemics. The predicted 1985 epidemic was not averted, although it was smaller than the previous two (see Figure 40).

Improving immunisation uptake
Research into non-vaccinated children suggests that there are two barriers still to be overcome. First, nearly four in ten parents in one study were still worried that pertussis vaccine caused brain damage and, equally important, some doctors (especially GPs) still advised against vaccination, even when there were no relevant grounds for doing so.[62,63] The 82 per cent uptake rate attained in the Scottish Borders Health Board should serve as a yardstick of what can be achieved, despite these difficulties. Research into the development of a new vaccine may help allay fears in the future.

Tuberculosis
A better nourished population living in less crowded housing, together with effective treatment and active immunisation pro-grammes, have ensured the continued decline of TB. Although there were still nearly 7,000 reported cases (and nearly 500 deaths) in

Figure 40   Whooping cough in England and Wales: trends in reported cases (1967–1987)

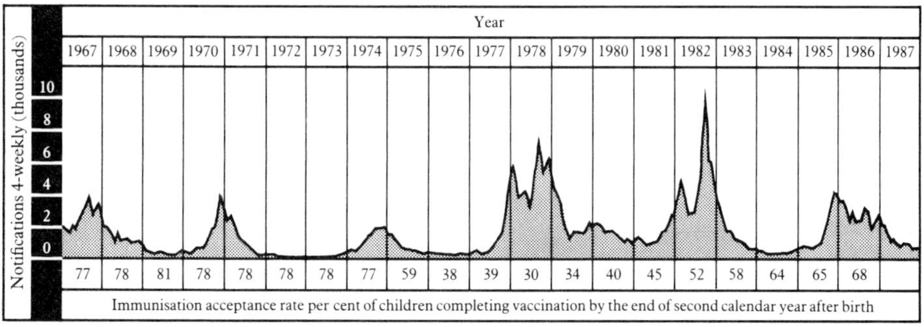

Source: Communicable Disease Surveillance Centre, 1988.

England and Wales in 1983, the cost-effectiveness of continued mass vaccination has been called into question.[64] It is current policy in nearly all health authorities to vaccinate schoolchildren between 11 and 13, together with all newborn babies in areas where TB incidence is high (case reports of TB are 14 times as common among people of Asian origin than of white origin). The DHSS's Joint Committee on Vaccination and Immunisation has estimated that between 1967 and 1981 eight million BCG vaccinations prevented only 500 cases of TB in white people. Predictions suggest that by the year 2001 mass vaccination will prevent only 45 cases. The MRC estimates that replacing mass vaccination with a selective approach will lead, in 1991, to only 40 cases per year requiring treatment that might otherwise have been prevented.[65]

Immunisation: implications for policy

Some countries have achieved more than the UK by adopting different immunisation policies, but others do better simply because their policy has been more effectively implemented. In the USA and eastern Europe, for example, immunisation is a compulsory requirement for school entry. These countries have been far more successful than the UK in approaching WHO targets. The Scandinavian countries have achieved better results than the UK[66] without using compulsion, but the centrally controlled services of the small Scandinavian countries may not be translatable to the UK. In the UK, a well-organised programme can achieve good results.[67] Evidence from the USA, Scandinavia and the UK suggests that some of the key features of a successful immunisation campaign include:

• mandatory immunisation of all children;
• a well-funded, coordinated effort between central government and responsible local authorities and professionals;
• sensitive publicity campaigns with local sources of advice (often

the community physician) aimed at both informing public and professionals;

- a single person at district or primary health care level (or both)[68] with overall responsibility for implementing the immunisation programme;
- an effective, but flexible, system – almost always computerised – for calling and following up different target populations,[69,70] and a reliable system for monitoring uptake within primary care;
- an additional intensive strategy for reaching highly mobile or socially deprived groups;[71]
- good liaison between community physicians, DHAs and primary health care staff and parents which has been shown to work well through immunisation advisory clinics,[72] or specially trained immunisation nurses;[73]
- audit of progress in primary care and a reliable system of feedback of information from DHAs to individual practices.

We believe that there is enough evidence to justify changing current immunisation policies and welcome the proposed introduction of measles, mumps and rubella (MMR) vaccination for under twos. Our belief is based on three premises.

- The UK may not be able to reach satisfactory immunisation targets for measles, pertussis and (especially) rubella without legislation.
- In those parts of the country which have achieved very high rubella vaccination rates (over 90 per cent) for both teenage girls and women after childbirth, CRS has not been eliminated.[74,75]
- The triple MMR vaccine has been shown to be effective in the USA (as a single dose in children aged 12–15 months) and Scandinavia where it is given in a two-dose schedule at 18 months and 12 years.[76,77] Analysis of 30 years' experience of using the mumps vaccine as part of the triple vaccine in the USA suggests that the benefit to cost ratio of mumps vaccination is high at 39:1.[78] In 1983 it was estimated that mumps vaccination reduced the number of cases from over two million to under 33,000.[79,80]

The future of immunisation Although immunisation policy has so far focussed on childhood, we also have effective vaccines against hepatitis B (a chronic and sometimes fatal liver disease) and pneumococcal pneumonia which can be fatal in elderly people. There is scope for improving the uptake of hepatitis B vaccine among at-risk hospital staff and extending it to homosexual men who are also a high risk group. Experience with the pneumococcal vaccine in the elderly is limited and requires further research. While we are still a long way from finding a vaccine that might be effective against AIDS (see Chapters

5 and 7) it is conceivable, although far from a reality, that a vaccine might be developed against a form of meningitis caused by an organism (meningococcus) that is resistant to many antibiotics, and finally, in the distant future, to cervical cancer.

Dental health The mouth is the gateway for what we eat, drink and smoke. It is not surprising, therefore, that it harbours two of the commonest, preventable diseases which reflect our modern lifestyle: tooth decay (caries) and chronic gum (periodontal) disease. Together they account for the extraction of eight million teeth every year, leaving a quarter of all British adults with no natural teeth. Most of the £800 million spent on dental health care each year is devoted to the treatment and alleviation of pain caused by these two diseases. Poor dental health starts early in childhood and, despite improvements in recent years, much remains to be achieved: in 1983 nearly half of our five year olds and 93 per cent of 15 year olds in England and Wales had evidence of tooth decay.

Promoting dental health A combination of a diet that is high in refined sugars (mainly sucrose) together with inadequate oral hygiene (irregular and

Table 24 **Fluoridation in the UK – its impact on dental decay in children**

(a) *Anglesey vs Arfon (Wales) (5/12 year olds)*

	Anglesey (fluoridated)	Arfon (non-fluoridated)
DMF score* (age 5)	1.58	3.55
Number of 'milk' teeth extracted per 100 children (age 5)	1	45
Number of permanent teeth extracted per 100 children (age 12)	13	74

(b) *Changes in the extent of decay among 5 years olds*

	Birmingham (Northfield) (fluoridated) DMF score*	Dudley (non-fluoridated) DMF score*
1967	4.88	5.19
1970	2.63	5.07
1980	1.22	3.45

*DMF score = Decayed missing or filled teeth.
Sources: Jackson D, James PMC and Thomas FD. Fluoride in Anglesey: a clinical study of dental caries. British Dental Journal 1985, 158, 2: 45–49.
Anderson RJ, Bradnock G et al. The reduction of dental caries prevalence in English school children. Journal of Dental Research 1982, 61 (special issue): 1311–1316.

181

incorrect toothbrushing) lead to the accumulation of dental plaque (a substance containing bacteria which coats the teeth and can lead to the destruction of enamel and gums) which causes tooth decay and gum disease.[81] Inadequate tooth brushing is the major determinant of chronic gum disease but is a poor predictor of tooth decay. High levels of dietary sugar are the main cause of tooth decay. These conclusions are supported in evidence summarised by numerous national and international expert committees.[82-86]

Fluoridation Fluoridation is one of the most effective ways of reducing tooth decay in the community. This conclusion is supported by the evidence considered by every major independent and government expert committee examining the role of fluoridation of the water supplies.[87-91] Moreover, in 1985 the Knox report [92] commissioned by the DHSS, together with the verdict of a court case concerning the safety of fluoridation, should have finally allayed any fears that fluoridation (at levels of one part per million) might pose a risk to health. Worldwide evidence, also confirmed in the UK, shows that fluoridation can reduce the prevalence of tooth decay in children by at least 50 per cent, and extractions by 15 per cent (see Table 24). Five year olds living in Anglesey (a fluoridated area) have 56 per cent fewer decayed, missing or filled teeth (DMF score) than their contemporaries living in non-fluoridated Arfon on the Welsh mainland (see Table 24(a)). Between 1974 and 1983 tooth decay fell 44 per cent among five year olds in Anglesey compared with only 22 per cent in Arfon.[93] Similar changes have occurred in Birmingham (Northfield) where the water was fluoridated in 1964.[94] The DMF score among five year olds was reduced by 75 per cent between 1967 and 1980 compared with only 34 per cent in Dudley, which is not fluoridated (see Table 24(b)). 1985 estimates of costs suggest that at 7p per person per year fluoridation in Birmingham is cheaper to implement than the £6 dental care costs incurred for the average five year old.[95] US experience also suggests that fluoridation leads, in the long term, not only to the preservation of healthy teeth, but to an increase in the number of children for whom an individual dentist can provide care.[96]

Even more importantly, experience from fluoridation in Newcastle shows that this measure reduces dental decay throughout all social classes and thus has the potential to help reduce the social class disparity in tooth decay.[97] Evidence from the trends so far, however, show that gains in dental health in both fluoridated as well as non-fluoridated areas are so far greatest among social classes I and II. This probably reflects the much higher sugar consumption among working class families (see page 186).

In 1985, about 5.5 million Britons – only 10 per cent of the

182

population – had fluoridated water supplies. Areas covered included the Midlands, north east England and parts of Wales. Implementation of fluoridation in the UK lags seriously behind other countries such as the USA, where 95 million people drink fluoridated water, and the Republic of Ireland where fluoridation is mandatory. Both public and professional support is substantial. Between 1974 and 1978, 90 per cent of the former area health authorities were in favour of fluoridation, together with 71 per cent of the public polled throughout the UK for the National Association of Health Authorities in 1985. Part of the delay was due to a legal technicality which was rectified in October 1985 through the Water (Fluoridation) Act. Health authorities everywhere (except Northern Ireland) are now free to ask water authorities to fluoridate local water supplies. Urban water supplies are, technically, the easiest to fluoridate. Smaller water supplies may prove to be more difficult and expensive.

Dental health and a healthier diet

Evidence from the USA – where fluoridation programmes are advanced – makes it clear that fluoridation alone will not eliminate tooth decay in the UK. For dietary sugar is the most important determinant of tooth decay. The average Briton consumes nearly twice the amount of sugar recommended by NACNE[98] and the BMA[99] to promote a reduction in tooth decay, as well as obesity and its associated ill health (see Chapters 3 and 7).

While the absolute amount of sugar in the diet is an indicator of the risk of tooth decay, the frequency of its consumption, and the way in which it is consumed, are more important predictors.[100,101] Those who eat sugary foods often, and especially between meals, are at greatest risk of tooth decay. This kind of eating pattern is predominant among pre-school[102] and secondary school children.[103] In a culture where the over-consumption of calories is a major problem, the current high intake of sugar represents unnecessary additional or 'empty' calories. These levels are not inevitable: the government's wartime nutrition policy led to much lower sugar consumption levels and a subsequent reduction in tooth decay of 30 per cent among five year olds and 43 per cent among 12 year olds.[104]

The consumption of sugar, like that of other products which can be hazardous to health, is determined by complex cultural, commercial, socioeconomic and individual factors. Little of the interplay between these factors has been adequately researched, but it is clear that the message to reduce sugar intake must make itself heard against a background of £400 million of confectionery advertising and a retail and entertainment sector where sweets and sugary foods are the most available snacks.

A study on feeding attitudes and practices among women and

their pre-school children has demonstrated that social and cultural factors are powerful determinants of what children eat and why, and that the offering and acceptance of sweet foods symbolises the power relationship between mother and child.[105]

The health consequences of current, high sugar consumption levels are much wider than dental health alone. The high prevalence of overweight, obesity and its attendant risks of diabetes and coronary heart disease (see Chapter 3) and low intakes of unrefined carbohydrates in the diet, are also related to high levels of sugar consumption.

Health education and oral health While a reduction in sugar consumption and the establishment of water fluoridation are central to the prevention of dental decay, they will not significantly affect chronic gum disease. This requires long-term education programmes to encourage regular toothbrushing in early childhood. There is good evidence from the UK and Scandinavia that health education programmes directed at both parents and children make an important contribution to dental health.[106] The Natural Nashers dental health education project for 13–14 year olds sponsored by the former HEC has demonstrated that it is possible not only to improve knowledge and attitudes towards oral hygiene but to reduce plaque scores.[107] The Natural Nashers programme (and the dental health component of SHEG's Be All You Can Be campaign) is now being successfully disseminated through cooperative efforts of district health authorities and local education authorities, and had reached 100 DHAs in England and Wales by 1985.[108]

The role of dentists and auxiliary staff While dentists have contributed towards the relief of pain and the preservation of teeth that are already decayed (especially among adults) there is no good evidence that visiting the dentist, even on a regular basis, has had any major impact on the prevalence of either tooth decay or gum disease.[109,110] As research has not been able to demonstrate any clear health benefits from six-monthly dental check-ups, there is good reason for extending the period between visits to 12 months.[111] The potential for turning the dental screening visit into a preventive rather than restorative event is currently limited by the under-use of dental auxiliaries and by existing methods of dental remuneration by fee for item of service. The effectiveness of the dental consultation in the promotion of dental health remains to be established. We know little, as yet, about attitudes among dentists and auxiliary staff to preventive work, although the nature of auxiliaries' work offers an obvious starting point. Recent experience with the use of fissure sealants among children suggests that when levels of overall decay are very low, a small proportion of decay

184

Figure 41   Tooth decay in the UK: 5–15 year olds (1983)

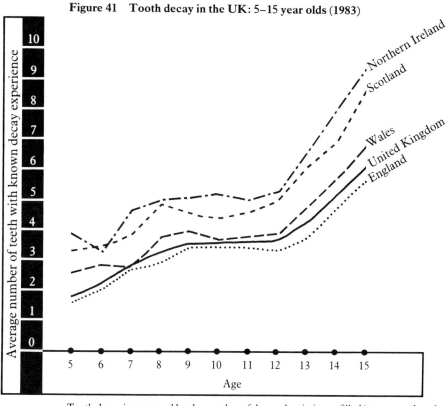

Tooth decay is measured by the number of decayed, missing or filled 'permanent' teeth (DMF ratio) plus the number of decayed or filled 'milk teeth' (df ratio).
Source: Todd J E, Dodd T. Children's dental health in the United Kingdom. OPCS. London, HMSO, 1985.

in remaining fissures may be prevented in a cost-effective way. This is currently the subject of a DHSS investigation.

Trends in dental health in the UK

Children, and to a lesser extent adolescents, enjoy better dental health today than at any time since the second world war. Although it is hard to find objective confirmation of changes in gum disease (which afflicts 99 per cent of adults), there is good evidence that tooth decay is decreasing among children. An OPCS survey of children's dental health in 1983 showed that, among 5–15 year olds, English children had the lowest levels of tooth decay in the UK, and Northern Ireland (followed by Scotland) the highest levels (see Figure 41).

Comparison with a survey in England and Wales a decade earlier showed that dental health had improved in all age groups. The improvement was most striking among five year olds where the proportion of children with decayed teeth fell by one-third (from 71 per cent to 48 per cent) over the decade (see Figure 42). Despite these encouraging trends, the prevalence of tooth decay is still unacceptably high in children as well as in adults and there is no evidence of a narrowing in the social class or geographical disparity in tooth decay.

Explaining trends in dental health

The reasons underlying the encouraging decline in tooth decay among children in the last decade are multifactorial and unlikely to be explained by either water fluoridation or dental care patterns, which have remained largely unchanged. The 18 per cent fall in per capita sugar consumption between 1970 and 1984 has almost certainly contributed to the decline (see Figure 43), although the higher levels of sugar consumption in social classes IV and V may in part explain the continuing social class disparity (see Chapter 8).

There are, however, two major changes over the last decade which go some way towards explaining the overall encouraging trends: the almost universal inclusion of fluoride in toothpaste[112] (use increased from five per cent in 1970 to 97 per cent in 1978), together with continuing efforts to improve oral hygiene through school health education. While clinical trials of fluoride toothpaste predict that tooth decay can be reduced by about a quarter over a short period,[113] the *actual* fall in tooth decay was much greater than the trials predicted. It has been argued that the effect of long-term fluoride toothpaste use, together with some retention and swallowing of the toothpaste, have probably boosted the effect of fluoride. In addition, fluoride toothpaste has a much bigger effect on newly erupted teeth in infancy and this may explain why the predictions underestimate the actual effects of fluoride toothpaste.

Improved health education is almost certain to be responsible for some of the improvement – especially in very young children. Nevertheless, the 1983 OPCS survey shows that the educational message is still misunderstood. Although three-quarters of parents knew that sugar causes dental decay, most said that *toothbrushing* rather than cutting down on sugar was the best way to reduce it.

186

Figure 42   Trends in tooth decay among children in England and Wales (1973–1983)

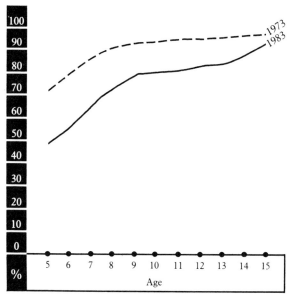

Tooth decay is measured by the number of decayed, missing or filled 'permanent' teeth (DMF ratio) plus the number of decayed or filled 'milk teeth' (df ratio).
Source: Todd J E, Dodd T. Children's dental health in the United Kingdom. OPCS. London, HMSO, 1985.

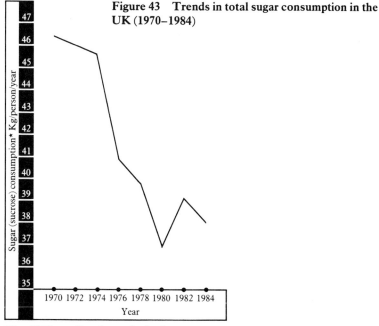

Figure 43   Trends in total sugar consumption in the UK (1970–1984)

*Total UK supplies of sugar for food use
Source: Ministry of Agriculture, Fisheries and Foods.

187

13 Health in adolescence

Children of the future Age,
Reading this indignant page;
Know that in former time,
Love! sweet love! was thought a crime.
                                        WILLIAM BLAKE

Introduction Adolescence is a time of uncertainty, experiment and change. We have chosen to focus on the health implications of two contrasting issues – sexuality and illicit drug use – not because they affect this age group alone, but because they illustrate the relationship between the inexperience of adolescence and some of its consequences for health. We have already assessed the public health implications of cigarette smoking and alcohol consumption – both of which usually start in adolescence or earlier (see Chapters 3, 4 and 7) – and have assessed ways of minimising ill health and premature death from two specific sexually transmitted diseases: cervical cancer and AIDS (see Chapters 4, 5 and 7). We now broaden our discussion of sexuality in three ways. We assess sexual health from the viewpoint of personal relationships, control of fertility, and sexually transmitted disease in general. We then consider trends in illicit drug misuse and their possible explanations. We conclude the chapter with an assessment of action to curb the use and minimise the harm caused by illicit drugs.

Sexuality: satisfaction and safety The sexual expression of love and tenderness is of profound importance in all our lives. It would thus be disingenuous to claim that our assessment of sexuality and its health consequences could be value-free. WHO has furthered our thinking by identifying three elements that should inform any discussion of sexuality and health:

- the capacity to enjoy and express sexuality, without guilt or shame, in fulfilling emotional relationships;
- the capacity to control fertility;
- freedom from disorders which compromise health, and sexual or reproductive function.

In our consideration of the prevention of cervical cancer and the spread of AIDS (see Chapter 7), we stressed the need to integrate policies for the prevention of sexually transmitted disease on the one hand, with those aimed at promoting freedom of sexual expression and control of fertility on the other. This is not merely because contradictory policies do not work, but because a properly coordinated common strategy is likely to be more cost-effective.

Sexuality and health

We can say little with certainty about how we, as a society, express ourselves sexually and the extent to which it brings us happiness. We know a little, but not much more, about how early in life we become sexually active and how many sexual partners we have. We are left to draw conclusions from scant research on selected groups of people. We have very little information on men, but a large, although unrepresentative, survey of 15,000 women readers of Woman magazine in 1982 concluded that over nine out of ten women saw sex as an important part of their relationships and three-quarters were either very happy or reasonably satisfied with their sexual relationships.[1] Despite this, a majority felt they could not talk freely with their partners; few saw themselves as good lovers; and less than half usually reached orgasm.

Some small scale qualitative research on teenage boys suggests that they still seem unwilling to share in the responsibility for their sexual activities,[2] but larger studies of older men in the US show that they have similar hopes and aspirations to those of women. Although boys and girls first become sexually active at earlier ages, most teenage girls still believe that partners should stay faithful to one another. We have no information on boys' views.

Fertility control

The reduction in perinatal and maternal mortality which resulted from better birth spacing was evident earlier this century.[3] But today's fertility rates are already very low; childbirth is a much less risky experience for both mother and child and there is a range of freely available, as well as relatively safe and effective, forms of contraception. Contraception can thus be seen for the potential it has to promote a better quality of life, and not only through the avoidance of ill health caused by too many unplanned pregnancies.[4–7]

Trends in fertility

Fertility rates in England and Wales have declined dramatically among women in all age groups – except among those in their 30s where there has been a steady increase since 1977. The total period fertility rate decreased from 2.5 children per woman in the later 1960s to 1.7 in the early 1970s.[8] The teenage birth rate, which comprises about eight per cent of the total period fertility rate, has followed a similar pattern over time: a decline of about 40 per cent occurred during the 1970s, with a levelling off at about 30 births per 1000 women aged 15–19 since 1977.

After the 1967 Abortion Act, the numbers of legally induced abortions performed on women resident in Great Britain rose rapidly and initially stabilised at between 110,000 and 120,000 a year. These rates – which are lower than those in much of northern Europe and north America – remained relatively stable until the 1970s, when contraception became much more widely available. They later rose again to about 150,000 in 1985. Moreover, the overall teenage conception rate (births plus terminations) decreased by almost 14 per cent between 1974 and 1984 (see Figure 44). Teenagers and young women are becoming pregnant less often, but when they do become pregnant they are more likely to have an abortion than older women (see Figure 44).

Figure 44   Trends in conception rates in England and Wales (1974–1984)

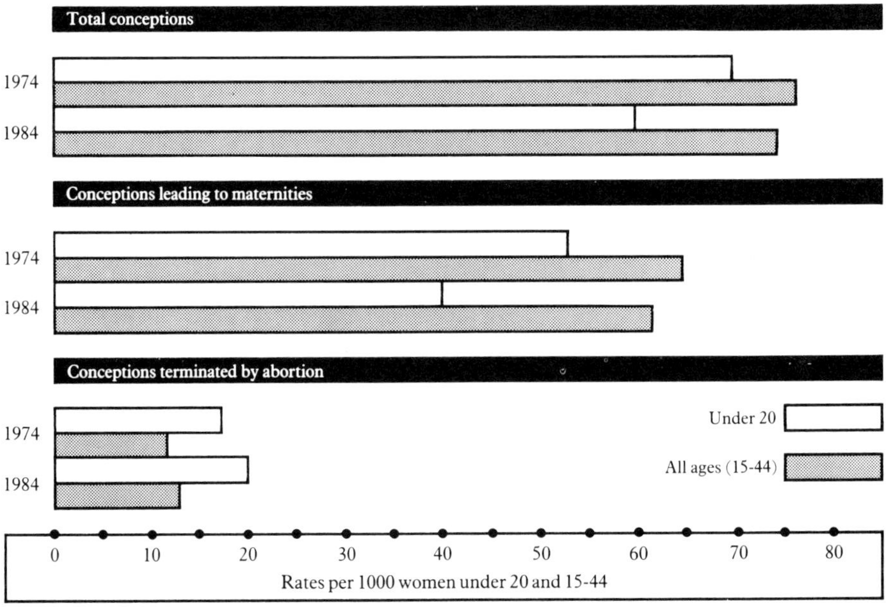

Under 20 includes women aged 15–19. All ages includes women aged 15–44.
Source: OPCS.

Young people and their fertility   Today's teenagers and young people are exercising more choice and control over their fertility than a decade ago. Teenage girls are less likely to become pregnant or to become mothers than they were ten years ago, and those that do are much more likely to do so from choice. This picture emerges from research commissioned by the Birth Control Trust in England and Wales as well as Scotland.[9] These trends have occurred *in spite* of other evidence from a national survey among Scottish teenagers[10] which showed that in 1986 teenagers were more likely to be sexually experienced, and to have become sexually active, than a decade ago.

Abortion among young women – a continuing challenge   There remains cause for concern since there has been a proportionately greater increase in abortion rates among teenagers and young women than for women in any other age group (see Figure 44). Between 1974 and 1984 abortion rates increased by one-fifth among

190

the under 20s compared with only 11 per cent among women as a whole (aged 15–44) in England and Wales. Moreover, women in the youngest age groups also experience the greatest delay in obtaining abortions. A study of abortions among women in Wessex in 1975 showed that less than half of those aged 17–18 obtained their abortions before the 12th week of pregnancy, compared with 70 per cent of women in other age groups.[11] The most recent review of late abortions in 1984 shows that this position has not changed.[12]

Sexually transmitted disease

Trends in sexually transmitted disease are often hard to interpret because we have to rely on selective national information from attendances at sexually transmitted disease clinics and genito-urinary medicine departments. Numerous factors, such as changing social perceptions, improved professional recognition and diagnosis, can artificially boost the numbers coming forward to such clinics.[13] Incomplete information has led to numerous claims concerning the existence of 'epidemics' of individual, sexually transmitted diseases such as herpes and non-specific urethritis. While the available

Table 25 Trends in the six most common sexually transmitted diseases in Great Britain

	Change in reported new cases 1978–83 (%)	STD clinics: increase in new attendances 1973–83 (%)	Assessment of trends
Non-specific genital infection	+38	+27	Exaggerated increase due to better detection
Candidiasis (thrush)	+47	+13	Often not sexually transmitted
Gonorrhoea	−14	Decrease	Real decrease, possibly due, in part, to fear of AIDS
Genital warts	+57	+11	Real increase; some due to growth of professional interest
Trichomoniasis	−10	Decrease	No change
Genital herpes	+98	+6	Most due to increased publicity, awareness and new treatment

Source: Adapted from Communicable Disease Surveillance Centre. Sexually transmitted disease surveillance in Britain. British Medical Journal 1985, 291: 528–530.

evidence confirms that there is a true epidemic of AIDS (see Chapter 5) and probably of genital warts (see Chapter 4) we urgently need to monitor representative samples of the *whole* community in order to be able to predict more accurately the future impact of some of these growing problems.

Analysis of the trends by the Communicable Disease Surveillance Centre (CDSC) shows that the big increases in both the numbers of reported new cases and new attendances for herpes and non-specific genital infections are exaggerated by other factors, and that the only real increases in incidence that have taken place are for genital warts and AIDS (see Table 25).

Sexuality: explaining the changing picture

The last two decades have seen a number of unprecedented social changes which have had a profound bearing on attitudes towards sexuality and the expression of sexuality. The growth of the women's rights and gay rights movements have prompted a more open assessment of the role of sex in human relationships. This, together with a liberalisation of attitudes to the sexual expression of love, the development of oral contraception and earlier physical maturity, has been influential in promoting greater confidence in the way sexuality – especially among women – is expressed. Growing fears about AIDS, however, have led to a reassessment of sexual attitudes and demonstrable changes in sexual behaviour in the homosexual community (see Chapter 7). The risk of AIDS, together with renewed calls for sexual fidelity, may have equally profound effects on attitudes to sex and sexuality in years to come.

The enabling family planning legislation of 1974, the provision of free contraception since 1975, and the 1967 Abortion Act (which applies everywhere in the UK except Northern Ireland) have had a central role, not only in the reduction of unwanted pregnancies and perinatal mortality (see Chapters 2 and 11), but also in helping to remove some of the fear and misery previously associated with the unwanted consequences of sexual activity. Although there are no national data, the bigger reductions in fertility among working class than middle class women suggest that public health legislation, combined with education and information programmes, can reach all classes. Sex education in schools has had a major contributory role, although its effect cannot be separated from that of the numerous other measures which have also been important. Fears that sex education leads to unacceptable early sexual experimentation are not supported by the evidence which suggests that there is little difference in the age of starting to have sexual intercourse among children who have had sex education compared with those who have not.

The patchy provision of abortion services, the lack of accurate, easily available pregnancy testing services, together with poorly developed family planning services for young people may, in part, explain why young women delay seeking an earlier abortion. But we need to know more about why such women avoid consulting a doctor earlier so that more appropriate services can be developed. The chances of a woman obtaining an early abortion still depend mainly on the beliefs of the doctors she consults. This partly explains why there are still more abortions performed outside than inside the NHS, although poorly organised services in the NHS – a lack of day care facilities and inadequately trained staff – often make an abortion in the charitable part of the private sector a quicker, more humane experience.

Table 26 Pregnancy rates among 15–19 year olds: an international comparison

	Pregnancy rate per 10,000
USA	96
England and Wales	45
Canada	44
France	43
Sweden	35
Netherlands	14

Source: Alan Guttmacher Institute. Report to the Ford Foundation on the findings and policy implications of a comparative study of teenage pregnancy and fertility in developed countries. New York, Alan Guttmacher Institute, 1985.

Towards healthier sexuality – how can progress be made?

Experience of the last two decades, together with detailed international research on the factors which influence fertility control, now offer more information on the components of an effective strategy for reducing unwanted pregnancies – especially among young people. The Lane committee,[14] which reviewed the workings of the 1967 Abortion Act in 1974, concluded that an efficiently functioning Abortion Act can form only a part of the strategy. Improved education about aspects of human sexuality, together with acceptable contraception, abortion and counselling services in the NHS, were also of central importance. The findings of a 37 country study by the US Alan Guttmacher Institute in 1985 show that high teenage pregnancy rates were not the inevitable accompaniment of liberal attitudes to sex and sexuality.[15]

Statistical analysis of six countries in the Guttmacher report showed that while England and Wales had teenage pregnancy rates that were half those in the USA, rates in Sweden and the Netherlands were much lower still (see Table 26). Analysis of all 37 countries identified the following factors to be significantly associated with high teenage pregnancy rates:

- low levels of socioeconomic development;
- implicit or explicit pronatalist policies;
- early marriage;
- generous maternity benefits and leave.

Other associated factors were:

- a lack of community openness about sexuality;
- inequitable income distribution;
- high levels of church attendance;
- restrictions on teenage access to contraceptive and education services.

The importance of education, together with the provision of accessible services, has been confirmed in other research which shows that long-term educational commitment among women is a key predictor of reliable contraceptive use.[16] The low teenage pregnancy rates in Sweden and the Netherlands were *not* associated with increased abortion rates or decreased rates of sexual activity. In Sweden this success has been associated with government-supported, local and national education programmes[17,18] and in the Netherlands with widespread, open discussion of sexuality together with high quality primary care services which are accessible to young people. The very high rates in the USA seemed to be associated with media which conveyed sex in an irresponsible fashion at the same time as the prevailing moral climate advocated abstinence. This hampered proper dissemination of information about sexuality and contraceptives.

Trends in contraceptive use There has been a steady increase in contraceptive use since 1970. By 1983, three-quarters of people aged 18–44 in Britain used some form of contraception. Use was highest among married or cohabiting couples (83 per cent) and lowest among single people (50 per cent); just over half of those in their late teens used contraception. When people who were sterile or trying to have a child were excluded, the proportion of sexually active people not using contraception fell to less than 10 per cent.[19] This contrasts favourably with the 45 per cent of Americans aged 15–44 who use no contraception.[20]

Although the pill is still the most popular form of contraception – and still increasing in popularity among young, single women – there has been a steady fall in its use over the last decade (see Figure 45). Worry about the increased risk of heart disease and stroke among older women, and among those who smoke and take the pill,[21] together with new evidence of a possible link between the pill and breast cancer (see Chapter 4) has been associated with this decline.

The most striking change in patterns of contraception has been the increase in the use of vasectomy and sterilisation, now the commonest forms of fertility control among older, married or cohabiting couples who have completed their families (see Figure 45). The previous resistance of men to vasectomy has largely disappeared. In 1983 there were equal numbers of men and women who had been sterilised.

By contrast, the use of barrier methods of contraception has continued to decline, with fewer than one in four couples using the sheath or diaphragm/cap in 1983. While the sheath was the most popular form of contraception until the 1960s, it was rapidly replaced by the pill. This has important health implications as those most at risk of sexually transmitted disease – including AIDS and cervical cancer – are in the youngest age groups where the use of non-barrier methods is actually *increasing*. These trends, together with the latest evidence that the active component of contraceptive jelly used with the diaphragm/cap may be able to neutralise the AIDS (and possibly other) virus (see Chapter 7), have implications for future family planning policy.

Family planning services Family planning has been demonstrated to be highly cost-effective: every £100 spent by the NHS on it can result in a £500 saving by preventing unwanted pregnancies.[22] Two surveys of DHA family

Figure 45   Trends in contraceptive use among women in Great Britain who have been or are married (1973-1983)

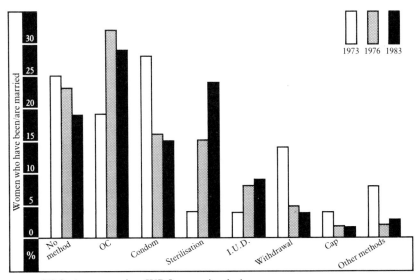

OC Oral contraceptive. IUD Intrauterine device.
Source: Wellings K. Trends in contraceptive method usage since 1970. British Journal of Family Planning 1986, 12: 15–22.

planning services in England and Wales in 1982 and 1984 showed that, despite financial stringencies, the services were well maintained throughout both countries and that doctors and nurses were receiving adequate in-service training – increasingly organised by individual DHAs.[23]

Current gaps in the provision of specialist services include a lack of female sterilisation and vasectomy services, with less than half providing special sessions for young people (see Table 27). This is an important omission as there is good evidence that young people are more likely to use such specialist services.[24,25] The DHSS provision of funds to set up three special schemes for young people are therefore welcome. We need to know more about the quality of the family planning service offered by general practice, used (but not preferred) by 60 per cent of people.

Sexuality and family planning: information and education

Despite its proven value, and the obvious support it receives from 96 per cent of parents and 95 per cent of teenage children, there have been numerous barriers to the effective dissemination of information and education about sexuality and family planning. The government's ambivalent stance was evidenced in its refusal to allow the former HEC to publish a leaflet on sexuality and contraception while recognising the need to promote the use of condoms and 'safe sex' in its campaign on AIDS (see Chapter 7). Condom advertising is not permitted in cinemas and the IBA did not permit television advertisements to promote condoms as a protection against sexually transmitted disease until August 1987. Some recent efforts by the Family Planning Information Service (FPIS) set up by the FPA and former HEC have met with opposition from the IBA which has insisted on amendments to a TV advertisement designed to promote more responsibility among men – on the unsubstantiated grounds that it would offend viewers.

The FPIS, established in 1977, has become the major source of information on family planning. Its aim to reach the widest possible audience is being realised through innovative schemes such as the Health Care in the High Street scheme which makes family planning leaflets available in 12,000 chemists. Its latest project, Men Too, focusses on the hitherto neglected role of men in family planning and sexual relationships. It has potential for expansion to deal with new challenges presented by sexually transmitted disease and AIDS.

The role of the media in shaping attitudes to sexuality is an important, under-researched field. British television documentaries have made a major contribution, while the most irresponsible programmes currently shown are imported from the USA.

The transfer of responsibility for sex education from local authorities to school governors in the 1986 Education Act was

Table 27 National summary of DHA family planning services, January 1983–January 1984, England and Wales

	DHAs providing service (%)	DHAs not providing service (%)	Services expanded (%)	Services maintained (%)	Service reduced (%)	NA*	HP**
Clinics	100	0	14	81	4	1	
Doctor sessions	100	0	12	82	5	1	
Post-coital service	83	17	31	50		19	
Vasectomy	35	65	5	29	1	38	27
Female sterilisation	12	88	1	13	1	50	35
Sub-fertility	28	72		31	1	57	11
Psycho-sexual sessions	77	23	14	59	3	23	1
Special sessions for young people	44	56	7	41	1	51	
Domiciliary family planning	63	37	13	50	3	34	

* no answer ** hospital provision
The percentages are based on the completed returns from 145 district health authorities out of a total of 162 DHAs approached.
Source: Family Planning Association. Report on district health authority family planning services in England and Wales. London, FPA, 1985.

primarily in response to a minority of MPs who wanted to give parents the right to remove their children from sex education lessons. However, much progress has been made in schools. Studies in the mid-1970s[26] suggested that sex education was sporadic, taught as an isolated, single topic, and restricted mainly to the 'mechanics' of animal and human reproduction. A similar survey of schools in three cities in 1986[27] showed that there have been the following major changes.

- Eighty-nine per cent of teenagers and 78 per cent of parents said that they had had some primary school education about sex and personal relationships.

- The range of topics covered at secondary school was much wider, including personal relationships, contraception and sexually transmitted disease; nearly 30 per cent had covered homo-sexuality.
- The teaching was firmly integrated into the curriculum rather than being treated as an isolated topic.

The survey also showed that there was little parental involvement in primary or secondary sex education. Nearly half the teenagers said they had not discussed sex with their mother, and nearly three-quarters had not talked to their father about it.

Future investigations Although a consideration of sub-fertility is beyond the scope of this report, it affects an estimated one in ten couples, is likely to grow in relative importance if fertility levels remain low, and if the trend among women to postpone pregnancy until their 30s continues. Little is yet known about the birth control or counselling needs of differing ethnic groups,[28] still less about sexuality in old age. These should become areas of future attention. The move from a narrow, family planning base towards a broader interest in psychosexual problems (see Table 27) in clinics may play an increasingly important role in these and other issues.

Illicit drug use The challenges presented by illicit drug use are complex and rapidly changing. Although the threat posed to the public health by legal drugs such as tobacco and alcohol is currently much greater, the evidence suggests that the use of potentially hazardous illicit drugs is growing rapidly. Furthermore, evidence is accumulating to suggest that the intravenous use of illicit drugs is likely to be the most important influence on the future size of the AIDS epidemic in the UK.[29]

Most recent surveys suggest that experimentation with illicit drugs by teenagers is still rare, that most use is occasional and does not lead to dependence.[30] Table 28 shows that the drug most commonly used is cannabis. Nevertheless, we cannot afford to be complacent since the most reliable estimates suggest that there were at least 50,000 people in the UK who were dependent on opiates (heroin and morphine-like drugs) in 1983. It is clear that use is not concentrated in London alone, for use of the whole range of illicit drugs may be just as extensive in Scotland.[31] We do not yet know how to assess the extent of damage associated with illicit drug use. The small numbers of UK deaths associated with opiate (82 in 1983) and solvent misuse (77 in 1983) tells us little about the social and psychological damage associated with their use, even though the vast majority of experimentation with illicit drugs does not result in long-term harm to the user or to society.

While we have some information on the extent of experimentation with illicit drugs among young people, much less is known about modes of drug use and the relationship between occasional use and persistent, often intravenous, use. The stereotype of the intravenous heroin user of the 1960s is probably no longer appropriate as most of today's illicit drug takers use more than one drug. Evidence from a study of heroin use in northern England suggests that heroin smoking has become a stable pattern in certain localities.[32] While heroin smoking is less hazardous than its intravenous use, we know little about the relationship between smoking and intravenous use, and whether smoking heroin is a transient practice.

Table 28 Recent estimates of the prevalence of illicit drug use among young people

STUDY	YEAR	AGE	PREVALENCE (per cent)		
			Cannabis	Solvents	Heroin
Schools in England and Wales	1986	Secondary School	17	6	2
NOP opinion poll	1982	15–21	13–28	2–4	1
Lothian school leavers	1983	19–20	22–35	1.6–2.3	0.6–0.7

Source: Plant MA. Drugs in perspective. London, Hodder and Stoughton, 1987.

Illicit drug use: recent trends

Trends in official data on convictions and seizures of illicit drugs and on hospital admissions for treatment of drug-related problems are difficult to interpret because they reflect changes in policies to control drug misuse as well as possible changes in actual use. Nevertheless, it is clear that there has been a rapid growth in drug use since the late 1970s, especially opiates, amphetamines and cocaine. The number of new narcotics addicts notified to the Home Office in the UK between 1975 and 1984 increased nearly six-fold. The number found guilty or cautioned for drug offences increased two-fold overall, with more than a six-fold increase in the number of offences associated with heroin. The number of police seizures for heroin and cocaine increased by more than 13-fold and five-fold respectively.

A more comprehensive assessment of the official statistics on opiate use in an inner London borough, together with information from surveys and from fieldwork by statutory and voluntary agencies in contact with drug users, confirms a real increase in opiate misuse (primarily heroin) in inner London between 1977 and 1983.[33]

Extrapolation from these figures in the whole of the UK suggests that Home Office figures represent a five to ten-fold underestimate of the actual prevalence, which may have risen by ten-fold between 1970 and 1983.[34]

The increase in experimentation and use of illegal drugs is also confirmed by the findings of community studies, although these are not fully comparable and may reflect patterns of drug use in a particular region. All the studies before the mid-1970s showed that only a small minority had ever used illegal drugs, that cannabis was the drug most commonly used (with amphetamine in the 1960s) and that use of heroin and cocaine was rare. Solvent misuse (including glues and other volatile solvents) was first documented in the mid-1960s. Although there are no reliable national data, individual studies now suggest that as many as 20–25 per cent of 13–15 year old boys in Glasgow have engaged in solvent misuse.[35] In the last decade the best data come from a prospective study which followed up Scottish 15–16 year olds in the Lothian region. In 1979, 15 per cent of the boys and 11 per cent of the girls reported using drugs 'for kicks'. At the age of 19–20 (in 1983) these figures had increased to 37 per cent for males and 23 per cent for females. Cannabis was still the drug most commonly used; the proportion having tried heroin, although higher than in the 1960s, was still small at less than one per cent.[36] A similar picture has emerged in other recent prevalence studies of teenagers and young people[37] and is supported by indirect evidence showing that the proportion of fourth year students in Wolverhampton schools who knew someone taking illegal drugs increased from 15 per cent in 1969 to 28 per cent in 1984.[38]

The relationship between the use of legal drugs (such as tobacco and alcohol) and illegal drugs merits further research. It has been argued that while increases in the price of tobacco and alcohol are associated with a fall in their consumption, this may result in a shift to greater use of illicit drugs such as heroin, whose street price is low,[39] and that this might most affect those who have least money to spend. The picture is probably more complex: while studies of teenagers confirm that the use of illicit drugs has risen faster than that of alcohol or tobacco, the recent downward trend in cigarette consumption among adults has not occurred among teenagers (see Chapter 4).

Explaining patterns of drug misuse

The misuse of illegal drugs is determined by a complex of individual, social and international factors. The use of illicit drugs is not confined to any particular lifestyle or socioeconomic group, although historical analysis suggests that those who are most at risk of misuse are a young, but changing group.

There are clearly a number of identifiable broad influences that

200

help to explain the sharp rise in opiate misuse since the mid-1970s. At that time, political changes in Iran led to the influx of large quantities of cheap, pure heroin which were smuggled into the UK and other parts of western Europe. Between 1978 and 1983 the 'street price' of heroin is estimated to have halved relative to inflation.[40] This extended the geographical and financial availability of heroin beyond those who could afford it in the 1960s.

There is a growing body of evidence which has linked the misuse of heroin with social deprivation[41,42] and with unemployment in particular.[43,44] This has been a persistent finding in recent surveys of drug use, and of some indicators of related harm. In the USA the rise and more recent fall in illicit drug misuse has been closely associated with similar changes in levels of unemployment. However, evidence from northern England suggest that unemployment only predicts high levels of misuse when associated with easy local availability.[45]

Drug misuse: minimising the harm

It is probably not feasible to eliminate all illicit drug use because there will always be a black market associated with drugs whose use is prohibited. Although the legalisation of drugs such as heroin might end the black market[46] we know of no evidence to suggest that misuse and related harm would be reduced. It is possible, however, to define three more realistic goals:

- to reduce experimentation with potentially hazardous illicit drugs;
- to help those who are dependent on such drugs to stop or reduce the harm associated with use;
- to minimise the harm associated with continued drug use.

We believe that these goals are likely to be achieved by a combination of measures designed to reduce the supply and demand for illicit drugs and discourage the more hazardous forms of drug use, together with supportive socioeconomic measures aimed at reducing the deprivation associated with a high risk of misuse (see Chapter 8). This is supported by the conclusions of the government's report on the prevention of drug misuse from the Advisory Council on the Misuse of Drugs (ACMD).[47]

Reducing the supply of drugs

Attempts have been made to control the supply of drugs at international level by crop substitution and control of trafficking, and at the national level by better policing and enforcement of the drugs laws together with tight controls on the prescription of narcotic drugs. In practice, the impact of such measures is likely to be different for those who experiment with drugs and those who are regular users. While it is true that the more a drug is available the more people are likely to experiment, small increases or decreases in supply are likely to have very little effect. By contrast, a small decrease in supply in an already tight market can lead to a dramatic shift among existing users from one illicit substance to another,[48] as has been shown to be the case in the USA.[49] Furthermore, efforts to reduce illegal trafficking and promote better enforcement, however enthusiastically supported, will never be complete. It has been estimated that no more than 10 per cent of the total amount of heroin available on the black market is confiscated,[50] and efforts have not yet succeeded in forcing up the street price of heroin.

Opiate and amphetamine prescribing patterns were a major source of illicit supply of these drugs before powers under the 1971 Misuse of Drugs Act restricted their prescription. While such restrictions have dramatically reduced the contribution of medical prescriptions to the black market, methadone prescribed by registered medical practitioners still finds its way there.

Reducing the demand for drugs The two approaches aimed at influencing demand involve education to reduce experimentation and treatment and support for those who wish to stop using drugs. Educational initiatives can be considered at several levels, ranging from mass media approaches to long-term drug education programmes aimed at young people, parents and professionals.

Extensive evaluation of drug education programmes has shown that education alone cannot be expected to change behaviour. Evaluation of drug education programmes for young people has been extensive – especially in the USA. The findings from such research have been remarkably consistent and have been summarised in the ACMD report.[51] Its main conclusions are given below.

- Knowledge about drugs can be increased[52] but changes in attitude are harder to achieve.[53] Indeed, there is some worrying evidence that the more young people are informed about illicit drugs, the safer they feel about using them.[54,55] Overall, drug education programmes have been ineffective in changing behaviour,[56,57] and sometimes even counterproductive.[58-60]
- Mass media campaigns that focus on single drugs and use shock tactics designed to influence young people are, at best, inappropriate and can actually lead to experimentation with drugs.[61-63] Isolated examples of careful use of the mass media to publicise campaigns directed at irresponsible prescribing by doctors (for example, the CURB campaign to reduce barbiturate prescription, (see Chapter 10) have been more successful in influencing their target audiences.
- The most useful drug education campaigns for young people are now thought to be those which put legal and illegal drugs into a

realistic social and cultural context, and attempt to encourage young people to develop sufficient knowledge and self-confidence to make appropriate decisions concerning their use.[64,65]

We have little reliable information on the effectiveness of treatment and rehabilitation in both reducing demand and minimising the more harmful consequences of drug misuse. Progress has been hampered by incomplete agreement on what the goals for treatment should be, and whether long-term abstinence is seen as the ultimate aim. This, together with ill-informed views on the nature of opiate dependence and withdrawal, has led to unnecessarily negative conclusions about the value of treatment and rehabilitation. Some US research suggests that the image of heroin use as the most intractable addiction is too pessimistic[66] and that more long-term follow-up studies of drug users are needed. An important study in the UK showed that as many as 35 per cent of opiate users attending a drug dependency unit were still abstaining after ten years.[67]

Most research has been conducted on a select minority of drug users who attend inpatient, hospital-based drug dependency units over a short period. Yet the available evidence suggests that inpatient treatment is not superior and is more costly than outpatient treatment.[68] Moreover, the findings from one Scottish practice show that users dependent on opiates are more likely to consult the GP than the hospital.[69] These findings may reflect the local situation and more research is urgently needed on how best to support dependent drug users in the community. The potential for developing such support in primary care is substantial and could operate alongside the well-established drug support network run by voluntary agencies. A survey of GPs in England and Wales in 1986 showed that one in five had seen patients with problems related to illicit drugs in the previous month.[70] Over half the patients were under 25 and two-thirds wanted help with withdrawal. The same survey showed that a majority of GPs believed that those dependent on opiates were difficult to treat and nearly half were either unprepared or unwilling to take responsibility for treatment.[71]

Reducing the harm among continuing drug users

The possibility of reducing drug-related harm without necessarily reducing drug use itself has recently gained considerable currency. While there is a danger that such an approach may seem to condone potentially hazardous use of illicit drugs, the need to minimise the spread of AIDS through intravenous drug misuse and the sharing of infected 'works' (see Chapter 5) has become urgent. The government has piloted 15 needle exchange schemes where intravenous drug users are given clean syringes in exchange for used ones in order to stop needle-sharing. The outcome of such a policy in terms of reducing the risk of spread of AIDS, hepatitis B and other infections is not yet known. We do not yet know enough about occasional or recreational drug use and its relationship to persistent misuse to recommend measures to prevent this transition. Any attempts to influence this transition will need to proceed with caution, but more research may throw light on this ill-understood aspect of drug misuse.

Drug misuse: progress in the UK

Despite a continuing lack of knowledge, the ACMD[72] and the more recent Social Services Committee report[73] concluded that the dramatic growth of drug misuse warranted a practical response. The ACMD recommended a comprehensive strategy which included controls on the drug supply through strengthening licensing and prescription controls; a balanced drug education programme which focussed on the integration of drug education in other aspects of the curriculum and avoided sensational mass media campaigns; improved professional training; and the development of community-based local initiatives by RHAs and DHAs. It envisaged that such a strategy would be coordinated by an interministerial committee, with a new national body to help monitor the activities of local drug advisory committees.

The national campaign against the misuse of illicit drugs was subsequently launched by the government in 1985. Despite claims to the contrary, it is still too early to tell whether it has had an impact. The government has not so far completely followed the advice of the ACMD. It has established an interministerial committee on drugs chaired by the Home Secretary which has outlined its general strategy but avoided setting any long-term objectives, emphasising the essentially unachievable aim of eliminating all illicit drug misuse. The committee has attempted to control illicit drug supplies by contributing to international projects on crop eradication and substitution and has strengthened police and customs enforcement activities. It has also expanded the provisions of the Misuse of Drugs Act to bring dipipanone, diethylproprion, barbiturates and benzodiazepines under stricter control. It also introduced legislation in 1986 which enables the assets earned by convicted traffickers to be confiscated.

National efforts to reduce demand through education and the provision of treatment and support services have been less satisfactory. Despite a substantial body of evidence pointing to the counterproductive effects of sensational mass media campaigns focussing on single drugs, a £2 million series of TV commercials (followed by a further £2 million series) under the banner Heroin Screws You Up was launched in England and Wales in 1985, directed mainly at teenagers and their parents. Despite government claims that the campaign was responsible for increasing awareness and negative attitudes to illicit drugs, its evaluation was in-adequate[74,75] and increases in awareness were equally likely to have resulted from a series of major, independent initiatives on television (such as the BBC's Drugwatch) and in other media. The equivalent campaign run in Scotland by SHEG was more in line with ACMD recommendations and included a low key approach: Choose Life not Drugs. The latest £5 million campaign is aimed at reducing the risk of HIV infection. More long term initiatives for both teachers and pupils have been prepared by SHEG and the former HEC working with TACADE and the Institute for the Study of Drug Dependence.

The planning and development of longer term, local treatment and rehabilitation services has been poor. Recommendations from both the ACMD and the Social Services Committee reports to provide continuing central funding to support the development of a diverse range of NHS and community-based services have not been fulfilled. Instead, a central fund of £17 million was established in 1986 which will support community-based initiatives for a maximum of three years only and £5 million has been allocated on an apparently one-off basis to RHAs to develop their drug dependency facilities. The provision of drug dependency units is still heavily concentrated in London; longer term rehabilitation is still left largely to the underfunded domain of voluntary agencies.[76] Although nearly all health authorities have now set up multidisciplinary drug committees, there has been little advice on how to proceed. The challenge for the future is to develop and expand a more equitably distributed network of diverse treatment and rehabilitation facilities to cater for a much wider range of drug users than has hitherto been considered.

14 Health in adulthood and old age

Start Young, Stay Active.
CICERO 44BC (*On old age*)

Introduction This chapter first assesses the influence of paid work on health and the opportunities for promoting health in the workplace. We consider progress in reducing work-related disease over the last decade and assess the implications of our findings for future policy. We then move on to assess whether goals for health promotion in old age are different from those in younger people, ways in which they might be achieved, and how much progress has been made in the UK.

Health in the workplace While it has long been recognised that the working environment, and work itself, can jeopardise health, the UK has been slow to act on this knowledge and even slower to see the opportunities that the workplace offers to promote health and to prevent disease. The workplace offers access to 26 million adults – the majority of whom are young and often difficult to reach through other means. As a major proportion of the workforce are manual workers, there are also special opportunities to reach many of the people who are most at risk, not only of work-related ill health, but of many other aspects of ill health (see Chapter 8).

Ill health at work Official figures suggest that about two per cent of all deaths in 15–64 year olds in Great Britain – 1,300 injuries and 1,000 'prescribed' (compensatable) industrial diseases – are directly attributable to work. In 1978 the Royal Commission on Civil Liability – the most recent report to produce such data – found that of 1.8 million non-fatal injuries, 45 per cent of those in men arose from work and 23 per cent in women. In 1979–80 the working population made more than nine million claims for new spells of sickness, of which 9,500 were deemed to be due to 'prescribed' disease. The limitations of the prescribed disease category prevent a full assessment of the burden of ill health attributable to the workplace, but the two commonest groups of occupational disease recorded in Great Britain in 1982 were hearing loss and skin problems (see Table 29).

While prescribed work-related injury and disease form only a small proportion of the total burden of ill health, they represent an underestimate of the true importance of occupational disease because they do not take account of many disorders which are not prescribed diseases. However, even when these factors are taken into

206

account, work-related disease still accounts for only a relatively small fraction of the total mortality in the community. Despite this, there is no room for complacency because our knowledge of workplace hazards is far from complete.

Table 29   Incidence of occupational disease in Great Britain (1979–1980)

Occupational disease	Numbers recorded
Infectious	27
Poisoning and other diseases	95
Repiratory system	935
Musculo-skeletal connective tissue	3,672
Skin	5,660
Hearing loss	5,900
TOTAL	16,289

Source: Schilling RSF. More effective prevention in occupational health practice. Journal of the Society of Occupational Medicine 1984, 34: 71–79.

Trends in occupational disease

Prescribed, work-related diseases and injuries are preventable almost by definition because they are caused by identifiable agents in, or aspects of, the working environment. It is difficult to assess progress in the UK because information on prescribed diseases is not available for individual causes. Over the last twenty years there appears to have been a steady fall in the incidence of work-induced injuries and prescribed diseases. While this may be partly due to declining hours of work (a shorter working life) and unemployment, the gradual implementation of the Health and Safety at Work Act (1974) has probably had an important long-term role in this reduction. The Act placed new, enforceable responsibilities on employers to provide a safe and healthy workplace as well as to maintain high standards of monitoring and evaluation of control measures.

In manufacturing industry, however, there has been a disturbing 24 per cent increase in the incidence of fatal and major injuries from 70.4 per 100,000 in 1981 to 87 per 100,000 in 1984.[1] The explanation for this increase is not clear.

Much of the progress in the reduction of occupational risks has come from the control of known occupational causes of life-threatening diseases, such as asbestos-related lung cancer and mesothelioma and bladder cancer caused by aromatic amines used in the rubber and dyestuffs industries. There are now stringent controls on the permitted concentration of asbestos fibres in the workplace and the use of blue asbestos is banned. The rubber industry's response to the evidence linking dust and fumes to

207

bladder, lung and stomach cancers has been swift and positive.[2] Two years after the Employment Medical Advisory Service (EMAS)[3] confirmed the findings of early research, the British Rubber Manufacturers Association, together with the relevant trade union and the Health and Safety Executive (HSE), published a guide[4] which recommended immediate control of all dust and fumes.

Towards the new occupational health

WHO and the International Labour Organisation (ILO) defined the aims of occupational health, as long ago as 1950, as 'the promotion and maintenance of the highest degree of physical, mental and social wellbeing of workers in all occupations by prevention of departures from health, and controlling risks'.[5] This principle is today embodied in WHO's European strategy for Health for All by the Year 2000.[6] Until recently, emphasis in the workplace has been on the provision of remedial services. In the last ten years there has been a growing awareness of the need for much broader preventive activity as the workplace has a significant role to play in promoting health both in relation to traditionally perceived occupational hazards and to more general health promotion issues. This trend was confirmed in the 1983–85 report of EMAS, the former medical arm of the HSE.[7]

The older idea that a work-related disease had to be one in which work exposure was a 'necessary' cause (that is, prescribed diseases) has given way to a wider concept of work-relatedness which derives from a better understanding of the multifactorial nature of disease. WHO has divided work-related disorders into four new categories (see Table 30) which give a better idea of the scope for prevention in the workplace.[8,9] This classification expands the opportunities for using the working environment as a focus for the promotion of health. Category II of work-related disease, for example, includes heart disease, which is the leading cause of death in the UK, and mental ill health which is the second most common reason why people consult their GPs (see Chapter 10).

Research has helped to identify work-related factors contributing to heart disease among viscose rayon workers.[10] A controlled, prospective study comparing Finnish rayon workers who were exposed to carbon disulphide with those who were not, showed that in the first five years of the study, exposed workers were nearly five times more likely to die of heart disease than non-exposed workers – even after accounting for other major risk factors. Measures were then taken to reduce carbon disulphide levels to below 10 parts per million and 10 years later death rates among the exposed rayon workers had fallen to the same level as those in the non-exposed group.[11]

Evidence is now accumulating that other work-related factors may contribute to, or aggravate, heart disease, including sedentary work (see Chapter 9) and job stress (see Chapter 3). Some of the components of job stress, such as 'moonlighting' or working overtime for long periods,[12] together with rigid work routines[13] and shift work,[14] are associated with an increased risk of heart disease. In the prospective Framingham study on heart disease, a combination of highly demanding work and poorly defined supervision was a powerful predictor of subsequent heart disease in women – even when adjusted for other major risk factors.[15] In Category IV disease (see Table 30), where access to potential dangers at work is the important factor, innkeepers and bartenders have been shown to have a higher risk of cirrhosis of the liver than any other occupation[16] and suicide in medical laboratory workers is much higher than in other occupations.[17] This clearly offers scope for developing preventive policies for the control of alcohol and drugs at work, as well as counselling and support programmes.

Table 30 Categories of work-related disease

Category	Definition	Examples
I	Work – the necessary cause	Lead poisoning
II	Work – a contributory causal factor, not a necessary one	Coronary heart disease, mental ill health
III	Work – provokes a latent or aggravates established disease	Peptic ulcer, eczema mental ill health
IV	Work – offers ready accessibility to potential dangers	Innkeeping (alcohol) Medicine (drugs)

Source: Schilling RSF. More effective prevention in occupational health practice. Journal of the Society of Occupational Medicine 1984, 34: 71–79.

The working environment and quality of life

Difficulties in definition and measurement are less easy to overcome in the study of the impact of work stress on mental health and the quality of working life. Few would doubt that underpaid work, authoritarian management, inflexible working hours and routines, and some modern production methods, diminish the quality of a working person's life, but we have no good means of measuring their impact on health. Concern has been expressed that today's working population may be experiencing the adverse psychosocial effects of new electronic technology and prolonged enforced leisure (in many cases unemployment),[18–20] but research has so far been inconclusive and uncertainty on the evidence[21] concerning the health effects of visual display units (VDUs), for example, continues. Trades unions have already adopted a preventive strategy on VDUs. They have negotiated agreements specifying lighting arrangements and limiting exposures to four hours a day.[22] The challenge now facing employers is to minimise these sources of occupational stress by planning work and work hours in such a way as to stimulate a participating workforce and maximise satisfaction among employees. The challenge to epidemiologists and social scientists is to find ways of measuring the effect of such interventions on the physical, mental and economic wellbeing of the workforce.

Progress in the workplace

To get a clearer picture of what is being done to promote health in the workplace, we and the former HEC commissioned a survey of major UK employers' associations and trades unions.[23] The sample was neither comprehensive nor representative of the whole of industry. The aim was to gain a general impression of the way in which occupational health was interpreted in practice by major public and private sector employers and trades unions. The pattern of results showed that, on the whole, public sector employers and trades unions were most likely to have developed policies and practical occupational health programmes. Private sector employers were doing less well.

Table 31   Ranking of priority issues for health in the workplace

Highest priority	*No priority*
Noise	Contraception
Safety	Sexually transmitted disease
Dusts	Personal development
Muscular/chemical hazards	
Alcohol	
Smoking	
Stress	
Nutrition	

Source: Webb T, Schilling R et al. Health at work? A report on health promotion in the workplace. Health Education Authority. Forthcoming.

It was clear that both employers and trades unions gave issues such as alcohol, smoking, stress and nutrition nearly as much priority as the traditional occupational concerns of noise, safety and dust control (see Table 31). Trades unions gave more priority than employers to nutrition and much more to family care issues, such as maternity/paternity leave and child care. Contraception, sexually transmitted disease and personal development were accorded very little priority by either trades unions or employers. Clearly, some of the major risk factors for coronary heart disease – with the notable exception of obesity – are now emerging as key issues for future action in the workplace. Among all trades unions and employers, those issues which have had the most significant influence on their occupational health programmes over the last decade were identified as government legislation (the Health and Safety at Work Act) and a number of specific health matters arising in the workplace. Health promotion agencies were seen to have little influence. Over 60 per cent of respondents saw government grants as the most useful way of encouraging the establishment of occupational health programmes in the future and nearly half wanted to see the secondment of skilled health promotion staff to industry.[24]

The role of occupational health services Unlike the situation in France and Germany, whose occupational health services are a statutory part of their health service, occupational health services in the UK remain mainly private and fragmented. In 1976, one-third of industrial workers had no occupational health cover.[25] By 1985 the HSE concluded that there had been little progress and expressed concern that up to half the workforce were likely to have no occupational health cover as they were employed in small firms with 250 employees or less, where services are virtually non-existent.[26] Moreover there has been little development of a coordinated occupational health service in the NHS – Europe's largest employer. Medical students and GPs generally receive very little occupational health training, and although there were good postgraduate nursing and medical courses, the majority of occupational health staff working in industry have no professional qualifications.[27] Training is not financed by government.

Any call for improvement or upgrading of the occupational health services should be based on evidence of their effectiveness. It is disappointing, therefore, that there has been so little research in this field in the UK.[28] The multifactorial nature of work-related health problems requires a realistic assessment of the role of occupational health staff together with other contributing influences.

The provision of, and research into, occupational health services and programmes in the USA is highly developed. This is partly because major employers bear the costs of health care of their employees. Many US employers also have evidence (often confidential) that such programmes help to provide a fitter, more productive and satisfied workforce.[29] But American economic analyses may not apply in the UK and we need more information on the costs and benefits of health promotion programmes in the UK. From the little we know, there seems to be obvious scope for the reduction of absenteeism and improvement of productivity, as well as for the promotion of a better quality of working life. The evidence suggests that smoking is responsible for the loss of 50 million working days a year – for smokers take, on average, twice as much sick leave as non-smokers.[30] Alcohol misuse has been estimated by the DHSS to cost industry £600 million each year.

We also lack good evidence of the effectiveness of coordinated health promotion policies and programmes in the workplace. Most of the available evidence is based on programmes designed to reduce the risk of coronary heart disease. A recent WHO collaborative study in the prevention of heart disease – in which the UK participated – was able to demonstrate that a simple, factory-based programme of advice on diet, smoking and exercise could significantly reduce heart disease.[31] The scope for this kind of intervention is actively being pursued in numerous industries in Wales as part of the Heartbeat Wales programme (see Chapter 7). Advice and education about a healthy lifestyle is being backed up with workplace policies which ensure that catering policy makes a wide range of healthy foods available and that smoking control policies, and the provision of exercise and showering facilities, make it easier for employees to act on the advice they are given.

There is now a growing body of evidence, mainly from the USA, that it is possible significantly to reduce smoking in a workforce[32] and generate substantial economic gains for employers.[33] These findings have not been confirmed in a UK context. The savings in terms of improved productivity due to reduced sickness and absenteeism alone are likely to be substantial. Surveys in the early 1980s suggest that nine out of ten employers still have no formal policies on smoking at work (except for safety reasons) and most thought that employees would object[34] – although the opposite is the case (see Chapter 7). Other research suggests that a lack of occupational health staff with appropriate communication skills is a major bar to developing such policies.[35] Yet many individual companies documented in the ASH/HEC guide to *Action on Smoking at Work* have not only been prepared to develop such policies, but have found them to be acceptable to employees.[36]

We have yet to see widespread implementation of the *spirit* of the Health and Safety at Work Act which clearly places a responsibility on employers to protect the 'health' and 'welfare' of their employees as well as their 'safety'. Our survey of workplace employers and trades unions shows that the interest is there, although the necessary will and support needed to translate this into practice is often lacking.

Health in old age One of the most obvious achievements of the last few decades has been the increase in size of the elderly population. Improved standards of living and child health earlier this century, together with better nutrition, prevention and health care, have all helped to ensure that by 1983 the average expectation of further life at 65 for a woman and man in England and Wales was 17 and 13 years respectively (see Chapter 2). The retired population now forms

212

Table 32 **Population projections in the elderly (Great Britain)**

Age	1971 (numbers in millions)	1984 (numbers in millions)	2001 (projection)	Projected percentage change (1984–2001)
65–74	4.8	4.8	4.7	−2.1
75–84	2.2	2.9	3.0	+3.4
85+	0.5	0.7	1.0	+43

Source: Central Statistical Office. Social trends 16. London, HMSO, 1986.

about one-fifth of the community. Population projections for the turn of the century suggest that the biggest expansion in numbers will take place in the oldest age groups: a 3.4 per cent increase in the 75–84s and a 43 per cent increase in the over 85s is expected between 1984 and the year 2001 (see Table 32).

A striking aspect of old age in the UK and the rest of the affluent world is that two-thirds of retired people are women and that 80 per cent of the people who care for the elderly are also women. By the age of 85, women outnumber men by four to one. The reasons why women outlive men have not been adequately researched, but are mainly because mortality rates for heart disease and lung cancer have, so far, always been lower in women than for men. This gap may well close as smoking takes its toll on women as it has on men (see Chapter 4).

e challenge – die young as e as possible While the postponement of premature death might be a valuable goal for the under 75s, it is less appropriate for older age groups. The realisation that the measurement of disease and death rates is an unsatisfactory way of assessing health in old age has led to the search for new indicators which could form a more helpful basis for policy and planning. The accurate assessment of health in old age requires the regular collection of national data on the prevalence of disease, disability and dependency if we are to build up a picture, not only of those who survive, but of the proportion of people who can expect to live 'autonomous' or disability-free lives.[37]

The multidimensional assessment of health in old age forms the cornerstone upon which policies need to be based – especially as multiple, chronic conditions[38] are more common in old age. There are five important dimensions of such an assessment: the ability to perform activities of daily living; mental health; physical health; and social and economic function.

A realistic objective is for the majority of us to live long, disability-free lives, to die ultimately at the limit of what is seen as our average biological lifespan (about 85). This position, represented graphically by the curve in Figure 46, is known as the 'rectangular curve'.[39] It has been suggested that, in ideal circumstances, curves B and C, representing disease and disability survival curves, would approach those of curve A. The hope would be to 'compress' or shorten the period towards the end of our lives when the risk of disability increases. This, according to WHO, would increase independence and autonomy.

We do not yet have enough UK or international information on whether the idea of dying a 'natural death' could be a reality and we await the outcome of Scandinavian research which is following a representative group of the elderly into advanced old age.

Figure 46   Towards a natural death: the rectangular human survival curve, 1900–1980 (US data)

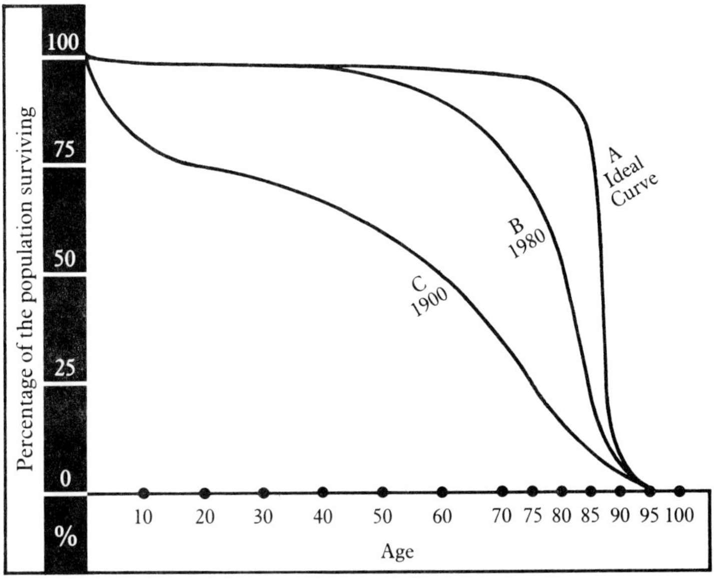

Source: Fries R, Crapo L. Implications of the rectangular curve. San Francisco, W H Freeman and Co, 1981.

The health of the elderly in the UK

Data now available in the UK have begun to permit a shift from disease measurement towards a fuller assessment of independence in old age. The available mortality data show that the major diseases which kill old people are the same as those which kill the middle-aged. Among 60–84 year olds, where the information is most accurate, coronary heart disease, cancers (lung, large bowel and breast in women) were responsible for 60 per cent of deaths among men and women in England and Wales in 1984.[40]

The prevalence of ill health increases with age. In England and Wales in 1983, seven out of ten people over 75 reported suffering chronic ill health (see Table 33). There is some suggestion of rising

Table 33   Ill health in old age (Great Britain)

Indicator	65–74	Age 75+	All ages	Trend 1972–83 (all ages)
Chronic sickness	61%	69%	32%	↑
Restricted activity number of days/person/ year	42	51	24	↑
GP consultations average no/person/year	6	7	4	No change

Source: Office of Population Censuses and Surveys. General Household Survey 1983. London, HMSO, 1985.

Table 34   Independence and health in old age: two community studies

The General Household Survey (1980)			The Scottish study in Clackmannan (1976)	
INDICATOR	AGE 65+ (%)	75+ (%)	INDICATOR	AGE 65+ (%)
General health Good/fair	76	72	*General health* 'Good for age'	61
Mobility Unable to go out alone	12	22	No disability	63
Self care Unable to wash all over alone	9	15	*Impairment* Trouble with joints Trouble with chest	17 16
Unable to feed alone	<0.5	1	Trouble with back	9
Domestic tasks Unable to shop	14	27	Functional incapacity	
Unable to cook	7	12	(appreciable or severe)	17
Use of services in last month			Independent in daily activities and mental function	54
GP's surgery	27	23		
Community nurse	6	12		
Chiropodist	11	17		
Home help	9	18		
Meals on wheels	2	6		

Sources: Office of Population Censuses and Surveys. General Household Survey 1980. London, HMSO, 1982.
Bond J, Carstairs V. Services for the elderly: a survey of the character and needs of a population of 5,000 old people. Scottish Health Services Study No 42. Edinburgh, SHHD, 1982.

215

trends in ill health over the last decade, but these are based on self-reported information which is subject to ill-understood fluctuations. The over 65s also suffer from multiple, chronic conditions, with arthritis and joint problems, followed by respiratory disease, most commonly reported.[41] Other problems such as cataracts and dementia tend to be under-emphasised. The presence of disease gives us little idea of the true level of incapacity or loss of independence it imposes. For example, while diabetes is a chronic disease it may result in little loss of independence, and it is this which is important in old age. The presence of multiple health problems need not *necessarily* compromise a person's functional status.

A more informative picture emerges from studies of the functional capacity of the elderly. Although methods differ and results often depend on self-reported data without accompanying objective testing, two major representative studies of the over 65s, one covering Great Britain[42] and one covering Scotland,[43] show that up to three-quarters of elderly people see themselves as healthy for their age and 63 per cent in the Scottish study had no evident disability (see Table 34). In the study of Great Britain, over 80 per cent were independent in 'activities of daily living' (ADL). The picture for the over 75s also shows that only a minority suffer severe functional incapacity (see Table 34). But when mental function was included in the assessment (as in the Scottish study) the majority among the over 65s who were independent in ADL was reduced to 54 per cent (see Table 34). Overall, therefore, the widely held negative view of old age is not substantiated by the evidence. A qualitative study showed that elderly people held a positive view of themselves and their abilities.[44] This is an important finding because other research suggests that *self-perception* of health among elderly people is a more accurate predictor of future mortality than other measures that may seem to be more objective.[45]

Progress towards 'natural death' in the UK

An assessment of how much progress we have made in the UK towards living disability-free lives and dying a 'natural death' (see Figure 46) depends on a number of assumptions. First, it implies that we know enough about the biology of old age to be able to predict with confidence that there is a natural limit to the lifespan of about 85 years. Second, it assumes the current reductions in death rates (see Chapter 2) will slow down in very old age – for which there is little evidence in the UK.[46] Third, it assumes that preventive measures will reduce the incidence of the major chronic diseases. While this is possible for some diseases, such as lung cancer and respiratory disease, it is likely that heart disease and stroke will continue to be major causes of mortality in a majority of elderly people for a long time to come, although future generations entering

216

old age may have less atherosclerosis. Moreover, we still do not know how to prevent arthritis and dementia (see Chapter 10) which are major causes of disability in old age and are likely to increase in prevalence as the numbers reaching old age also increase. Despite these uncertainties, it is possible that some of the loss of functional capacity associated with ageing is avoidable. This should act as a stimulus to develop appropriate policies for both elderly people and their carers rather than a justification for not pursuing strategies to prevent premature death earlier in life.

Towards a policy for promoting health in old age One of the biggest barriers to effective health promotion in old age is the negative attitude to old age that prevails among the public, the media and some professionals. Not only is ageing seen as a period of inevitable decline, the terminology we use to describe old age often has a negative, pejorative meaning.

It is government policy to support elderly people so that they may live independent lives in their own homes.[47] This is also the goal of statutory and voluntary agencies concerned with old age (and the BMA) and is assumed to be the aspiration of most elderly people themselves. WHO has recently translated this overall goal into six more specific objectives:[48]

- to prevent unnecessary loss of functional capacity;
- to maintain the quality of life in old age by preventing distressing symptoms;
- to assist elderly people to live in their own homes and to prevent unnecessary admissions to residential care;
- to prevent the breakdown of informal networks of care, particularly families;
- to prevent unnecessary decline in functional capacity and quality of life if admission to long-stay care is essential;
- to prevent iatrogenic (doctor-induced) disease, including the distress that can be caused by inappropriate interventions in old age.

Such ambitious goals for the promotion of health in old age demand a broad response. Three overall approaches are open to us:

- social and welfare policy;
- support for a healthy lifestyle;
- health care policy.

These three approaches are clearly interdependent and we assess each in turn.

In this report our terms of reference have so far precluded a detailed discussion of the contribution of medical care to the promotion of health. Conventional wisdom suggests that it is small.

But this assumption needs re-examination in the context of old age, where the primary goals are the promotion of autonomy and independence and *not* simply the postponement of premature death. The successful integration of prevention, treatment and rehabilitation in British geriatric practice should prompt a reassessment of the role of medical intervention in the promotion of health in old age.

The potential of the hospital and specialist services to preserve and improve functional capacity in old people is considerable. Among those aged 65 and over in England there are over 1,000 operations a week for cataract, 500 prostatectomies and 500 hip replacements, while large numbers of patients receive surgical or gynaecological repair, are being treated for angina and diabetes, or are being rehabilitated from stroke. Yet, despite considerable expenditure on these specialist services, there are no representative national or regional data on their outcomes and effectiveness. For example, although we know that hip replacement surgery is cost effective[49] in terms of quality of life gained, waiting lists vary widely from district to district. Information on the role of other medical treatments in maintaining the functional wellbeing of elderly people is almost completely lacking.

Social and welfare policy

The promotion of autonomy in old age requires action on many fronts. While there has been little direct research on the impact of income, housing, transport and communication policies on wellbeing, it is obvious that they have considerable bearing on the ability of elderly people to function independently in the community. State pensions form the major source of income for retired people. While they have increased in real terms since 1976, pensioners still formed 27 per cent of the poorest fifth of the community in 1982 (see Chapter 8). One fifth of pensioners are so poor that they require a supplementary pension. British pensioners also fare much worse than many of their European contemporaries whose pensions begin to approach a replacement rather than a subsistence income.[50]

Housing

There is considerable scope for the promotion of independence through safe and sensitively designed housing. Elderly people are more likely than others to live in old, dilapidated housing: they occupy nearly one-third of houses deemed to be unfit. Against a background of major reductions in public expenditure on housing, it is hard to see how the necessary improvements can be made. About half of elderly people are owner occupiers, and it is this sector which contains some of the poorest housing stock. There was a 38 per cent increase in the number of owner-occupied homes designed as unfit between 1971 and 1981, yet improvement grants to owner occupiers decreased by 28 per cent between 1974 and 1985. This Scottish study of the elderly at home showed that nearly 60 per cent of their houses had no aids such as handrails or non-slip mats, and nearly half of the occupants had no obvious way of signalling in an emergency[51] – a finding confirmed in the 1980 study of elderly people throughout Great Britain[52] in which only 61 per cent of households had a telephone.

Housing and cold-associated ill health

The potential for adequately heated and insulated housing to prevent unnecessary extra ill health in the elderly has not been fully assessed,[53] but research on the role of low indoor temperatures in precipitating disease as well as discomfort suggests that they are important. While community[54] and hospital studies[55] show that severe hypothermia affects only a small proportion of the elderly[56] (there are about 500 deaths from hypothermia recorded by OPCS in England and Wales each year) recent research has highlighted the much bigger problem of what is now known as 'cold-associated disease'. Analysis of weekly death rates between 1974 and 1984 shows that 80 per cent of weekly fluctuations can be explained by changes in temperature. From these figures it has been estimated that there are about 40,000–75,000 cold-associated deaths in the UK every year.[57] This represents 12 per cent of all deaths and is two to three times as high as in America and in other parts of Europe where winter temperatures are much lower.[58]

The impact of cold-associated disease is felt most in elderly people and is apparent in major increases (about 50 per cent) in mortality from respiratory disease, heart disease and stroke (about four per cent) during severe winters.[59] Although there has been a fall in the number of cold-associated deaths over the last 25 years, countries like Sweden and the USA have reduced these seasonal swings more effectively than the UK – despite bigger drops in average winter temperatures.[60] A national hypothermia study in the UK[61] showed that those at highest risk were likely to live alone, have no central heating, unheated bedrooms and no community services. Based on these findings it recommended:

- effective insulation in elderly people's homes;
- an adequate heating allowance;
- the issue of low wattage electric blankets to those at high risk.

Other international research has shown that the spread of central heating has made an important contribution to the fall in cold-associated deaths throughout Europe, Japan and the USA.[62] The minimum recommended indoor temperature for adults in the UK is 18.3°C and WHO has recommended that 21°C should be viewed as a minimum for elderly people.[63] Yet indoor temperature surveys in 1972 showed that three-quarters of their living rooms were below the

UK minimum for adults [64] when the outside temperature was 5°C. There is no evidence that the situation has improved since then.[65] Government policy on the prevention of cold-associated problems in the elderly is contradictory. Severe weather payments are available when outside temperatures are very low, but the termination of the system of insulation grants has made it difficult for all but better off individuals and the most imaginative local authorities to improve insulation in elderly people's homes.

Sheltered housing Although only a tiny proportion of elderly people live in sheltered housing (1.3 per cent in a Scottish study), the growth of the elderly population in the 1970s led to an expansion in the building of sheltered housing. Such building in the public sector is now at a standstill, although it continues in the private sector.

There has never been a clear policy of eligibility for sheltered accommodation and local authority provision varies widely,[66] although the average – 27 per 1000 elderly – is below the arbitrarily designated ideal of 50 per 1000. Limited funds have led many authorities to develop alternative schemes of sheltering with 'mobile wardens', 24 hour on-call systems, and alarms. But they still await evaluation.

Planning transport and leisure Two-thirds of households with elderly people have no access to a car. Thus cheap and accessible public transport is a central factor in determining whether old people can continue to participate in the life of the community. The recent deregulation of buses and increases in fares (see Chapter 6) disregard this requirement. According to the 1980 General Household Survey, nearly a quarter of the over 75s did not use public transport because of physical difficulties. Although there has been little research in the UK, the findings of major prospective health studies of over 70s and over 80s in Sweden and Denmark suggest that bus design and traffic control systems need amending as the landing platform on buses was too high for many old people and timespan between changing traffic lights was not long enough for an elderly person to cross the road safely.[67,68] The Department of Transport is currently examining the UK position. Many local authorities have adopted sensitive policies for maximising the social integration of old people, such as door to door bus services, mobile day centres, improved concessionary fares, and easy access to shopping, health centres and public buildings.[69] Such policies, together with well thought out recreational and sports facilities and adult education courses, can help elderly people to reach their potential.

Supporting a healthy lifestyle in old age

Good health in old age depends, in part, on the avoidance of diseases when younger. We have already discussed the measures needed to reduce smoking and to encourage healthy eating, moderate drinking and regular physical activity among younger people (see Chapters 7 and 9). Research on whether similar measures *in old age* have any beneficial effect is lacking. One community survey in Cardiff showed that older people – especially the over 75s – have lower smoking rates, drink less and take much less regular exercise than younger adults.[70] At present we have no good information on the effect of changing smoking, drinking and eating habits in old age, although one American study has shown that people who stop smoking in old age have lower subsequent rates of heart disease.[71] The promotion of physical activity in old age is one area where the evidence for its beneficial effects justifies action. For research now shows that much of the loss of fitness in old age is not inevitable and results from disuse – rather than from the ageing process itself (see Chapter 9).

General nutrition in elderly people has been the subject of considerable concern. Major community surveys show that most have an adequate diet,[72] although about one or two per cent (about 200,000 people) suffer from serious subnutrition. While detailed assessment of under-nutrition has shown that deficiency of nutrients, such as folic acid and vitamin D, are associated with ill health, supplementation has not been shown to be beneficial.[73] The evidence that abnormal bone thinning (osteoporosis), which affects 25 per cent of women by the age of 60, can be delayed by calcium supplementation is mixed.[74] But hormone replacement therapy (oestrogens combined with progestogens) is demonstrably effective in preventing osteoporosis.[75] Although the increased risk of heart disease associated with this treatment is not as great as assumed hitherto[76] the question of whom to select for treatment is not yet resolved.

Care in the community – supporting self care and community care

In our enthusiasm to promote health in old age, we often forget that old people themselves, together with their families, relatives and friends, have a key role in maintaining a good quality of life. The present challenge to community agencies and to health and other professionals is to find a balance between actions designed to support (rather than undermine) the efforts of elderly people and their families to look after themselves, without at the same time neglecting their welfare needs.

Although a detailed account of how voluntary and statutory provisions in the community have contributed to their autonomy is beyond the scope of this report, active partnership between elderly people and voluntary agencies such as local Age Concern groups is widespread.[77] In 1985, Age Concern and the former HEC launched a

221

joint initiative, Age Well, which aims to support and raise the profile of existing initiatives organised by elderly people and by local agencies. The Age Well campaign forms part of the former HEC's Health in Old Age programme which received six per cent of the HEC's total programme budget for 1986/7. SHEG and the Welsh Office have also launched their own small initiatives on health in old age, but financial support has been limited. Age Concern already provides a number of training courses for professionals with an interest in old age, but research commissioned by the former HEC shows that undergraduate, in-service and continuing education for health workers is seriously lacking.[78]

Despite many innovative schemes, statutory provision of services, such as leisure facilities, adult education activities, day centres and lunch clubs, tend to be neglected in favour of the provision of meals on wheels. There is now increasing recognition of the emotional and social support that district nurses, social workers and home helps can give elderly people and some authorities ensure they are adequately trained. Better coordination and interdisciplinary training of such 'paid carers' will lead to a more sensitive distribution of services where they are needed.[79]

Supporting informal care Debate on the provision of community support for the growing number of elderly people is often inappropriately focussed on an assumed huge burden of resources that will have to be shifted into statutory and residential services. While the need for such services will undoubtedly increase among the over 85s, 95 per cent of elderly people continue to live in their own homes and between 1975 and 1985 there was only a six per cent increase in their numbers in residential care (relative to a 26 per cent increase in the total number of over 75s between 1971 and 1981).

Although we await the publication of a major national study by OPCS, it is clear from the Scottish study in Clackmannan[80] and from more selected community studies in general practice,[81,82] that the mainstay of support for old people continues to come from self-care and unpaid female relatives.[83,84] Despite changes in the social roles of women, they continue to shoulder this responsibility willingly,[85] often with very little outside support and at great personal cost,[86] including restrictions in personal freedom[87] and high levels of anxiety and depression.[88] The major studies point to the following conclusions.

- The main supporters identified by elderly people themselves are wives, daughters or daughters-in-law.
- The main kinds of material support offered are help with housework, shopping, mobility and, to a lesser degree, personal care.

222

- An inverse care law appears to operate whereby the more disabled the elderly person, the lower is the likelihood that her supporter will receive help from the statutory services.
- Most statutory support is concentrated among those elderly who live alone and have no immediate informal network.

Despite the minimal demands of informal carers, most remain unfulfilled: about a third would like some short, occasional respite, yet in one study less than half reported having had a few days off in the previous year.[89] In the same study, relief care had been organised by the health or social services in only seven per cent of cases. Many schemes like the Crossroads Care Attendant Schemes have established national networks that provide trained, paid carers, but such efforts cannot be expected to bridge the gap.[90] This is regrettable as there is now some evidence that respite care can postpone institutionalisation and increase the quality of life of carers.[91]

The full value, extent and personal costs of informal care are only just being realised. Few cost benefit studies of various types of community care include a proper assessment of the costs of informal care.[92]

Preventing disability, promoting functional dependence – the role of the NHS

We have already referred to the potential role of the hospital services in promoting health in old age. The primary health care team also has a major potential contribution to make.

Avoiding iatrogenic action While overprotective behaviour by health and other professionals can be a problem, iatrogenic, or doctor-induced health problems, are probably one of the commonest preventable problems in old age. The overprescription of drugs to old people is a complex and poorly documented field. While we know that the elderly receive a disproportionate amount of all drug prescriptions, we do not know exactly what proportion is appropriate. There is a higher prevalence of ill health and a higher incidence of GP consultations than in young people. Elderly people are especially vulnerable to doctors who overprescribe medicines. They are more likely than other groups to receive repeat prescriptions[93] and in one study up to 28 per cent of repeat prescriptions to the elderly were deemed unnecessary.[94] Studies of admissions of elderly people to hospital suggest that at least 10 per cent are associated with the overprescription of drugs.[95] Drug groups commonly overprescribed include benzodiazepines, diuretics and digoxin.[96] Measures to minimise overprescription and unnecessary multiple drug prescribing have been recommended by the RCP[97] and RCGP,[98] and include:

- regular feedback on prescribing practices;
- better education and information for both prescribers and clients

from independent sources;

- clear, computerised recording systems for drugs and repeat prescriptions.

Geriatric screening Research that has demonstrated an iceberg of undetected disease in elderly people has raised some unresolved questions about the value[99] and practicability[100] of establishing screening programmes (the early detection of undiagnosed disease) for them. Evidence supporting screening for disease is mixed. While screening for breast cancer in women aged 50–74 demonstrably reduces mortality (see Chapter 7), biochemical and x-ray screening tests in elderly people have no demonstrable role outside the hospital. The value of screening for high blood pressure is, at present, uncertain. The European Working Party on High Blood Pressure in the Elderly, which conducted the first randomised controlled trial of treatment for high blood pressure in the over 60s,[101,102] has demonstrated a 52 per cent reduction in the incidence of non-fatal strokes as well as a 60 per cent reduction in fatal heart attacks, and this has been confirmed in general practice.[103] The Canadian Task Force on Periodic Screening has recommended two-yearly screening for high blood pressure in the over 65s,[104] but the side effects of treatment and interactions with other drugs present special problems in elderly people.[105] We await a further assessment of risk and benefit in the current MRC trial of high blood pressure in the elderly.

Interest in screening has now broadened from the detection of disease to assessment of functional capacity and social need. Results from the limited number of trials[106–108] so far, suggest that health visitor assessment and intervention on an annual or quarterly basis does not have much impact on levels of disability but can increase use of appropriate services and may reduce the need for hospitalisation. Although screening is assumed to add to an elderly person's quality of life there is no firm evidence yet. Even if this were regarded as a sufficient basis for setting up a screening programme, a general practice with a population of 4,000 would require 18 extra hours of health visitor time per week for the first year alone.[109] While the case for establishing a full screening programme for elderly people is not yet convincing, there is scope for using the consultation itself as an opportunity to detect hitherto unrecognised problems ('case-finding'). As 90 per cent of the over 75s will consult their GP at least once a year[110] and the minority who do not appear to be in good health,[111] attention has now been focussed on the use of the consultation itself ('anticipatory care') to detect unrecognised problems. A short questionnaire which is designed to assess key *functional* problems (such as mobility, foot care, hearing and vision)

224

is now being investigated.[112] The benefits to old people themselves are obvious and are supported by the RCGP and Age Concern.[113] The demands made on the GP's workload have yet to be assessed.

Dying with dignity   Three out of four people now die in hospital. This profound shift from home to hospitals is sometimes seen as an unwelcome medical intrusion into a natural process. But many elderly people and their families and friends are glad of the option. In many cases, sudden fatal illness precludes any other choice, but an elderly person and his or her family should, where possible, be offered a choice of where to die. Dying in hospital undoubtedly increases the risk of unnecessary medical intervention and emotional neglect, but dying at home with inadequate care and support is not necessarily preferable. The increasing trend away from dying at home has left many GPs inexperienced and unsure as to how best to support the dying and their relatives at home.[114] At a time of financial stringency it has proved difficult to provide the necessary nursing support services – especially night nurses – whose contribution has been regarded as essential.[115] Six out of ten GPs in one survey were keen to look after more dying patients at home, but nearly as many wanted further training – especially in communication skills and bereavement counselling. If this survey reflects attitudes among GPs in general, then there is clearly the will in primary care to support the dying and the bereaved at home. What is needed is a reorientation of training and services so that GPs and other primary care staff can help their patients to die well.

PART III: TOWARDS A STRATEGY FOR THE 1990s

15 The basis of the strategy

'Discern the Past
Understand the Present
Declare the Future.'
SOCRATES

Introduction In this chapter we identify 17 priorities for public health action which emerge from our review of public health in Parts I and II of the report. We discuss the justification for our choices, and set out the framework within which we shall develop our detailed strategy in Chapters 16 and 17.

Priorities for public health action Our analysis in Parts I and II of the report shows that we can identify a number of public health priorities where there is sufficient evidence to conclude that action would have a significant benefit on health. The following 17 areas for action emerge.

The reduction of tobacco consumption This mainly concerns cigarettes, but also relates to other forms of tobacco consumption such as sucking tobacco (see Chapters 3, 4, 7, 13).

The promotion of a healthy diet This primarily requires a decrease in the consumption of saturated fats, sugar and salt and an increase in dietary fibre intake (see Chapters 3, 4, 7, 12).

The reduction of alcohol consumption This involves reducing average alcohol consumption for the whole population and is not simply a matter of reducing the prevalence of heavy drinking (see Chapters 5, 6, 7).

The promotion of physical activity There is a need for an increase in regular physical activity in all age groups (see Chapters 9, 14).

The promotion of road safety This aims at a further reduction in the numbers of road accidents and their consequences (see Chapters 6, 7).

The promotion of health at work This concerns the promotion of health and the reduction of health risks at work (see Chapters 4, 14).

Effective maternity services This concerns interventions, the care of both the mother and the child during pregnancy and labour, and around birth (see Chapters 2, 11).

Child health surveillance This includes both immunisation against infectious disease (see Chapter 12) and the early detection of remediable ill health.

Early cancer detection At present, this mainly relates to screen-

Table 35 Choosing public health priorities and their justification

I: *Priorities where the evidence justifying detailed action is strong*

Priority	Evidence for action	Feasibility/ effectiveness of action	Public support	Professional support	Political support	Possible economic benefits
Tobacco	★★★★★	★★★★	★★★★	★★★★★	★★★	?[1]
Diet	★★★★	★★★★	★★★	?	?	?
Alcohol	★★★★	★★★★	★★	★★★	★	?
Physical activity	★★★★	★★	?	?	★★	?
Sexuality	★★★★★	★★★★	★★★★	★★★★	★★★★	★★★[2]
Road safety	★★★★★	★★★★★	★★★★	?	★★	?
Maternity	★★★★★	★★★★	★★★★★	★★★★★	★★★★★	★★★★[3]
Immunisation	★★★★★	★★★★★	★★★★	★★★★★	★★★★	★★★[4]
Dental health	★★★★★	★★★★★	★★★★	★★★★★	★★★★	?
Early cancer detection	★★★★★	★★★★	?	★★★★	★★★★	★★[5]
Hypertension reduction	★★★★	★★★★	?	★★★★	?	★★[6]

1 It is probably not possible to do a full benefit to cost analysis of the impact of tobacco prevention policy, but GPs' advice to patients to stop smoking is highly cost-effective.
2 This refers to the positive benefit to cost ratio for family planning services.
3 This refers to the positive benefit to cost ratio of antenatal screening for Down's syndrome and neural tube defects.
4 This refers to the positive benefit to cost ratio of immunisation programmes in the USA.
5 This refers to the accepted cost-effectiveness of breast screening, and to what, in the committee's view, could be a cost-effective cervical screening programme.
6 This refers to the known cost-effectiveness of screening for high blood pressure in primary care.

II: *Priorities where the case for action is strong but where more evidence for effective intervention is needed*

Priority	Evidence for action	Feasibility/ effectiveness of action	Public support	Professional support	Political support	Possible economic benefits
Psychoactive drugs	★★★★	★	?	?	★★★★	?
Health at work	★★★★	★	?	?	None	?
Social support	★★★	★	?	?	?	?
Child health surveillance	★★★★	★★	★★★	★★★★	★★	?

III: *Priorities where the case justifying action is strong, but where the expertise or scope of the committee is limited*

Priority	Evidence for action	Feasibility/ effectiveness of action	Public support	Professional support	Political support	Possible economic benefits
Services for the elderly	★★★★★	★★	?	?	★	?
Adequate income	★★★★	★★★	★★	?	?	?
Safe housing	★★	★★★★	★★★★	★★★★	★	?

★★★★★	Very strong evidence or support
★★★★	Strong evidence or support
★★★	Fairly good evidence or support
★★	Some evidence or support
★	Poor evidence or support

ing for breast cancer and cervical cancer (see Chapters 4, 7).

High blood pressure detection and prevention This concerns blood pressure screening as well as the promotion of dietary improvement (see Chapters 3, 9, 14).

The reduction of psychoactive drug misuse This concerns reduction both in the misuse of prescribed psychotropic drugs and in the use of illicit drugs (see Chapters 5, 10, 13).

Services for the elderly This includes social, welfare, education and leisure as well as health services for the elderly (see Chapter 14).

The maintenance of social support This concerns the preservation and maintenance of supportive social networks (see Chapters 9, 10, 11).

The promotion of dental health This involves fluoridation as well as dietary change and the reduction of tobacco use (see Chapters 3, 12).

The promotion of a healthy sexuality This includes the promotion of rewarding sexual relationships, the control of fertility and the prevention of sexually transmitted disease, including cervical cancer (see Chapters 4, 5, 7, 13).

Adequate income This concerns increasing national wealth, reducing income inequalities and reducing unemployment (see Chapter 8).

Safe housing This concerns the provision of enough, well-designed and soundly constructed housing (see Chapters 8, 10, 14).

While there is sufficient evidence to warrant action in each of these areas, our review shows that the evidence supporting a *detailed* strategy for action is stronger in some cases than others. Moreover, we believe that it is better to limit our detailed recommendations to those areas where we feel confident that the evidence, and our understanding, is strong enough to justify doing so. We also believe that it is important to make explicit the basis for a rational strategy. We have, therefore, identified six criteria upon which our recommendations are based:

- the strength of the evidence supporting the need for action;
- the strength of the evidence supporting the feasibility or effectiveness of action;
- the degree of public support or acceptability;
- the degree of professional support;
- the degree of political support;
- the economic benefits.

Although we lack good information in relation to many of these criteria, we have attempted throughout our foregoing analysis to document the degree of public, professional and political support for public health measures that have been shown to be effective. After considering these six criteria we have divided our 17 public health priorities into three groups.

1 Those where both the evidence and the support for action is strong.
2 Those where the case for action is strong, but more evidence of the feasibility of implementation is still needed.
3 Those where the case for action is strong, but where detailed recommendations are beyond the scope or expertise of this committee.

1 Public health priorities where the evidence and support for action is sufficient

Tobacco	Maternity services
Diet	Dental health
Alcohol	Early cancer detection
Physical activity	High blood pressure reduction
Sexuality	Immunisation
Road safety	

As guidance for the reader we set out in Table 35 the justification for selecting these priorities based on the six criteria we have tried to use throughout the report. Although the quality and reliability of the evidence concerning public, professional and political support is much greater in some areas (such as tobacco) than others, we believe that the evidence supporting the development of a detailed strategy in each case is strong. We set out our detailed recommendations for each in Chapters 16 and 17.

2 Public health priorities where the case and/or support for action is strong, but where more evidence of the effectiveness of action is needed

Psychoactive drug misuse
Health at work

Child health surveillance (other than immunisation)
Social support

Despite the government's highly visible, mass media initiatives to reduce **illicit drug misuse**, we believe that the disproportionate attention devoted to heroin in the mass media at the expense of other drugs may prove to be counterproductive. We believe that much more effort should be directed towards testing the effectiveness of community and individually oriented support. While national and international measures are clearly needed to help control the trafficking of opiates, we would like to see more research devoted to the consequences of the heavy focus on heroin for other patterns of drug misuse before unreservedly endorsing current strategies. We do, however, welcome recent initiatives to control the spread of AIDS through the provision of exchangeable syringes and hope that community-based programmes tailored to specific, local drug problems, together with innovative forms of support for drug users who wish to end their dependence, prove to be successful.

Other, promising opportunities for the prevention of **psychoactive drug misuse** lie in the further reduction of inappropriate benzodiazepine prescription. While policy in this field is still in the early stages of development, the considerable media attention given to the topic seems to have contributed to the downward trend in prescriptions for sedatives.

While the **workplace** offers obvious opportunities for reducing ill health and preventing disease, the committee did not feel there was sufficient evidence available upon which to base a detailed strategy for the promotion of occupational health. Although the control of well-known hazards in the rubber and asbestos industries and, to a lesser extent, smoking and diet are well-researched and implemented, these are the exceptions to the general lack of research and evaluation of workplace health promotion in the UK. We need to know much more about the effects of such activity on employees' health, and how occupational health staff might best be deployed in such initiatives, before we can recommend detailed action.

In the case of **child health**, the way forward is hampered by a lack of knowledge of the value of interventions, such as advice on a healthy lifestyle, and inadequate research on how to make worthwhile interventions (such as screening for hearing and visual deficits) effective and efficient. With the exception of **immunisation**, therefore, the committee did not feel able to make detailed recommendations for an overall child health programme. We hope that local efforts that are currently being researched will fill this unacceptable information gap.

Although evidence is now accumulating that **social support** may be important in the protection of physical, and possibly mental health, we have little information on how it might be most helpful to intervene. With the exception of isolated, although important, trials of social support in pregnancy and early childhood, there is little research which points the way forward for effective intervention elsewhere. Indeed the scope for intervention may be very limited, as it is not simply the amount of social support which counts, but its quality. In our view, the best opportunities – although largely unresearched – lie in areas where intervention might be best directed towards maintaining rather than supplanting *existing* networks for the elderly with much more priority being given to support for informal carers.

3 Public health priorities where the case for action is strong, but where detailed recommendations are beyond the remit or the expertise of the committee

Services for the elderly
Adequate income
Safe housing

In the case of **services for the elderly** there are two main difficulties which confronted the committee. First, it is obvious from our discussion of the promotion of health in old age (see Chapter 14) that action is needed on a wide number of fronts, ranging from social welfare and housing policy to education, leisure and health promotion services. We feel that others may be more competent to make detailed recommendations on these issues. Second, many of the measures likely to have a significant impact on the health of the elderly concern the delivery of effective treatment, such as hip replacement, cataract and gynaecological surgery, and support services from local and health authorities. While we remain convinced of the value of these services, it is beyond the primary remit of this report to discuss treatment and support services in any detail. We know others are working in this field and look forward to the results of their deliberations.

While we believe that the provision of an **adequate income** for everyone, together with a reduction in unemployment, is likely to have major benefits on wide-ranging aspects of health (see Chapter 8), it is beyond the expertise of this committee to propose a detailed strategy for how such objectives may be realised by government and others. Nevertheless, we reiterate the central importance of ensuring that the health effects of socioeconomic policy are taken into account. We also emphasise throughout our detailed strategy the need to develop measures to reduce inequalities in specific aspects of health and its determinants. Indeed the success of any strategy designed to promote health or to prevent disease is dependent on the simultaneous development of socioeconomic policies that are conducive to the reduction of inequalities in income and to the creation of wealth.

In the case of **housing**, the evidence linking bad housing to poor health is tenuous, although the improvement of our housing stock is clearly a priority in itself and would be likely to result in improvements in the quality of life for many of the most deprived in the community. The health benefits of a more sensitive housing policy for the elderly are likely to confer major gains in health. Nevertheless we believe that others are more qualified to advise on how housing policy should be developed in the interests of promoting good health.

The elements of the strategy   In keeping with our analysis in Parts I and II of the report, we can identify three overall health goals which form the cornerstones of our approach:

Goal 1: to promote longevity;
Goal 2: to promote a better quality of life;
Goal 3: to promote equal opportunities for health.

The strategy itself can be divided into three interconnected parts:

- resources for health;
- lifestyles for health;
- preventive services for health.

We next consider the framework for the strategy together with a brief discussion of what resources might be needed to support public health action. We devote each of the remaining chapters to developing the other two components of the strategy. In order to set out a coherent plan of action we have adopted a uniform way of dealing with each of the public health priorities. For each we set out the following elements:

- general objectives;
- quantified targets to be achieved by the year 2000 or earlier;
- expected or possible health outcomes;
- recommendations for implementation to identifiable national and local agencies: we concentrate our recommendations on those agencies and organisations which have clear responsibilities for health.

While we consider it essential that each of these agencies should be responsible to the interests of public, community and voluntary agencies, it is not the role of this report to recommend to either individuals or community agencies what their contribution to public health should be.

Resources for health

Our foregoing analysis has made it clear that a comprehensive strategy to promote public health needs to be underpinned by the following elements:

- good organisation;
- adequate funding;
- long-term commitment and programme planning;
- well-defined research and evaluation.

We have already pointed to some of the strengths and deficiencies in these elements in the UK and compared our position with that of other countries. It is beyond the scope of this report to undertake a major review of organisation, funding, programme planning and research, as much of the necessary information was not available to us. We have chosen instead to concentrate on how these issues relate to the specific public health priorities we have defined. Nevertheless it is obvious from our review that the following elements should form the foundation of an effective public health strategy – irrespective of the issue concerned:

- high-level ministerial responsibility and accountability for public health;
- interministerial liaison that permits the health aspects of all public policy to be taken into account;
- good channels of communication between central government and local health service and other agencies, with sensitive consultation of community and professional opinion;
- adequate central government funding to support the implementation and research components of a long-term strategy at national, regional and local levels, with specifically allocated local funds;
- a national plan for health with a set of clearly defined, quantified targets (where possible) for the nation that is reflected in the plans of national health promotion agencies, health and local authorities, and primary care;
- an annual mechanism of reporting back to the nation on progress, at national and local levels.

Towards a new UK approach

In the last chapter we referred to WHO and to some health authorities in the UK which have set numerical targets for the promotion of health and reduction of disease. In the interests of promoting a clearer set of recommendations for action on each of our identified issues, we have chosen to adopt an approach which is complementary to, but distinct from, the setting of disease reduction targets.

We focus instead on setting targets for influencing the *determinants* of disease and health which we define numerically where the data allow. We believe that this shift in emphasis will not only help to

236

define health responsibilities both inside and outside the NHS, but will also enable us to set realistic targets which are achievable in policy terms. It will allow agencies to develop appropriate tools for monitoring the implementation process as well as the health outcomes. Most important of all, however, this approach allows for the logical expression of the fact that most avoidable diseases have many causes and that each individual cause or determinant of health and disease will in turn contribute to a range of different diseases. In this way we avoid making predictions about disease and health outcomes that are notoriously difficult to make and are also subject to medium-term fluctuation.

For example, while we consider that the reduction of mortality from lung cancer and coronary heart disease is likely to result from measures to reduce smoking, we cannot yet predict accurately what the disease outcomes might be over the next decade. In the case of smoking-induced disease, this is because smoking is only one of many factors involved in the causation of coronary heart disease and today's lung cancer rates reflect smoking patterns of more than two decades ago which were very different among men and women. This serves to complicate any predictions about future trends as lung cancer will continue to rise among women for many years, even if we are successful at reducing the current smoking rate among women as well as men. For these reasons, it seems wiser to set targets for the reduction of smoking in various sectors of the community and to measure the health outcomes, rather than to set the health outcomes in the first place and to monitor smoking rates.

Setting targets Target-setting has long been seen as an essential part of the formulation of any strategy in the commercial sector. It has increasingly become part of the planning process in the NHS as well. Pressure on the new generation of NHS managers to choose between and monitor different aspects of policy in the NHS has led to an increasing tendency to define policy targets in numerical terms and to monitor progress accordingly. More than half of the English regional health authorities in our own survey in 1985 had adopted a set of numerical targets for the promotion of health. This method of setting objectives has the following advantages.

- The setting of a clearly defined numerical target offers a clear means of monitoring progress.
- It can act as a stimulus for the provision of an appropriate local database on the health of the community which might not otherwise be available.
- It offers a way of highlighting key aspects of health promotion policy which are distinct from, but complementary to, other aspects of NHS policy.

237

- Target-setting can offer a way of ensuring better commitment and implementation of health policy.

Target-setting has also some disadvantages.

- It tends to focus exclusively on what is easily quantifiable and often omits aspects of health that are difficult to quantify.
- It sometimes encourages an unjustifiably didactic approach, especially if not accompanied by sufficient public debate.
- Careless target-setting based either on inadequate data or unrealistic short-term objectives can be counterproductive, and lead to unnecessary stresses being placed on those expected to achieve them.

In our strategy, therefore, we have attempted to quantify only those targets for which we have a sufficient past database to predict potential future achievement. We have also identified other targets for action which may not yet be quantifiable, but which represent areas of policy in which progress can usefully be made. The aim of target-setting, in our view, is not to use it as a method of penalising policy makers if they fail to reach targets, but rather as a positive source of inspiration for those concerned with promoting the health of the nation.

16 Lifestyles for health

Give me neither poverty nor riches;
feed me with food convenient for me.
PROVERBS XXX, 8

Introduction In the previous chapter we briefly outlined the first part of our proposed strategy. This concerned the 'resources' necessary to support the overall strategy. We also identified 11 of 17 public health priorities for which we believe detailed plans for action can be justified. These now form the basis of the second and third parts of the strategy for which we develop detailed recommendations in this and the final chapter. They can be grouped as follows:

Lifestyles for health
- Tobacco
- Diet
- Physical activity
- Alcohol
- Sexuality
- Road safety

Preventive services for health
- Maternity
- Dental health
- Immunisation
- Early cancer detection
- High blood pressure detection

In this chapter we give detailed recommendations for action in the six priority areas we have defined as 'Lifestyles for health'.

Tobacco

General objectives
1 To create a physical and social environment where non-smoking is the norm.
2 To support the creation of a generation of non-smokers.
3 To maximise public awareness of the risks of smoking across all sectors of the community.
4 To support the efforts of those who wish to stop smoking.

TARGETS TO BE ACHIEVED BY THE YEAR 2000
(OR EARLIER)

1 To increase the percentage of adult non-smokers (including ex-smokers) in the community to at least 80 per cent.
2 To increase the proportion of children under 16 who are non-smokers to at least 95 per cent, and to reverse the trend towards increased smoking in girls.
3 To reduce the gradient in smoking rates between manual and non-manual classes.

4 To ensure that at least 95 per cent of children and adults understand the risks of smoking.

EXPECTED HEALTH OUTCOMES

Physical health 1 A reduction in coronary heart disease mortality in the under 65s and a reversal of the upward trend in mortality from this disease among manual workers (Chapter 3).

2 A reduction in mortality from lung cancer in men under 65 and a reversal of the upward trend in incidence of lung cancer among women over 55.

3 A further decline in chronic lung disease. A reduction in the contribution made by passive smoking to lung cancer (Chapter 4).

4 A small contribution towards a reduction in the numbers of low birthweight babies and in perinatal mortality, and a reduction in the incidence of stroke and coronary heart disease associated with the use of oral contraception (Chapters 4 and 13).

Mental and 1 Increased fitness (Chapter 9).
social wellbeing 2 Increased productivity at work and a reduction of absenteeism due to smoking-related disease (Chapter 14).

RECOMMENDATIONS FOR IMPLEMENTATION

Government 1 Cigarette taxation should be increased annually to keep pace with inflation.

2 An advertising levy (a 10 per cent levy would raise approximately £10 million) should be imposed on total expenditure on tobacco promotion to finance additional public education programmes.

3 A legislative plan should be set out with the aim of banning all forms of tobacco advertising and sponsorship over a two-year period.

4 The ceiling for maximum permitted tar yield of cigarettes should be gradually reduced to 10 milligrams of tar.

5 Two new tar bands should then be created:
'Dangerous' – under five milligrams tar per cigarette;
Very dangerous' – five to ten milligrams tar per cigarette.

6 There should be a changing series of strengthened and enlarged health warnings on cigarette packs (and on advertising until it is banned).

7 There should be an immediate ban on the sale or promotion of chewing and sucking tobacco. No new tobacco product should be introduced into the market without a major inquiry into its health effects.

8 Government funding for the national smoking education programme should be increased.

240

9 Government funds should not be used to support the growth or manufacture of tobacco at home or abroad.

Health promotion

1 New emphasis should be given to more recently discovered health effects of tobacco such as passive smoking, the combined risks of smoking and oral contraceptive use and the relationship of smoking to cervical cancer, coronary heart disease and the loss of fitness.

2 Programmes should be designed to reach those groups where smoking prevalence is static or increasing – including children, especially girls, and those in manual work.

3 There should be better consultation and coordination between government and local and voluntary agencies to support smoking control policy.

Cigarette and tobacco retailing industry

1 Attempts should be made to diversify into non-tobacco products.

2 Attempts to create new markets abroad should cease.

3 The industry should endeavour to retrain employees likely to be made redundant as the tobacco trade continues to decline.

The communications media

1 Continual efforts should be made to ensure adequate coverage of both new and well-known health aspects of tobacco.

2 Editors and programme makers should be free to comment on matters relating to smoking, despite possible pressure from advertising and promotional interests in tobacco.

3 Fictional characters should, whenever possible, reflect the non-smoking majority in the population.

Training institutions

1 The influence of smoking on health should be adequately presented in the training and education of doctors, dentists, nurses, health educators, paramedical professionals and environmental health officers.

2 Students should be taught appropriate communication and other skills necessary to support efforts to reduce smoking in the community and in individuals.

Local authorities

1 There should be a clearly stated policy on smoking and health in each local authority.

2 The following elements should be covered:

- smoking at meetings held on local authority premises;
- tobacco sponsorship or advertising on local authority owned premises or billboards;
- enforcement of the law governing the sale of cigarettes to minors;
- plans for developing and monitoring smoking policy and

smoking education programmes in primary and secondary schools;

- plans to use the strengths of environmental health officers to promote smoking and health policies in restaurants and shops.

Health authorities

1 The reduction of smoking and smoking-related diseases should form part of a clearly stated strategy for the promotion of health at both district and regional levels.

2 The elements of the smoking control strategy should include:

- a non-smoking norm at all health authority meetings;
- a clearly signposted non-smoking norm in all health premises with special areas set aside for smokers;
- a ban on the sale of cigarettes on health premises;
- support for patients and staff in their efforts to stop smoking.

3 There should be a named community physician or health education officer with responsibility for overseeing the implementation and monitoring of the smoking and health policy.

Primary health care

1 Family practitioner committees (and their Scottish equivalents) should develop clear objectives for the reduction of smoking in the community as part of the overall long-term strategy for primary health care.

2 There should be an agreed method in general practice for encouraging and supporting the reduction of smoking among individual patients.

Employers and trades unions

1 There should be a clearly stated signposted smoking control policy in the workplace that has been jointly agreed between employers and trade union representatives.

2 Facilities should be made available to employees to assist them in their efforts to stop smoking.

3 Occupational health staff should be involved in this enterprise.

Nutrition

General objectives

1 To create an environment in which healthy food is accessible to all sectors of the community.

2 To create a climate in which the nutritional aspects of food are taken into account in the development of food policy.

3 To increase public, professional and political awareness of what constitutes a healthy diet.

242

TARGETS TO BE ACHIEVED BY THE YEAR 2000 (OR EARLIER)

1 To reduce the proportion of total energy intake derived from fats to 30 per cent.

2 To reduce the proportion of energy derived from saturated fats from 17 to 10 per cent.

3 To reduce the average blood cholesterol level in the community to 5.2 millimoles per litre in the over 30s and to 4.7 millimoles per litre in the under 30s.

4 To reduce total sugar intake from 38 kilograms per head per year to 20 kilograms per head per year and to minimise the eating of sugary foods between meals.

5 To increase the total dietary fibre intake – especially cereal fibre – from approximately 20 grams per person per day to 30 grams per person per day.

6 To reduce the average salt intake from approximately 10 grams per person per day to 5 grams per person per day.

7 To reduce the socioeconomic disparity in intake of high fibre foods and sugar intake.

EXPECTED HEALTH OUTCOMES

hysical health
1 A reduction in incidence and mortality from coronary heart disease. An increase in expectation of life, especially at the age of 45 (Chapters 2 and 3).

2 A possible reduction in incidence of bowel and breast cancers (Chapter 4).

3 A reduction in the incidence of inflammatory bowel disease, constipation, obesity and diabetes (Chapter 4).

4 A reduction in the incidence of dental decay in children (Chapter 12).

Mental and
:ial wellbeing
Increased productivity due to prolongation of life in middle age and reduction in disability (Chapters 2, 3 and 4).

RECOMMENDATIONS FOR IMPLEMENTATION

Government
1 Government should develop a clearly stated national nutritional policy based on the above targets.

2 The DHSS should be responsible for ensuring that the nutritional aspects of food policy in other departments are adequately reflected.

3 The Ministry of Agriculture, Fisheries and Foods (MAFF) should implement a comprehensive food labelling system which clearly informs the consumer of the fat (saturated and polyunsaturated),

sugar, fibre and salt content of all foods. A simple 'traffic lights' system of identifying foods that are high, medium or low in the above substances should be adopted.

4 MAFF should make representations to the EEC to modify policies which run counter to the guidelines recommended in the NACNE and COMA reports.

5 To restore the balance of information to the consumer, a levy on the advertising and promotion of foodstuffs (a 0.1 per cent levy would raise approximately £4 million) should be imposed to help finance public education and information programmes on nutrition.

6 Steps should be taken to return to agreed minimum nutritional standards in schools.

Health promotion

1 The long-term nature of any programme to promote healthy eating should be set out in a clearly stated strategy that reflects the above quantified targets.

2 The promotion of healthy eating should form part of a more comprehensive approach to promote healthy living.

3 Health promotion agencies should assist with information and monitoring support to promote healthy eating within local health and other authorities.

4 Priority and funding support for regional and local programmes should be given to those parts of the UK (for example, Scotland) where diet-related disease (especially coronary heart disease) levels are highest.

Training institutions

1 The study of diet-related disease and nutrition should form an integrated part of the undergraduate, postgraduate and continuing education programmes for doctors, nurses, health educators, dieticians, teachers and environmental health officers.

2 Professionals should be encouraged to develop skills to help put this special knowledge into practice.

Food and drug industry

1 Retailers should develop a policy of maximising access and information to consumers of a wider choice of healthy foods – especially in parts of the country where it is poor.

2 Attempts should be made by food manufacturers to minimise the amount of salt and sugar added during food processing.

3 Food manufacturers and government should agree on an implementable code of practice for the responsible advertising of food and confectionery.

4 This should be monitored by a body independent of the food and advertising industries and representing consumer and health interests.

244

5 The growing emphasis on the advertising of healthy foods should be encouraged.

6 Drug manufacturers should avoid adding sugar to medicines.

Local authorities

1 There should be an explicit policy within the authority to promote healthy nutrition.

2 This policy should include:
- provision of adequate information;
- provision of a range of healthy food at local authority-organised functions;
- encouragement by environmental health officers to promote the growth of 'healthy menus' in restaurants and catering establishments;
- development of healthy catering policies and nutritional standards in schools;
- development of nutrition education programmes in the curricula of both primary and secondary schools;
- the appointment of a local education authority adviser with special responsibility for nutrition education;
- the development of nutrition education courses for adults, including the Look after Yourself package.

Health authorities

1 The promotion of healthy nutrition and the reduction of diet-related disease should be a clearly stated part of regional and district health promotion plans.

2 This strategy should include:
- provision of healthy food alternatives for patients and staff in health authority premises;
- provision of informative material about healthy nutrition through menus and leaflets addressed to patients and staff;
- provision of dietary advice in suitable health authority settings, including antenatal and child health clinics.

Primary care

1 There should be an agreed means of assessing, recording and monitoring diet and weight in the whole practice population.

2 A named person within each practice should be responsible for agreeing long-term targets for monitoring and promotion of healthy nutrition with the FPC (or Scottish equivalent).

3 Agreement should be reached on which primary care staff are to be involved in counselling to promote healthy nutrition, and how such work might be evaluated.

Employees and trades unions

1 A conscious effort should be made to provide healthy food alternatives in staff canteens and restaurants.

2 Complementary information on diet and health should be made

245

available to staff.

3 Occupational health staff and trade union health and safety representatives should be jointly involved in the development of programmes and advice concerning healthy nutrition.

4 Occupational health staff should establish a nutritional surveillance system including weight monitoring, dietary profiles and blood cholesterol measurements.

Alcohol

General objectives

1 To promote patterns of alcohol consumption that minimise its harm without jeopardising its benefits.

2 To create an environment which minimises pressures to drink excessively and maximises choice of non-alcoholic alternatives.

3 To improve understanding of the adverse medical, psychological and social effects of excessive drinking and to promote a better understanding of what constitutes 'safe' drinking patterns.

4 To support the efforts of those with alcohol problems who wish to cut down on their drinking or remain abstinent.

TARGETS TO BE ACHIEVED BY THE YEAR 2000 (OR EARLIER)

1 To halt the rise in per capita alcohol consumption by 1989 and to reduce it by 20 per cent by the year 2000.

2 To halt the rising consumption of alcohol among women.

3 To reduce high levels of alcohol consumption and harm among high risk occupational groups, including those in the alcohol production and retailing industry, managerial and business executives, and journalists.

4 To reduce by at least 20 per cent the proportion of men who drink over 20 standard units of alcohol per week and the proportion of women who drink over 14 standard units of alcohol per week.

5 Substantially to reduce drinking and driving – especially among the under 25s.

6 To reduce the numbers of heavy drinkers, problem drinkers and those dependent on alcohol.

EXPECTED HEALTH OUTCOMES

Physical health

1 A reduction in alcohol-related disease, including cirrhosis of the liver, high blood pressure, cancer of the oesophagus and digestive tract, obesity, and deaths and injury from accidents at work, at home, and on the roads (Chapters 5, 6 and 14).

246

Mental and social wellbeing

1 Economic benefits, such as increased productivity, and reduced absenteeism (Chapters 5 and 14).
2 Reduction in domestic violence, child abuse and assault (Chapters 5 and 10).
3 Reduction in public drunkeness and criminal damage (Chapter 5).
4 Reduction in admission for hospital treatment for alcohol dependence (Chapter 5).

RECOMMENDATIONS FOR IMPLEMENTATION

Government

1 Taxation on all alcoholic drinks should be adjusted annually to keep pace with the retail price index.
2 It should be mandatory for all alcohol advertising and containers to display clear information on the alcoholic content of the product being sold or advertised.
3 There should be warnings to consumers on all advertising material on what constitutes excessive or unsafe patterns of drinking.
4 There should be an annual levy imposed on alcohol advertising (a three per cent levy would raise approximately £5 million) which should be used to help finance public and community education and information programmes.
5 Present funding for national alcohol education programmes should be increased to £10 million per annum.
6 There should be no further relaxation of the licensing laws.
7 The law relating to roadside breath testing legislation should be clarified so that it is clear that the police are legally allowed to breathalyse motorists at any time.
8 It should be an offence to sell alcoholic drinks to persons under the age of 18 (not merely those *known* to be under age) and this legislation should be enforced.

Health promotion

1 There should be a clearly defined long-term strategy for the reduction of alcohol consumption. Its objectives and targets should be numerically defined.
2 Funds for supporting alcohol education programmes should be allocated separately from those devoted to illicit drug education.
3 There should be better integration of the currently sporadic drink and drive campaigns, together with the national alcohol education programme.
4 More effort should be made to support and evaluate activities aimed at reducing alcohol consumption among individuals in primary care, the workplace, and voluntary and community groups.
5 The content of national alcohol education programmes should be linked to specific government initiatives such as drinking and

driving, the labelling of alcohol containers and advertising.

The communications media

1 More conscious effort should be made to present the harmful effects of alcohol.
2 The images of drinking presented in the press, radio and television should be realistic reflections of the negative as well as the positive effects of alcohol.
3 There should be a code of practice governing the way in which alcohol is presented on television to young audiences.

Alcohol and advertising industries

1 There should be a stricter code of advertising practice that is enforceable by a newly appointed independent body. The code should proscribe the use of alcohol advertising and promotion which associates drinking, especially excessive drinking, with glamour or sexual prowess.
2 Better information and confidential help with alcohol problems should be available for employees in the alcohol industry.
3 More visible efforts should be made to support campaigns promoting safer drinking.

Local authorities

1 There should be an overall commitment to minimise alcohol related harm.
2 Local authority policy should deal with the following areas:
   - local authority meetings and entertaining should offer non-alcoholic drink in preference to alcohol during the working day;
   - health considerations should be taken into account when new licences to sell alcohol are granted;
   - non-alcoholic drinks should be offered at local authority leisure and recreation premises in preference to alcoholic drinks;
   - alcohol education should form an integrated part of primary and secondary school curricula and there should be an education adviser with overall responsibility in this field;
   - the police should make efforts to create a climate where drinking and driving is regarded as unacceptable and to enforce the existing drinking and driving laws.
3 Local authorities should offer confidential alcohol counselling or referral services, and occupational health staff should be involved in running such programmes.

Health authorities

1 The reduction of alcohol consumption and its related damage should form a specific part of strategic and DHA plans.
2 Health authorities should have clearly defined policy objectives concerning alcohol and health, including:

248

- a ban on the sale of alcoholic beverages on health authority premises during working hours;
- a ban on alcohol drinking among all health authority employees who are involved in direct patient contact in clinical work;
- several options for referral of patients for alcohol counselling;
- better coordination of policy on the referral of patients with alcohol problems between psychiatry, social work and other medical departments.

3 More support should be given to community agencies concerned with helping those who wish to reduce their drinking.

Primary care

1 There should be an agreed method of assessing, recording and monitoring the drinking habits of all patients.
2 There should be agreed objectives for the reduction of alcohol consumption within each practice population.
3 Primary health care staff should have an agreed system of referral and support of patients with drinking problems.

Employers and trades unions

1 There should be a clearly defined policy on the sale and drinking of alcohol during working hours among employees whose safety and health as well as that of others may be put at risk.
2 Non-alcoholic beverages should be offered in preference to alcoholic ones at meals and social functions organised during working hours.
3 There should be a confidential counselling programme available for employees who wish to seek help in overcoming an alcohol problem.
4 Occupational health staff, where possible, should be involved in organising and administering such a programme.

Physical Activity

General objectives

1 To encourage participation in appropriate, regular physical activity in all age groups and sectors of the community.
2 To provide cheap, accessible sport and recreation facilities for all members of the community.
3 To increase public and professional understanding of the importance of physical activity to the maintenance of health.
4 To create a social climate in which regular physical activity is seen as a normal part of work and leisure.

TARGETS TO BE ACHIEVED BY THE YEAR 2000
(OR EARLIER)
1 To increase the proportion of ten to 15 year old schoolchildren

participating in regular, vigorous exercise to at least 90 per cent.

2 To increase the proportion of the population participating in regular aerobic physical activity to 30 per cent between ages 16–64.

EXPECTED HEALTH OUTCOMES

Physical health

1 Increase in physical fitness (Chapter 9).
2 Prevention of the loss of stamina, strength and suppleness – especially in old age (Chapters 9 and 14).
3 Decrease in obesity, blood pressure and diabetes, with concomitant decrease in coronary heart disease in the long term and probable increase in lifespan (Chapters 3 and 9).
4 Possible reduction in osteoporosis (Chapter 14).
5 Increased risk of sport-related injuries and possible small increased short-term risk of heart disease (Chapter 9).

Mental and social wellbeing

1 Increase in sense of mental wellbeing and possible antidepressant effect (Chapter 9).
2 Improved self image (Chapter 9).
3 Increase in social contact (Chapter 9).
4 Increased independence and autonomy in the elderly (Chapters 9 and 14).

RECOMMENDATIONS FOR IMPLEMENTATION

Government

1 Financial support for the Sports Council should be increased in real terms.
2 Tax incentives for employers should be introduced to encourage the building of better sports and recreational facilities at work.

Health promotion

1 Efforts should be made to work closely with the Sports Council to highlight the link between health and sporting activities.
2 The promotion of physical activity should form a clearly defined part of an overall, long-term health promotion strategy.
3 A narrow focus on the role of physical activity in the prevention of coronary heart disease should be avoided; new efforts should be made to focus on the importance of physical activity for wider aspects of health, particularly in old age.
4 The enjoyment of non-competitive sport and the social contact it offers should be given more emphasis in future information and education programmes.
5 More effort should be made with the Sports Council to find ways of making physical activity more attractive to women of all ages, to the elderly, and to those on low incomes.

250

Training institutions

1 The physical education training curriculum should be widened to encourage the development of skills in non-competitive sporting activities such as movement, dance and aerobic activities.

2 The broader implications of physical activity for health and disease should be covered as a formal part of the training of physical education and health professionals.

Local authorities

1 There should be a long-term plan for improved provision of sports and recreational facilities that is in keeping with the ten year plan for Sport for All.

2 Special provisions should be made to cater for the target groups identified in the Sport for All strategy, including women, the over 50s, lower socioeconomic groups and school leavers.

3 The promotion of physical activity should form part of a comprehensive programme of education and information, including plans for adult education courses.

4 Levels of physical activity in schools should be monitored and the range of activity offered should reflect the interests of those who do not wish to participate in competitive sport as well as those who do.

5 There should be better liaison with local industry and employers to promote better sports facilities in the workplace.

6 School sports and recreational facilities should be accessible to the rest of the community out of school hours.

7 Sport and recreational activities should be adequately advertised in the local community.

8 There should be plans to develop safe cycleways and exercise facilities in local parks to promote physical activity.

Health authorities

1 The promotion of physical activity should be part of health authorities' strategic and district plans.

2 Health authority premises should make adequate provision for sporting and exercise facilities.

3 Health authorities should collaborate with local industry, local authorities and community agencies in promoting better provision and participation in physical and sporting activities, such as local health fairs.

Primary care

1 Assessment of levels and advice on physical activity to patients should become part of good practice in primary care. The responsibilities for doing this should be clearly agreed between GPs and other primary care staff.

2 An agreed method should be devised for recording habitual physical activity in patients' notes.

3 Information should be made available to patients on the health

251

benefits of exercise and on the availability of sport and recreational facilities.

4 Patients who are overweight should be routinely advised to take more exercise. Efforts should be made to support and encourage such activities.

Employers and trades unions

1 Exercise facilities should be made available in the workplace. If the workplace itself is too small, there should be liaison with other local workplaces to provide joint facilities.

2 Workplace exercise programmes should be used as an opportunity to raise other aspects of health, including nutrition – such as the Look after Yourself programmes.

3 Occupational health staff should be involved in the organisation and monitoring of exercise programmes.

4 Adequate shower facilities should be available for staff who cycle to work or who wish to take exercise during their breaks.

Sexuality

General objectives

1 To promote the rewarding expression of sexuality to help fulfil emotional relationships.

2 To promote individual control over fertility.

3 To minimise the adverse health consequences of sexual activity.

4 To support those in need of help and advice with sexual or reproductive problems.

TARGETS TO BE ACHIEVED BY THE YEAR 2000
(OR EARLIER)

Sexual expression

1 To increase the proportion of adolescents who are adequately informed about the social, psychological and medical implications of sexual intercourse.

2 To increase to at least 95 per cent the proportion of adolescents who feel free to discuss their sexual feelings openly with their teachers in a school sex education programme.

Control of fertility

To increase to at least 95 per cent the proportion of women and men at risk of unwanted pregnancy who use safe and effective forms of contraception.

Prevention of sexually transmitted disease

1 To ensure that more than 95 per cent of all those who are sexually active understand the medical, psychological and social consequences of multiple sexual partners.

2 To reverse the downward trend in the use of barrier contraception

among those under 25.

3 To increase the responsible use of barrier contraception among men and women under 30 who are likely to have more than one sexual partner in a year.

4 To increase the proportion of boys and girls who understand and feel confident about the proper use of barrier contraception.

5 To increase understanding among women of the value and purpose of cervical screening.

6 To increase to at least 60 per cent the proportion of all women aged 20–65 who have a cervical smear every five years.

7 To increase the proportion of women aged 45 to 65 who have regular cervical smears, and to reduce the social disparity in patterns of cervical smear testing in all age groups under 65.

EXPECTED HEALTH OUTCOMES

Physical health
1 A reduction in the transmission of the AIDS virus and an eventual reversal of the epidemic rise of the disease (Chapters 5, 7 and 13).

2 A substantial reduction in the incidence and mortality from cervical cancer (Chapters 4, 7 and 13).

3 A reduction in other sexually transmitted diseases (Chapters 7 and 13).

Mental and social wellbeing
1 A reduction in unwanted pregnancies and the accompanying increased risk of mental ill health and marital disharmony (Chapters 10 and 13).

2 Increased self confidence and satisfaction in personal relationships (Chapter 13).

3 Increased control over fertility (Chapter 13).

RECOMMENDATIONS FOR IMPLEMENTATION

Government
1 The current, isolated programme to control AIDS should be integrated into a more coherent strategy for the prevention of AIDS and of other sexually transmitted diseases, including cervical cancer, together with plans to reduce unwanted pregnancy – especially among teenagers.

2 The provision of contraceptive services by general practitioners should be extended to condoms.

3 DHSS should take a lead in encouraging much wider availability of condoms, especially through retailers, in pubs and in other places frequented by young people.

4 All imported condoms should undergo mandatory quality testing.

5 The 1967 Abortion Act should be maintained and extended to Northern Ireland.

6 The expertise of the Family Planning Information Service (FPIS) in public education and information on a wide range of issues related to sexuality and health should be supported by increasing its annual budget (£5 million should provide an adequate starting basis).

7 Extra central funds should be given to health authorities and family practitioner committees for the adequate funding of a comprehensive cervical screening and follow-up service throughout the UK.

Health promotion

1 An attempt should be made to rationalise the hitherto disparate, but common, strands of health promotion activity concerned with responsible use of safe contraception, the prevention of cervical cancer and other sexually transmitted disease, together with the prevention of the spread of AIDS.

2 There is a need to focus on the risks of multiple partners, not only in the prevention of AIDS, but also in the prevention of cervical cancer and other sexually transmitted disease.

3 The value of barrier contraception for women as well as for men in the prevention of sexually transmitted disease needs to be emphasised.

4 Ways of overcoming uncertainties, distaste and a lack of understanding of how to use barrier contraception need to be found.

5 Separate sub-programmes need to be directed to specific target groups with different needs. This can best be achieved through detailed research and consultation with groups and organisations representing their interests in the community.

6 Effective use of mass media campaigns should avoid arousing a combination of fear and helplessness, but should focus instead on giving unambiguous, direct information on sexual practices that confer a high or low risk of sexually transmitted disease, including AIDS and cervical cancer.

7 Mass media campaigns should avoid making unacceptable moral judgments, but should endeavour to create a climate in which the expression of sexuality is seen to be an integral part of an emotional relationship.

8 Magazines and newspapers directed at specific target audiences, including young people, young women and homosexual men, should be used to test the kinds of messages that are likely to be effective in these groups.

The communications media

1 Manufacturers should advertise and promote condoms as a means of protecting against pregnancy and sexually transmitted disease in as informative a manner as possible.

2 There should be a code of practice governing misleading TV

254

advertising for condoms, monitored by the IBA.

3 Ways should be found of maintaining the current interest and focus on informative and non-sensational coverage of AIDS and ways of reducing the risk of its spread.

Training institutions

1 Undergraduate, postgraduate and continuing education programmes for doctors, nurses, health educators and social workers should include adequate information about the importance of sexuality in human relationships and its possible adverse outcomes.

2 GPs and other primary health care staff should be trained in the communication and counselling skills necessary to deal with the diverse health problems posed by sexuality in everyday practice.

3 Training courses should encourage counsellors to explore their own beliefs and prejudices about sexuality.

Local authorities

1 The promotion of good personal relationships and the prevention of sexually transmitted disease should be a fundamental part of primary and secondary school education.

2 There should be a named education adviser with specific responsibility for ensuring that sex education is a part of school curricula.

3 Specialist or community groups whose aim is to offer advice and counselling in the prevention of sexually transmitted disease or unwanted pregnancy should be given financial support.

4 Local authority initiatives should be linked with those of health authorities and other community organisations so that free confidential advice is available by telephone on all questions related to sexuality, contraception and health.

5 Local authority premises, such as youth clubs and recreational facilities, should be used to make condoms more accessible.

Health authorities and primary care

1 The prevention of sexually transmitted disease and unwanted pregnancy should form part of an integrated approach to the promotion of healthy sexual relationships.

2 Health authorities and FPCs (and their Scottish counterparts) should have clearly quantified objectives for the promotion of safe and effective forms of contraception, the provision of adequate day care and inpatient abortion services, together with the reduction of sexually transmitted disease, including AIDS and cervical cancer.

Family planning services

1 There should be a comprehensively equipped family planning, abortion and sexual counselling service in every health authority.

2 This service should offer both male and female sterilisation.

3 Pregnancy testing services should be more accessible.

4 There should be adequate day care abortion services.

5 Staff in these units should be trained to be sensitive to the needs of pregnant women – especial adolescents seeking abortion.

6 Family planning clinic staff, and doctors and nurses in primary care, should encourage greater use of barrier contraceptive methods among people under 25.

7 There should be a special family planning service for adolescents.

Prevention of sexually transmitted disease

1 DHAs should liaise with local authorities and other community agencies in planning information and advisory services on AIDS and in initiatives to minimise the risk of its spread.

2 These services should be well publicised locally.

3 AIDS counselling services should be expanded from the hospital and clinic settings to a broader service that is directed more towards the *prevention* of AIDS, and based in more accessible parts of the community.

Prevention of cervical cancer

1 Sufficient funds should be allocated by RHAs and DHAs to support efforts by health education officers in the *primary* as well as secondary prevention of cervical cancer.

2 Information should be available to women on the primary and secondary prevention of cervical cancer through the workplace, in general practice, and at family planning and gynaecology clinics.

3 Every DHA should have an adequately equipped and staffed laboratory cytology service, a colposcopy service, and the full range of treatment services for the prevention, detection and treatment of all stages of cervical cancer and pre-cancer.

4 There should be an agreed local programme for the prevention of cervical cancer that clearly delineates responsibilities of the DHA and of medical and other practitioners.

5 There should be a designated manager – preferably a community physician – whose responsibility it is to oversee and monitor the successful implementation of the programme to prevent cervical cancer.

6 Every health authority should provide an efficient five-yearly call/recall system for all women aged between 20 and 65.

7 Programmes should be organised so that joint responsibility and participation in the programme by patients and their GPs is possible.

Employers and trades unions

1 Employees should be informed about the value of safe and effective contraception and regular cervical screening for women.

2 Occupational health staff should be involved in monitoring cervical testing among female employees and in the provision of a cervical screening service.

3 If there is no established cervical screening service at the workplace, the mobile screening services of the Women's National Cancer Control Campaign should be invited to visit.

Road safety

General objectives

1 To minimise the risk of accident and injury to pedestrians and other road users.
2 To provide safe and accessible forms of public transport for all sectors of the community.
3 To make the roads in the UK as safe for pedestrians and cyclists as for other road users.

TARGETS TO BE ACHIEVED BY THE YEAR 2000 (OR EARLIER)

1 To decrease the proportion of car, van, coach and lorry drivers who exceed the speed limit.
2 To at least maintain the current 95 per cent of front seat car and van drivers who wear seat belts.
3 To increase the use of rear seat belts to at least 90 per cent.
4 To increase the use of appropriate forms of baby restraint in rear car and van seats to at least 90 per cent.
5 To reduce the number of local accident black spots by at least 60 per cent.
6 To at least treble the number of miles of segregated inner city cycleways.
7 To increase the roadside testing of blood alcohol levels and reduce by at least 50 per cent the proportion of drivers with blood alcohol levels exceeding the legal limits.
8 To maximise public understanding of the effects of excessive speed and of drinking and driving.
9 To maximise public understanding of the components of road safety and the effects of excessive speed and excessive drinking on the risk of injury and premature death on the roads.

EXPECTED HEALTH OUTCOMES

Physical health

1 A reduction in premature death and disability due to road injuries. This will be particularly apparent in the under 25s, and among young men (Chapters 6 and 7).
2 A reduction in premature death and serious injuries – especially head injuries – among cyclists (Chapters 6 and 7).
3 A reduction in injury and death rates among back seat passengers in cars and light vans (Chapters 6 and 7).

Mental and social wellbeing Possible increase in productivity due to a reduction in premature death among young people.

RECOMMENDATIONS FOR IMPLEMENTATION

Government
1 There should be clarifying legislation to allow 'random' roadside breath testing for alcohol.
2 The use of rear seat belts should be mandatory in all cars and light vans.
3 Public transport should be encouraged because it is the safest form of travel.
4 There should be more financial support for experimental cycleways and pedestrian precincts.
5 There should be stiffer penalties for drinking and driving offences.

The motoring industry
1 Manufacturers should avoid the use of advertising which glamorises speed.
2 There should be greater design emphasis on safety, including the development of standard, reinforced passenger boxes, improved bonnet design to minimise injury and improved seat belt design.
3 The promotion of safety rather than speed, and the marketing of safety devices, should be given more emphasis in marketing. Manufacturers should experiment with the use of an automatic flashing lights system which helps to alert the driver to excess speed in built up areas.

Health promotion
1 The national health promotion agencies should develop a new expanded road safety public education programme.
2 The programme should receive extra funding from the government.
3 The programme should be coordinated with government's legislative plans on various aspects of road safety, and with local road safety initiatives.
4 The aims of the new programme should include increasing public awareness of the effects of excessive speed and drinking and driving, and the needs of cyclists and pedestrians.

The communications media More attention should be devoted to coverage of road safety as a public health issue.

Training institutions Road safety education and policy should form part of the formal training for doctors, nurses and paramedical professionals, police and publicans.

258

Local authorities

1 There should be adequately funded accident investigation and prevention activity in every local authority.
2 Road safety officers should liaise with local health education units and draw on their expertise.
3 There should be a mechanism for the regular review of accident black spots and of action taken to reduce road injuries at these sites.
4 The needs of pedestrians and cyclists should be taken into account in local planning.
5 Plans should be made to increase segregated cycleways and pedestrianised areas in residential parts of cities.
6 Road safety education should be standard practice in all primary and secondary schools.
7 The police should promote better enforcement of drinking and driving legislation.
8 Local authorities should have a plan for increasing local awareness of the problem of drinking and driving.
9 More efforts should be made by the police to communicate and liaise with publicans to alert people who are at risk of drinking and driving.

Health authorities

1 The promotion of road safety and the reduction of injury on the roads should form part of every DHA and RHA health promotion strategy.
2 Every DHA should have a scheme for linking the loan of secure, low priced, baby seats in cars to either antenatal or postnatal clinics.
3 Casualty and other hospital staff should advise drivers with blood alcohol levels over the legal limit about the dangers of drinking and driving.

Employers and trades unions

1 If driving forms an essential part of employment, employees should be adequately trained for driving their vehicles.
2 There should be a policy to ensure that all employees driving cars or light vans owned by the employer should use adequately fitted seat belts.
3 There should be a policy of no drinking and driving among employees where vehicles are used as part of work.

17 Preventive services for health

Procrastination is the thief of time.
EDWARD YOUNG

Introduction This chapter outlines the third and final component of the proposed strategy to promote public health in the UK. We now make recommendations in the five priority areas we have grouped together as 'preventive services for health'.

- Maternity services
- The promotion of dental health
- Immunisation
- Early cancer detection
- High blood pressure reduction

Maternity services

General objectives
1 To promote a safe and satisfying experience of pregnancy and childbirth.
2 To promote an environment in which parents-to-be can participate actively during pregnancy and in the birth of their children.
3 To minimise unnecessary medical intervention during pregnancy and labour.
4 To maximise easy access to maternity services in all ethnic and social groups.

TARGETS TO BE ACHIEVED BY THE YEAR 2000
(OR EARLIER)

Antenatal care
1 To increase to at least 90 per cent the proportion of women making their first antenatal booking by the twelfth week of pregnancy and to decrease the social and ethnic disparity in early antenatal attendance.
2 To offer all women with low risk pregnancies the possibility of antenatal care that is shared between midwives, GPs and hospital consultants.
3 To increase to at least 90 per cent the proportion of pregnant women who are offered antenatal classes.
4 To offer all pregnant women support and advice in their efforts to stop smoking.

Antenatal
screening

1 To increase to at least 95 per cent the proportion of women over 35 who are adequately counselled and offered amniocentesis or an equivalent investigation.

2 To increase to at least 95 per cent the proportion of pregnant women who are offered antenatal screening for alphafetoprotein levels.

3 To inform and to offer screening to all pregnant women for pre-eclampsia, iron deficiency, syphilis and HIV antibody status.

4 To offer all women of Cypriot, Indian and Pakistani origin screening and counselling for the detection of thalassemia major.

5 To offer to all those at risk of haemophilia and Huntington's chorea adequate genetic counselling services.

Labour and
birth

1 To offer all women for whom it is appropriate, the opportunity to choose a home or hospital delivery in their second pregnancy.

2 To reduce the episiotomy rate to at least the level prevailing before 1960.

3 To ensure that every woman who has a hospital delivery can have a companion of her choice present during labour.

4 To restrict electronic and PH monitoring of the fetus to women in prolonged labour and at high risk of fetal distress.

5 To increase the proportion of mothers who are given their babies to hold immediately after birth in hospital units.

6 To increase the proportion of women breast feeding for six weeks to at least 75 per cent, and to reduce the social and regional disparity in breast feeding rates.

EXPECTED HEALTH OUTCOMES

Physical health

1 A reduction in the prevalence of babies born with neural tube defects and Down's syndrome (Chapter 11).

2 A possible small decrease in the proportion of low birthweight babies (Chapter 11).

3 A decrease in the rate of caesarean sections (Chapter 11).

4 A major reduction in prevalence of thalassemia major, haemophilia, and Huntington's chorea (Chapter 11).

Mental and
social wellbeing

1 An increase in parental satisfaction and a decrease in anxiety-related to the antenatal period (Chapter 11).

2 Reduced requirements for pain relief and a shorter labour (Chapter 11).

3 Better bonding between mother, father and child, and an increased likelihood of attempting breast feeding (Chapter 11).

261

RECOMMENDATIONS FOR IMPLEMENTATION

Government 1 The DHSS should issue guidelines to health authorities to ensure that there is adequate provision for women who wish to have a home delivery.

2 The policy of closure of small GP units should be reviewed.

3 The Maternity Services Advisory Committee should be asked to review the extent to which its recommendations have been implemented on a national basis.

4 Funds should be made available to ensure that genetic counselling services are available in every region. This should be based on a proper assessment of differential regional needs.

Health promotion 1 Efforts to promote health and minimise all drug use during pregnancy should be sensitive to the competing demands on pregnant women and should avoid using a guilt-inducing approach.

2 Efforts should be made to achieve the widest possible distribution of multilingual educational material in primary care, community centres and organisations – especially those which cater for Asian women.

3 The information covered should explain the value and purpose of the components of antenatal care, emphasising:
- maternity entitlement and benefits;
- the importance of early attendance in screening for congenital abnormalities and genetic diseases;
- the role and value of antenatal classes;
- the tests and monitoring used during antenatal care;
- the value of an equal partnership between the user and doctor or midwife.

Local authorities Education about preparation for parenthood should form part of an integrated course on health education in all secondary schools.

Health authorities and primary care 1 A clearly defined, long-term strategy for the improvement of maternity services should form part of every district and FPC's (and Scottish equivalents) plans.

2 There should be a maternity services committee in every district responsible for coordinating policy implementation.

3 The Maternity Services Advisory Committee's recommendations should be implemented, and there should be an explicit mechanism for monitoring implementation.

4 Adequate arrangements should be made to ensure that women in low risk categories are able to have a home delivery.

262

Employers and trades unions

1 Workplace policy should ensure that pregnant women are not exposed to unnecessary, potential hazards.
2 Efforts should be made to inform and encourage pregnant women employees about the benefits of early registration for antenatal care.
3 Working hours and shifts should be arranged so that attendance at antenatal clinic is made easy.
4 Trades unions and employers should negotiate adequate pay during maternity leave.

Immunisation

General objectives

1 To offer an immunisation programme to protect all children from polio, diphtheria, pertussis, measles and mumps. This should form part of a child health surveillance system which promotes joint participation between parents, children and health professionals.
2 To ensure that all children in high risk groups are immunised against TB.
3 To promote a better understanding of the value of immunisation to parents and health professionals.

TARGETS TO BE ACHIEVED BY THE YEAR 2000 (OR EARLIER)

1 To maintain diphtheria, tetanus and polio immunisation uptake rates at 85 per cent or higher.
2 To increase pertussis and measles vaccine uptake to at least 90 per cent.
3 To immunise at least 90 per cent of all boys and girls under two against rubella.
4 To immunise at least 90 per cent of all under-twos with the triple measles/mumps/rubella vaccine.

EXPECTED HEALTH OUTCOMES

Physical health

1 A reduction to negligible levels of measles and of measles encephalitis (Chapter 12).
2 The virtual elimination of congenital rubella syndrome and its associated deafness, blindness and severe intellectual impairment (Chapter 12).
3 A major reduction in the incidence of rubella (Chapter 12).
4 The reduction of whooping cough incidence and its complications to negligible levels (Chapter 12).
5 The virtual elimination of mumps and its adverse effects on fertility (Chapter 12).

263

RECOMMENDATIONS FOR IMPLEMENTATION

Government
1 Progress towards immunisation targets in the UK should be reviewed in 1990. If uptake levels are not satisfactory, then consideration should be given to make immunisation mandatory for children without contra-indications.
2 The triple measles/mumps/rubella vaccine should be introduced as soon as possible as part of the immunisation programme for children under two years of age.
3 Education and information campaigns should reinforce government policy in the achievement of stated targets and should aim to inform professionals and public about any changes in policy. The mass media do not always provide the best channel for communicating sensitive information intended to allay professional and parental fears about perceived hazards of immunisation.

Health authorities and primary care
1 Specific immunisation targets should form part of district and strategic plans.
2 A nominated member of the health authority staff should be given overall responsibility for overseeing and implementing the immunisation programme.
3 Each authority should operate a child health computing system which allows flexible call and recall of children requiring immunisation.
4 Authorities should offer an immunisation advisory service for parents who wish to discuss their concerns with a trained nurse or community physician.
5 There needs to be an immunisation strategy within primary care.
6 A person in every general practice should be designated to be responsible for coordinating and ensuring accurate monitoring of immunisation plans.
7 Separate responsibilities for immunisation should be agreed among participating professional groups in general practice.
8 Accurate updated immunisation records should be kept for every child registered in a general practice.
9 There should be a mechanism for audit or review of progress in achieving agreed immunisation targets in individual practices.

Dental health

General objectives
1 To prevent dental ill health and promote dental health throughout all sectors of the community.
2 To help create a new generation of children free from dental decay.

264

3 To promote a better understanding of the determinants of oral and dental health among children, their parents and professionals.

TARGETS TO BE ACHIEVED BY THE YEAR 2000 (OR EARLIER)

1 At least 75 per cent of the community should have fluoridated water supplies.
2 Per capita sugar consumption should be reduced from 38 kilograms per year to 20 kilograms per year with a reduction of the consumption of sugary foods between meals (see also Strategy for Nutrition, pages 242–246). The social disparity in sugar consumption should be reduced.
3 At least 95 per cent of children and adults should brush their teeth regularly.
4 At least 95 per cent of primary and secondary school children should understand the causes of tooth decay and chronic gum disease.
5 All children should be encouraged to use fluoride toothpaste – especially in non-fluoridated areas.
6 At least 95 per cent of parents should understand the role of sugar in causing tooth decay.

EXPECTED HEALTH OUTCOMES

ysical health
1 An increase in the proportion of five year olds who are free from tooth decay (Chapter 12)
2 An increase in the proportion of twelve year olds with less than three decayed, missing or filled teeth (Chapter 12).
3 A decrease in the social disparity in the prevalence of tooth decay – especially in fluoridated areas (Chapter 12).
4 An increase in the proportion of those under 40 who retain all their own teeth (Chapter 12).
5 An increase in the proportion of 65–75 year olds who retain enough teeth to avoid the need for dentures (Chapters 12 and 14).
6 An increase in the proportion of people in all age groups – especially the over 65s – who are able to eat a wider range of foods containing complex carbohydrates, for example, fresh fruits (Chapters 3 and 12).
7 A decrease in the prevalence of gingivitis – the precursor to periodontal (chronic gum) disease – among young people.
8 A reduction in the amount of pain experienced in relation to tooth decay and its treatment in childhood and adolescence.

Mental and al wellbeing
1 A decrease in the proportion of people – especially the elderly – who are embarrassed by having to wear dentures.

2 A possible decrease in the cost to the NHS of supplying dentures.

RECOMMENDATIONS FOR IMPLEMENTATION

Government 1 The government should adopt a clearly defined strategy for promoting dental health, the components of which should be linked to the promotion of a healthier diet and measures to reduce smoking and tobacco use. (See Strategies for Tobacco and Nutrition pages 239 to 246).

2 The health departments should take a lead in stimulating activity between health authorities and water authorities to speed up fluoridation of water supplies.

3 The legislation enabling health authorities to ask water authorities to fluoridate water supplies should be extended to Northern Ireland.

4 This process should be supported and coordinated with local health education drives to alert parents and children to ways in which they can contribute towards dental health.

5 The dental health service should be more directly linked with primary health care services. The remuneration system should avoid payment on an exclusive fee-for-item-of-service basis.

6 A mechanism should be found for remunerating preventive as well as restorative care.

Health promotion 1 The programme for the promotion of dental health should be closely linked with that of promoting healthy nutrition and reducing tobacco consumption.

2 The role of sugar in causing dental decay needs more emphasis in public education programmes and should be closely linked to mass media approaches designed to promote a healthier diet.

3 Joint initiatives to train local teaching staff and incorporate dental health education programmes into school curricula should continue to be supported.

Training institutions 1 The prevention of dental disease and the promotion of oral health should form a major part of the teaching curriculum for dentists, dental hygienists and other auxiliary dental staff.

2 Dentists and auxiliary staff should be taught to encourage and develop the necessary communication skills to teach and support patients' efforts to protect their dental health.

3 The prevention of dental disease and the promotion of oral health should be formally assessed as part of dental training.

4 The training curriculum for doctors and nurses should cover the promotion of dental health; the links between the promotion of good oral health and good nutrition should be clearly made.

266

Local authorities

1 There should be a concerted effort by environmental health departments, health liaison committees and health authorities to encourage water authorities to fluoridate local water supplies.

2 Local authority nutrition policy should reflect (see Strategy on Nutrition page 242) the importance of promoting the consumption of complex carbohydrates rather than sugary foods.

3 A local education adviser should be designated as responsible for coordinating the integration of dental health education into primary and secondary school curricula.

Health authorities

1 Fluoridation of the local water supply should form part of health authority strategic and district plans.

2 A person with sufficient expertise (usually the community dental officer) should be designated as responsible for overseeing local policy to promote dental health, in particular the fluoridation programmes.

3 If the local water supply is not already fluoridated, negotiations should be started with the local water authority in order to implement fluoridation.

4 A liaison group should be established to coordinate dental health activities between the local authority, health authority and water authority.

5 The school health service should be directly involved in the promotion of dental health in the schools.

Early cancer detection services

General objectives

1 To offer comprehensive breast (and cervical) cancer screening services (see also Strategy on Sexuality, pages 252–257) to all eligible women.

2 To promote public and professional understanding of the benefits of regular screening for breast (and cervical) cancer (see also Strategy on Sexuality).

TARGETS TO BE ACHIEVED BY THE YEAR 2000
(OR EARLIER)

1 To screen at least 60 per cent of all women aged between 50 and 64 for breast cancer.

2 To increase the understanding of all adult women of the need for regular breast screening.

3 To increase the awareness of the medical profession of the benefits of breast screening.

267

4 To provide all women who are screened with adequate counselling and advice facilities.

EXPECTED HEALTH OUTCOMES

Physical health A reduction in mortality from breast cancer (among women aged 50–64) by up to one third (Chapters 4 and 7).

Mental and social wellbeing It is possible that screening could either increase or reduce anxiety related to breast cancer.

RECOMMENDATIONS FOR IMPLEMENTATION

Government 1 Sufficient central funding should be allocated to fully support health authorities in the implementation of a comprehensive breast screening service.

2 The age eligibility range for breast screening should be kept under review so that if new evidence suggests that the programme can be extended either to younger or older women, this can be implemented.

3 A pilot study of the effectiveness and long-term consequences of extending the upper age limit for screening from 65 to 74 should be conducted.

Health promotion 1 The gradual run-up to implementation of the current breast screening programme should be used as an opportunity to increase awareness of the purpose and advantages of the programme among women over 50.

2 Funds should be specifically set aside for a new information and education programme on breast screening aimed at women over 50 and their general practitioners.

3 Health promotion authorities should take a lead in assembling and disseminating examples of good organisational practice that emerge from those health authorities and general practices currently piloting the new breast screening programme. The aim should be to promote and monitor good practice elsewhere and avoid the inefficiencies of the cervical screening programme so far.

4 The gradual implementation process should be used as an opportunity to identify information and counselling needs for women attending breast screening clinics, and anything that might discourage women from attending.

5 Based on such findings, literature should be sensitively designed and made widely available to women through the workplace, and at primary care and gynaecology clinics. An attempt should be made to answer women's questions about breast screening and the

treatment of breast cancer.

6 The effectiveness of a mass media campaign designed to encourage attendance at breast screening clinics should be carefully piloted and evaluated before being launched on a national basis.

Health authorities and primary care

1 Targets for achieving medium-term screening rates among women aged between 50 and 64 should be set.

2 The recommendations of the Forrest report should be adopted including:

- the establishment nationwide of multidisciplinary screening units across approximately two DHAs (health boards) covering a population of about 50,000 women each;
- the equipment of each unit with adequately trained staff and appropriate mammographic equipment;
- the designation of a community physician responsible for the implementation and monitoring of the service;
- the compilation of an up-to-date call/recall system from FPC registers to call women aged between 50 and 64 for screening every three years;
- personal invitations to all eligible women to attend a screening clinic.

3 Information and counselling should be seen as an integral part of every district/health board screening service – although the manner in which this should be set up has yet to be established.

4 Every general practice should designate one person to be in charge of overseeing, monitoring and auditing breast screening in the practice.

5 Every practice should have a clearly established procedure through which results of breast screening are conveyed to women and should make provisions for dealing with any further queries and follow-up that might be needed.

Employers and trades unions

1 Efforts should be made to increase awareness among women employees of the value of breast screening for those over 50.

2 Occupational health staff should monitor the screening status of women staff over 50 and investigate the costs and benefits of developing on-site screening facilities.

High blood pressure reduction

General objectives

1 To promote regular screening for high blood pressure among all adult men and women.

2 To promote a better understanding among professionals and public of the factors which contribute to high blood pressure.

269

3 To promote a better understanding of the importance of blood pressure screening in the prevention of disease.

TARGETS TO BE ACHIEVED BY THE YEAR 2000 (OR EARLIER)

1 To reduce the average blood pressure of the population.
2 To increase to at least two-thirds the proportion of people aged between 35 and 64 who have their blood pressure checked every five years.
3 To increase to at least 80 per cent the proportion of people with high blood pressure who are adequately treated and followed up.
4 To increase the proportion of health professionals and public who are aware that a diet high in salt, physical inactivity and obesity contribute to high blood pressure.
5 To reduce the average daily intake of salt (see Strategy on Nutrition, pages 242–246).

EXPECTED HEALTH OUTCOMES

Physical health 1 A reduction in the incidence and mortality from stroke (Chapters 3 and 14).
2 A possible reduction in coronary heart disease incidence (Chapter 3).
3 A possible reduction in disability and dependence in old age.

RECOMMENDATIONS FOR IMPLEMENTATION

Government 1 The government should take a lead in the campaign to prevent the health consequences of high blood pressure by emphasising its importance in existing programmes to reduce heart disease and in a new programme to reduce stroke.

Health promotion 1 New emphasis should be given to the control of high blood pressure in relevant existing health promotion programmes, including the prevention of heart disease and the promotion of a healthy lifestyle – especially in relation to diet and the prevention of obesity.
2 A new public and professional information programme should be established with the aim of increasing awareness of the health consequences of high blood pressure. Special emphasis should be given to the less well-known risk factors for high blood pressure, such as heavy alcohol consumption, obesity, physical inactivity and a high salt diet.
3 A new national plan should be established for increasing professional and public commitment to five-yearly screening for high blood pressure for all adults aged between 35 and 64 in primary

270

care and at the workplace. Consideration should be given to the promotion of self-monitoring for high blood pressure and actively involving pharmacies in this enterprise.

4 Examples of well-organised screening and follow-up programmes, both in primary care and at the workplace, should be widely disseminated to promote effective and efficient practice throughout the country.

5 The value of non-pharmacological approaches to the treatment of high blood pressure should be given wider publicity.

Health authorities and primary care

1 Every health authority, FPC and general practice should set clearly defined targets for both the reduction in the proportion of the population with high blood pressure and screening rates to be achieved in this population over a five year period.

2 A manager should be designated in every general practice with responsibility for overseeing and monitoring the efficiency of the blood pressure screening programme.

3 Responsibility for conducting screening in every practice should be clearly agreed between the health professionals involved.

4 Every practice should have a clearly defined, preferably computerised, system for recording, monitoring and following up patients who are screened and require treatment. This should include a means of regular review of treatment as well.

5 Doctors and nurses involved in the screening programme should not lose the opportunity of a screening session or interview to advise and monitor the primary prevention of high blood pressure and other aspects of lifestyle, including the avoidance of obesity and a high-salt diet, reduction of heavy drinking and physical inactivity. Active and informed participation by patients should be encouraged.

6 There should be better liaison and information exchange between primary care and specialist services concerning the initial diagnosis and subsequent treatment of high blood pressure, either in general practice or in hospital.

Employers and trades unions

1 Information should be made widely available to all staff of the importance of preventing high blood pressure, how this might be achieved and the contribution to be made by five-yearly blood pressure check-ups.

2 Occupational health staff should, in consultation with employees and health and safety representatives, establish a workplace blood pressure screening and monitoring programme for all staff.

References

Chapter 1

1 Robbins C, ed. Health promotion in North America: implications for the UK. London, King Edward's Hospital Fund for London, 1987.
2 Department of Health and Social Security. Public health in England. London, HMSO, 1988.
3 King's Fund Institute. Healthy public policy: a role for the HEA. London, King's Fund Institute, 1987.
4 Castle P, Jacobson B. The health of our regions: an analysis of the strategies and policies of regional health authorities for promoting health and preventing disease. A report for the Health Education Council. Birmingham, NHS Regions Health Promotion Group, 1988.
5 Pavitt L. NHS expenditure on disease prevention and health promotion. Written answer PQ533, 1 December, 1986/87.
6 Cohen R, Henderson J R. A minister for prevention. An initiative in health policy. Discussion paper 2/83, Health Economics Research Unit, University of Aberdeen, 1983.
7 See 4.
8 Department of Health and Social Security. Health promotion in the NHS: a report on visits by a DHSS task force. Health Trends, 1987, 19: 27–29.
9 World Health Organization. Targets for health for all – targets in support of the European regional strategy for health for all. Copenhagen, WHO, 1985.
10 Department of Health and Human Services, Public Health Services. Promoting health/preventing disease – objectives for the nation. Washington DC, DHHS, 1986.
11 Epp J. Achieving health for all: a framework for health promotion. Ottawa, Ministry of National Health and Welfare, 1986.
12 World Health Organization. Ottawa charter for health promotion. An international conference on health promotion. Copenhagen, WHO, 1986.
13 Faculty of Community Medicine. Health for all by the year 2000. Charter for action. London, Faculty of Community Medicine, 1986.
14 Ashton J. Healthy cities. Health Promotion, 1986. 1,2: 319–324.
15 Department of Health and Social Security. Prevention and health: everybody's business. London, HMSO, 1976.
16 Department of Health and Social Security. Care in action. A handbook of policies and priorities for health and social services in England. London, HMSO, 1981.
17 House of Commons Committee of Public Accounts. 44th report: preventive medicine. Session 1985–1986. London, HMSO, 1986.
18 See 3.
19 Parliament. The National Health Service, England and Wales. The Welsh Health Promotion Authority (Establishment and Constitution) order, 1980. London, HMSO, 1987. Statutory instrument no 151.
20 Welsh Office. Welsh Health Promotion Authority: policy memorandum. Cardiff, Welsh Office, 1987.
21 Welsh Office. A corporate management programme for the health service in Wales. Development and change 1987–1992. A consultation document. Cardiff, Welsh Office, 1987.
22 Whitehead M. Education for health: achievements of a decade. Scottish Health Education Group, 1988 (in press).

23 See 22.
24 Directorate of the Welsh Heart Programme. Take heart. Consultative document. Heartbeat report no 1. Cardiff, Heartbeat Wales, 1985.

Chapter 2

1 Office of Population Censuses and Surveys. Studies in sudden infant deaths. Studies on medical and population subjects no 45. London. HMSO, 1982.
2 Office of Population Censuses and Surveys. Sudden infant death syndrome 1983, 1984. OPCS Monitor, reference DH3 85/4, 13 August 1985.

Chapter 3

1 Wells N. Coronary heart disease: the need for action. London, Office of Health Economics, 1987.
2 Rose G, Marmot M G. Social class and coronary heart disease. British Heart Journal, 1981, 45: 13–19.
3 Coronary Prevention Group. Coronary heart disease and Asians in Britain. A report prepared by the CPG for the Confederation of Indian Organisations. London, CPG, 1986.
4 World Health Organization. Prevention of coronary heart disease. Report of a WHO expert committee. Technical report series 678. Geneva, WHO, 1982.
5 World Health Organization. Community prevention and control of cardiovascular diseases. Report of a WHO expert committee. Geneva, WHO/DVD85.2: 1984.
6 National Heart Foundation Australia. Dietary fat and heart disease: a review. Medical Journal of Australia, 1974: 575–579; 616–620; 663–668.
7 Department of Health and Welfare. Report of committee on diet and cardiovascular disease. Ottawa, DHW, 1976.
8 American Heart Association. Special report. Inter-society commission for heart disease resources. Circulation 1984: 70(1): 153A–205A.
9 European Atherosclerosis Society. Strategies for the prevention of coronary heart disease. European Heart Journal, 1987, 8: 77–88.
10 World Health Organization. Healthy nutrition: preventing nutrition-related disease in Europe. Copenhagen, WHO, 1988 (in press).
11 Anon. Consensus conference on lowering blood cholesterol to prevent heart disease. Journal of the American Medical Association, 1985, 253: 2080–86.
12 Royal College of Physicians and British Cardiac Society. Prevention of coronary heart disease. London, BCS, 1976.
13 British Cardiac Society. Report of British Cardiac Society working group on coronary disease prevention. London, BCS, 1987.
14 Committee on medical aspects of diet. Diet and cardiovascular disease. Report on health and social subjects no 28. London, HMSO, 1984.
15 National Advisory Committee on Nutrition Education. Proposals for nutritional guidelines in Britain: a discussion paper. London, Health Education Council, 1983.
16 Royal College of Physicians. Health or smoking? A follow-up report. London, Pitman Medical, 1983.
17 See 16.
18 US Surgeon General. The health consequences of smoking: cardiovascular disease, a report of the US Surgeon General. Washington DC, DHHS, 1983.
19 US Surgeon General. The changing cigarette. A report from the Surgeon General.

Washington DC, DHHS, 1981.

20 Rose G, Shipley M. Plasma cholesterol concentration and death from coronary heart disease: 10 year results of the Whitehall study. British Medical Journal, 1986, 293: 306–307.

21 Shaper A G, Pocock S J et al. Risk factors for ischaemic heart disease: the prospective phase of the British Regional Heart Study. Journal of Epidemiology and Community Health, 1985, 39: 197–209.

22 Anon. The value of preventive medicine. The CIBA Symposium 110. London, Pitman, 1985.

23 Peto R. Blood cholesterol, CHD and non-CHD mortality: evidence from all available randomised trials, reviewed in their epidemiological context (in press).

24 See 23.

25 See 20.

26 Martin M J, Hulley S B et al. Serum cholesterol, blood pressure and mortality: implications from a cohort of 361,662 men. The Lancet, 25 October 1986: 933–936.

27 Shaper A G. British blood cholesterol values and the American consensus. British Medical Journal, 1985, 291: 480–481.

28 Lewis B, Mann J I et al. Reducing the risks of coronary heart disease in individuals and the population. The Lancet, 1986, i: 956–959.

29 See 4.

30 See 13.

31 See 14.

32 See 28.

33 Cannon G. The politics of food. London, Century Hutchinson, 1987.

34 See 28.

35 Wenlock R W, Disselduff M M et al. The diets of British schoolchildren. London. Department of Health and Social Security, 1986.

36 Herfst H et al. The nutritive value of school and hospital meals. In: The proceedings of the Nutrition Society. Cambridge, University Press, 1984.

37 Raheja B S. Indians, diet and heart disease. The Lancet, 26 July 1986: 228.

38 McKeigue P M, Marmot M G et al. Diet and risk factors for coronary disease in Asians in northwest London. The Lancet, 16 November 1985: 1086–1090.

39 Silman A, Loysen E et al. Diet and risk factors for coronary heart disease in Asians in northwest London. Journal of Epidemiology and Community Health, 1985, 39: 301–303.

40 Peterson D B, Dattain J T et al. Dietary practices of Asian diabetics. British Medical Journal, 18 January 1986: 170–171.

41 See 4.

42 World Health Organization. Primary prevention of essential hypertension. WHO technical report series no 686. Geneva, WHO, 1983.

43 See 4.

44 Rose G. Strategy of prevention: lessons from cardiovacular disease. British Medical Journal, 1981, 282: 1847–1851.

45 Rose G. Sick individuals and sick populations. International Journal of Epidemiology, 1985, 14, 1: 32–38.

46 See 42.

47 Health Promotion Committee, Faculty of Community Medicine. Dietary salt and health (in press).

48 Cox B D, Blaxter M et al. The health and lifestyle survey. London, Health Promotion Research Trust, 1987.

49 Directorate of the Welsh Heart Programme. Pulse of Wales. Preliminary report of the Welsh heart survey. Heartbeat report no 4. Cardiff, Heartbeat Wales, 1986.

50 Cruickshank J K, Jackson S H D et al. Similarity of blood pressure in blacks, whites

and Asians in England: the Birmingham factory study. Journal of Hypertension 1985, 3: 365–371.

51 James W P T, Ralph A et al. The dominance of salt in manufactured food in the sodium intake of affluent societies. The Lancet, 21 February 1987: 426–429.

52 Medical Research Council Working Party. MRC Trial of treatment of mild hypertension: principle results. British Medical Journal, 13 July 1985: 97–104.

53 Breckenridge A (editorial). Treating mild hypertension. British Medical Journal, 13 July 1985: 89–90.

54 Patel C, Marmot M G et al. Trial of relaxation in reducing coronary risk: four year follow up. British Medical Journal, 13 April 1985: 1103–1106.

55 Royal College of Physicians. Obesity. A report. Journal of the Royal College of Physicians of London, 1983, 17, 1.

56 See 55.

57 Gatling W, Houston A C et al. The prevalence of diabetes mellitus in a typical English community. Journal of the Royal College of Physicans of London, 1985, 19, 4: 248–250.

58 Yudkin J. Nutritional factors in the aetiology of diabetes. (In press).

59 Anon. (editorial). Insulin-dependent? The Lancet, 12 October 1985: 809–810.

60 Anon. (editorial). Coronary heart disease in Indians overseas. The Lancet, 7 June 1986: 1307–1308.

61 Beckles G L A, Kirkwood B R et al. High total and cardiovascular disease mortality in adults of Indian descent in Trinidad, unexplained by major coronary risk factors. The Lancet, 7 June 1986: 1298–1300.

62 Padhani A, Dandona P. Diabetes and coronary heart disease in north London Asians. The Lancet, 25 January 1986: 213–214.

63 Mather H M, Keen H. The Southall diabetes survey: Prevalence of known diabetes in Asians and Europeans. British Medical Journal, 1985, 291: 1081–1084.

64 See 2.

65 Marmot M G (editorial). Type A behaviour and ischaemic heart disease. Psychological Medicine, 1980, 10: 603–606.

66 Mitchell J R A (editorial). Hearts and minds. British Medical Journal, 8 December 1984: 1557–1558.

67 Marmot M G. Look after your heart: stress and cardiovascular disease. Health Trends 1987, 19, 3: 21–25.

68 Theorell T. Stress at work. In Proceedings: Stress and Coronary Heart Disease. Coronary Prevention Group, London, 1986.

69 Shaper A G, Pocock S J et al. British Regional Heart Study: cardiovascular risk factors in middle-aged men in 24 towns. British Medical Journal, 1981, 283: 179–186.

70 Anon. (editorial). Coffee and cholesterol. The Lancet, 7 December 1985: 1283–1284.

71 LaCroix A Z, Mead L A et al. Coffee consumption and the incidence of coronary heart disease. New England Journal of Medicine, 1986, 315, 16: 977–982.

72 Marmot M G. Alcohol and coronary heart disease. International Journal of Epidemiology, 1984, 13, 2: 160–167.

73 Shaper A G, Philips A N et al. Alcohol and ischaemic heart disease in middle aged British men. British Medical Journal, 21 March 1987: 733–736.

74 See 22.

75 Puska P, Salonen J T et al. Change in risk factors for coronary heart disease during 10 years of a community intervention programme. British Medical Journal, 1983, 287: 1840–1844.

76 WHO Collaborative Group. European collaboration trial of multi-factorial prevention of coronary heart disease: final report on the six year results. The Lancet, 19 April 1986: 869–872.

77 See 44.
78 See 49.
79 D'Arcy Masius Benton & Bowles. The DMB & B Healthy Eating Study. London, Benton & Bowles, 1986.
80 Marmot M G. Interpretation of trends in coronary heart disease mortality. Acta Medica Scandinavica supplement, 1985, 701: 58–65.
81 Epstein F H. Lessons from falling coronary heart disease mortality in the United States. Postgraduate Medical Journal 1984, 60: 15–19.
82 Stamler J. Coronary heart disease: doing the 'right thing'. New England Journal of Medicine, 312, 16: 1053–1055.
83 Marmot M G. Life style and national and international trends in coronary heart disease mortality. Postgraduate Medical Journal 1984, 60: 3–8.
84 See 82.
85 Anon. The public and high blood pressure. Six year survey of public knowledge and reported behaviour. Washington DC, US DHHS, 1981.
86 See 82.
87 Kurji K H, Haines A P. Detection and management of hypertension in general practices in north west London. British Medical Journal, 24 March 1984: 903–906.
88 Coope J, Warrender T S. Randomised trial of hypertension in elderly patients in primary care. British Medical Journal, 1986, 293: 1145–1146.
89 Fullard E, Fowler G et al. Promoting prevention in primary care: controlled trial of low technology, low cost approach. British Medical Journal, 1987, 294: 1080–1082.
90 Hall J A. Audit of screening for hypertension in general practice. Journal of the Royal College of General Practitioners, May 1985: 243.
91 Hart J T. The management of high blood pressure in general practice. Journal of the Royal College of General Practitioners, 1975, 25: 160–192.
92 See 87.
93 See 85.
94 See 55.

Chapter 4

1 Doll R, Peto R. The causes of cancer. Oxford, Oxford University Press, 1981.
2 See 1.
3 See 1.
4 Health or Smoking. A follow-up report of the Royal College of Physicians. London, Pitman Medical, 1983.
5 Action on smoking and health. The economic consequences of smoking in Northern Ireland: a cost benefit analysis of tobacco production and use in the province. Belfast, ASH, 1986.
6 Department of Health and Human Services. The health consequences of involuntary smoking. A report of the Surgeon General. Washington DC, US DHHS, 1986.
7 National Health and Medical Research Council. Effects of passive smoking on health. Camberra, NH & MRC, 1987.
8 Wald N J, Namchahal K et al. Does breathing other people's tobacco smoke cause lung cancer? British Medical Journal, 1986, 293: 1217–1221.
9 US Department of Health and Human Services. The health consequences of using smokeless tobacco. A report of the Advisory Committee to the Surgeon General. Washington DC, US DHHS, 1986.
10 Harrison D F N. Dangers of snuff both 'wet' and 'dry'. British Medical Journal, 1986, 293: 405–406.

11 Jones P. Awareness of skoal bandits. British Medical Journal, 1986, 292: 1201.

12 Parkin D M, Stjernsward J. Cancer control, estimates of the world frequency of twelve major cancers. Bulletin of WHO, 1984, 62, 2: 163–182.

13 Boyle P, Zaridze D G et al. Descriptive epidemiology of colectoral cancer. International Journal of Cancer, 1985, 36: 9–18.

14 National Cancer Institutes. Cancer prevention research summary – nutrition. Washington DC, US DHHS, 1985.

15 Armstrong B, Doll R. Environmental factors and cancer incidence and mortality in different countries, with special references to dietary factors. International Journal of Cancer, 1975, 15: 617–631.

16 Royal College of Physicians. Medical aspects of dietary fibre: a report of The Royal College of Physicians. London, Pitman Medical, 1981.

17 See 1.

18 See 1.

19 Bingham S A, Williams D R R et al. Dietary fibre consumption in Britain: new estimates and their relation to large bowel cancer mortality. British Journal of Cancer, 1985, 52: 399–402.

20 See 13.

21 Bristol J B, Emmett P M et al. Sugar, fat, and the risk of colorectal cancer. British Medical Journal, 1985, 291: 1467–1470.

22 Hardcastle J D, Armitage N C. Early diagnosis of colorectal cancer: a review. Journal of the Royal Society of Medicine, 1984, 77: 673–674.

23 Nichols S, Koch R et al. Randomised trial of compliance with screening for colorectal cancer. British Medical Journal, 1986, 293: 107–110.

24 Gilbertson V A, McHugh R et al. The earlier detection of colorectal cancers. A preliminary report of the results of the occult blood study. Cancer, 1980, 45: 2899–2901.

25 Hardcastle J D, Farrands P A et al. Controlled trial of faecal occult blood testing in the detection of colorectal cancer. The Lancet, 1983 ii: 1–4.

26 Michalek A M. Occult blood screening. The Lancet, 1986, 19 April 1986: 907–908.

27 Winawer S J et al. Screening for colorectal cancer. In: Miller A B, Screening for cancer. London, Academic Press, 1985.

28 Anon. (editorial). Questions about occult blood screening for cancer. The Lancet, 4 January 1986: 22.

29 Frank J W. Occult blood screening. The Lancet, 24 May 1986: 1204.

30 Pike M C, Ross R K. Breast cancer. British Medical Bulletin, 1984: 351–354.

31 Kalache A, Vessey M. Risk factors for breast cancer. Clinics in Oncology, 1982, 3: 661–667.

32 See 30.

33 See 1.

34 See 14.

35 Meirik O, Lund E et al. Oral contraceptive use and breast cancer in young women. The Lancet, 20 September 1986: 650–653.

36 Pike M C, Henderson B E et al. Breast cancer in young women and use of oral contraceptives: possible modifying effect of formulation and age at use. The Lancet, 1983, ii: 926–30.

37 Olsson H, Landin Olsen M et al. Oral contraceptive use and breast cancer in young women. The Lancet, 1985, i: 748–49.

38 Stadel B V, Rubin G L et al. Oral contraceptives and breast cancer in young women. The Lancet, 1985, ii: 970–73.

39 Rosenberg L, Miller D R. Breast cancer and oral contraceptive use. American Journal of Epidemiology, 1984, 119: 167–76.

40 McPherson K, Neil A et al. Oral contraceptives and breast cancer. The Lancet, 1983, ii: 1414–15.

41 Paul C, Skegg D C G et al. Oral contraceptives and breast cancer: a national study. British Medical Journal, 20 September 1986: 723–726.
42 Anon. (editorial). Oral contraceptives and breast cancer. The Lancet, 20 September 1986: 665–666.
43 McPherson K (editorial). The pill and breast cancer: why the uncertainty? British Medical Journal, 20 September 1986: 70–71.
44 Osmond C, Gardner M J et al. Trends in cancer mortality 1951–1981. London, HMSO, 1983.
45 Singer A et al. Genital wart virus infections: nuisance or potentially lethal? British Medical Journal, 1984, 288: 735–737.
46 See 45.
47 British Medical Association. Cervical cancer and screening in Great Britain. London, BMA, 1986.
48 Anon. (editorial). Genital warts, human papilloma viruses and cervical cancer. The Lancet, 9 November 1985: 1045–1046.
49 Harris R W C et al. Characteristics of women with dysplasia or carcinoma in situ of the cervix uteri. British Journal of Cancer, 1980, 42: 359–369.
50 Skegg D G et al. Importance of the male factor in cancer of the cervix. The Lancet, 1982, ii: 581–583.
51 Austin D F. Smoking and cervical cancer. Journal of American Medical Association, 1983, 250, 4: 516–517.
52 Hellberg D et al. Smoking as a risk factor in cervical neoplasia. The Lancet, 24/31 December 1983: 1497.
53 Thomas D B, Holck S et al. Invasive cervical cancer and combined oral contraceptives. British Medical Journal 1985, 290: 961–965.
54 Wright N H et al. Neoplasia and dysplasia of the cervix uteri and contraception – a possible protective effect of the diaphragm. British Journal of Cancer, 1978, 38, 2: 237–239.
55 Beral, V, Booth M. Predictions of cervical cancer incidence and mortality in England and Wales. The Lancet, 1 March 1986: 495.
56 Black Sir Douglas (chair). Investigation of the possible increase incidence of cancer in West Cumbria. Report of the Independent Advisory Group. London, HMSO, 1984.
57 Jakeman D. Notes on the level of radioactive contamination in the Sellafield area arising from discharges in the early 1950s. Dorchester, UK Atomic Energy Establishment, 1986.
58 Heasman M A, Kemp I W et al. Incidence of leukaemia in young persons in west of Scotland. The Lancet, 1984, i: 1188–89.
59 Barton C J, Roman E et al. Childhood leukaemia in west Berkshire. The Lancet, 1985, ii: 1248–49.
60 Heaseman M A, Kemp I W et al. Childhood leukaemia in northern Scotland. The Lancet, 1986, i: 266.
61 Cook-Mozaffari P J, Vincent T et al. Cancer incidence and mortality in the vicinity of nuclear installations. England and Wales, 1959–1980. Studies in medical population subjects no 51. London, HMSO, 1987.
62 Beral V. Cancer near nuclear installations. The Lancet, 7 March 1987: 556.
63 Darby S C, Doll R. Fallout radiation doses near Dounreay and childhood leukaemia. British Medical Journal, 1987, 294: 603–607.

Chapter 5

1 Peterson B, Kristensson H et al. Alcohol-related death: a major contributor to mortality in urban middle-aged men. The Lancet, 13 November 1982: 1088–1090.

2 Royal College of Physicians. The medical consequences of alcohol abuse: a great and growing evil. London, Tavistock, 1987.
3 Royal College of General Practitioners. Alcohol – a balanced view. London, RCGP, 1987.
4 Anon. Putting alcohol onto the agenda. The Lancet, 22 November 1986: 1230.
5 McDonnell R, Maynard A. Estimation of life years lost from alcohol-related premature death. Alcohol and Alcoholism, 1985, 20, 4: 435–443.
6 World Health Organization. Problems related to alcohol consumption. Report of a WHO expert committee. Technical report series no 650. Geneva, WHO, 1980.
7 Office of Health Economics. Alcohol: reducing the harm. London, Office of Health Economics, 1981.
8 Plant M L. Women, drinking and pregnancy. London, Tavistock, 1985.
9 Rubin P C et al. Prospective survey of use of therapeutic drugs, alcohol and cigarettes during pregnancy. British Medical Journal, 11 January 1986: 81–83.
10 Kreitman N. Alcohol consumption and the preventive paradox. British Journal of Addiction, 1986, 81: 353–363.
11 See 6.
12 Royal College of Psychiatrists. Alcohol our favourite drug. London, Tavistock, 1986.
13 See 2.
14 See 3.
15 British Medical Association. Young people and alcohol. London, BMA, 1986.
16 Shaper A G, Phillips A N. Alcohol and ischaemic heart disease in middle-aged British men. British Medical Journal, 1987, 294: 733–736.
17 Marmot M G. Alcohol and coronary heart disease. International Journal of Epidemiology, 1984, 13, 2: 160–167.
18 See 6.
19 See 12.
20 Goddard E. Drinking and attitudes to licensing in Scotland. OPCS social survey division. London, HMSO, 1986.
21 Plant M A, Peck D F. Alcohol, drugs and school leavers. London, Tavistock, 1986.
22 Marsh A, Dobbs J et al. Adolescent drinking. A survey carried out on behalf of the Department of Health and Social Security and the Scottish Home and Health Department. London, HMSO, 1986.
23 See 6.
24 See 12.
25 Central Policy Review Staff. Alcohol policies in the United Kingdom. Stockholm, University of Stockholm, 1982.
26 Kendell R E. The beneficial consequences of the United Kingdom's declining per capita consumption of alcohol in 1979–82. Alcohol and Alcoholism, 1984, 19, 4: 271–276.
27 Wells N. The AIDS virus. Forecasting its impact. London, Office of Health Economics, 1986.
28 See 27.
29 Adler M. ABC of Aids. Development of the epidemic. British Medical Journal, 1987, 294: 1083–1085.
30 Anderson R, May R. Plotting the spread of AIDS. New Scientist, 26 March 1987: 54–59.
31 Anon. Latest UK figures on AIDS. British Medical Journal, 1987, 295: 1004.
32 See 27.
33 Anon. AIDS – a public health crisis. Population Reports, Series L, no 6. Baltimore, John Hopkins University, July–August 1986.
34 Geddes A M. Risk of AIDS to health care workers. British Medical Journal, 1986, 292: 711–712.

35 Friedland G H, Brian M D et al. Lack of transmission of HTLV-III/LAV infection to household contacts of patients with AIDS or AIDS-related complex with oral candidiasis. New England Journal of Medicine, 1986, 314, 6: 344–349.

36 See 34.

37 See 33.

38 See 33.

39 McEvoy M, Porter K et al. Prospective study of clinical laboratory and ancillary staff with accidental exposure to blood or body fluids from patients infected with human immunovirus. British Medical Journal, 20 June 1987: 1595–1597.

40 Acheson E D. AIDS: a challenge for the public health. The Lancet, 22 March 1986: 662–665.

41 See 29.

42 See 27.

43 See 29.

44 Melbye M. The natural history of human T lymphotropic virus-III infection: the cause of AIDS. British Medical Journal, 4 January 1986, 292: 5–11.

45 See 40.

46 See 27.

47 Kingsley L A, Detels R et al. Risk factors for seroconversion to human immunodeficiency virus among male homosexuals. The Lancet, 14 February 1987: 345–348.

48 Evans B A, Dawson S G et al. Sexual lifestyle and clinical findings related to HTLV-III/LAV status in homosexual men. Genito-urinary Medicine, 1986, 62, 6: 384–389.

49 Darrow W W, Echenberg D F et al. Risk factors for HIV infection in homosexual men. American Journal of Public Health, 1987, 77, 4: 479–483.

50 Anon. Who will get AIDS? The Lancet, 25 October 1986: 953–954.

51 Winkelstein W, Samuel M et al. Selected sex practices of heterosexual men and risk of infection by the HIV. Journal of the American Medical Association, 1987, 257: 1470–1471.

52 Melbye M, Bayley A et al. Evidence for heterosexual transmission and clinical manifestations of human immunodeficiency virus infection and related conditions in Lusaka, Zambia. The Lancet, 15 November 1986: 1113–1116.

53 Van de Perre P, Carael M et al. Female prostitutes: a risk group for infection with human T-cell lymphotropic virus type III. The Lancet, 7 September 1985: 524–526.

54 Skidmore C. AIDS and intravenous drug users. Health Education Journal, 1987, 46, 2: 56–57.

55 Bradbeer C. HIV and sexual lifestyle. British Medical Journal, 3 January 1987, 294: 5–6.

56 UK Haemophilia Centre Directors. Prevalence of antibody to HTLV-III in haemophiliacs in the UK. British Medical Journal, 19 July 1986, 293: 175–176.

57 Moss A R. AIDS and intravenous drug use: the real heterosexual epidemic. British Medical Journal, 1987, 294: 389–390.

58 Robertson J R, Bucknall A B et al. Epidemic of AIDS related virus (HTLV/LAV) infection among intravenous drug abusers. British Medical Journal, 22 February 1986, 292: 527–529.

59 Marmor M, Des Jarlais D C et al. Risk factors for infection with human immunovirus among intravenous drug abusers in New York City. AIDS, 1987, 1: 39–44.

60 Fuchs D, Dierich M P et al. Are homosexuals less at risk of AIDS than intravenous drug abusers and haemophiliacs? The Lancet, 16 November 1985: 1130.

61 Brettle R P, Bisset K et al. Human immunodeficiency and drug misuse: the Edinburgh experience. British Medical Journal, 15 August 1987, 295: 421–424.

62 Robertson J R, Bucknall A B V. Regional variations in HIV antibody seropositivity in British intravenous drug users. The Lancet 1986, i: 1435–14.

63 Ancelle-Park R, Brunet J B et al. AIDS and drug addicts in Europe. The Lancet, 12

September 1987: 626–627.
64 See 63.
65 See 58.
66 See 27.
67 See 27.
68 Anderson R M, Blythe S P et al. Is it possible to predict the minimum size of the AIDS epidemic in the UK? The Lancet, 9 May 1987: 1073–1075.
69 Carne C A, Johnson A M et al. Prevalence of antibodies to human immunodeficiency virus, gonorrhoea rates and changed sexual behaviour in homosexual men in London. The Lancet, 21 March 1987: 656–658.
70 See 27.
71 See 30.
72 See 27.
73 See 29.
74 See 57.
75 See 54.

Chapter 6

1 Sabey B E, Staughton G C. Interacting roles of road environment, vehicle and road user. Proceedings of 5th conference of International Association for Accidents and Traffic Medicine, 1975.
2 Staughton G C, Storie V J. Methodology of an in-depth accident investigation survey. Transport and Road Research Laboratory report no 762. Crowthorne, TRRL, 1977.
3 Smeed R J. Some statistical aspects of road safety research. Journal of Royal Statistics Society, 1949, 1: 112.
4 Sabey B E. Accident situations. Presented to the Berzelius Symposium VIII Cars and Casualties. Crowthorne, TRRL, 1985.
5 Plowden S, Hillman M. Danger on the road: the needless scourge. London, Policy Studies Institute, 1984.
6 Borkenstein R F et al. The role of the drinking driver in traffic accidents. Indiana, Indiana Department of Police Administration, 1964.
7 Sabey B E. Drinking and driving: options for the future. Crowthorne, TRRL, 1985.
8 British Medical Association. Young people and alcohol. London, BMA, 1986.
9 Department of Transport. Road accidents in Great Britain 1985. London, Department of Transport, 1986.
10 See 5.
11 Sabey B E. Experience of speed limits in Great Britain. Paper to International Symposium on Traffic Speed and Casualties. Gammel Avernaes, Denmark, April 1975. Crowthorne, TRRL. 1975.
12 Scott P P. Speed limits and road accidents. Paper to 'TRAFFEX 77' Traffic Engineering and Road Safety Conference, Stoneleigh, Warwickshire, April 1977. Crowthorne, TRRL, 1977.
13 See 5.
14 See 5.
15 Hillman N. Lowering the speed of traffic. In: Road safety what next? Conference proceedings. London, Policy Studies Institute, 1986.
16 Ashton S J, Thomas P D et al. The effects of mandatory seat belt use in Great Britain. Presented at 10th International Conference of Experimental Safety Vehicles. Crowthorne, TRRL, 1985.

Chapter 7

1 Rose G. Strategy of prevention: lessons from cardiovascular disease. British Medical Journal, 1981, 6: 1847.
2 Rose G. Sick individuals and sick populations. International Journal of Epidemiology, 1985, 14: 32–38.
3 Oliver M. Strategies for preventing and screening for coronary heart disease. British Heart Journal, 1985, 54: 1–5.
4 Lewis P, Mann J I et al. Reducing the risks of coronary heart disease in individuals and in the population. The Lancet, 26 April 1986: 956–959.
5 See 1.
6 World Health Organization. Smoking and its effects on health. WHO technical report series no 568. Geneva, WHO, 1975.
7 World Health Organization. Controlling the smoking epidemic. Report of the WHO expert committee on smoking control. WHO technical report series no 636. Geneva, WHO, 1979.
8 House of Commons Expenditure Committee. First report: preventive medicine. Session 1976–77. London, HMSO, 1977.
9 Black Sir Douglas (Chair). Inequalities in health. Report of a research working group. London, Department of Health and Social Security, 1980.
10 Royal College of Physicians. Smoking and health. A report. London, Pitman Medical, 1962.
11 Royal College of Physicians. Smoking and health now. A report. London, Pitman Medical, 1971.
12 Royal College of Physicians. Health or smoking. A follow-up report. London, Pitman Medical, 1983.
13 Peto J. Price and consumption of cigarettes: a case for intervention? British Journal of Preventive and Social Medicine, 1974, 28: 241–245.
14 Atkinson A B, Townsend J L. Economic aspects of reduced smoking. The Lancet, 1977, 3: 492–495.
15 Townsend J. Economic and health consequences of reduced smoking. In: Williams A (ed). Health and economics. London, Macmillan, 1987.
16 Lewit E, Coate D et al. The effects of government regulations on teenage smoking. Journal of Law and Economics 1981, 24, 3: 17.
17 See 14.
18 Townsend J. Cigarette tax, economic welfare and social class patterns of smoking. Applied Economics, 1987, 19: 355–69.
19 See 18.
20 Anon. An evaluation of the effects of an increase in the price of tobacco and a proposal for the tobacco price policy in Finland in 1985/87. Helsinki, Advisory Committee on Health Education.
21 Godfrey C. Employment in the alcohol and tobacco industries and its relationship to prevention polities. Economic and Social Research Council Addiction Research Centre, 1986. Unpublished.
22 Crofton J, Wood M (eds). Smoking control, strategies and evaluation in community and mass media programmes. London, Health Education Council, 1985.
23 Amos A. Women's magazines and smoking. Health Education Journal 1984, 43, 2, 3: 45–50.
24 Russell M A H, Wilson C et al. Effects of general practitioners' advice against smoking. British Medical Journal, 1979, ii: 231–5.
25 Jamrozik K, Vessey M. Controlled trial of three different anti-smoking interventions in general practice. British Medical Journal, 1984, 288: 499–503.
26 Richmond R L, Austin A, Webster I W. Three year evaluation of a programme by general practitioners to help patients to stop smoking. British Medical Journal,

1986, 292: 803–806.

27 Department of Health and Human Services. The health consequences of smoking. Cancer and chronic lung disease in the workplace. Washington DC, US, DHHS, 1985.

28 Rose G et al. A randomised controlled trial of anti-smoking advice: 10 years' results. Journal of Epidemiology and Community Health, 1982, 36: 102–108.

29 Gillies P, Wilcox B. Reducing the risk of smoking amongst the young. Public Health, 1984, 98: 49–54.

30 Åaro L E, Bruland E, Hawknes A. Smoking among Norwegian school-children 1975–80, III. The effect of anti-smoking campaigns. Scandinavian Journal of Psychology, 1983, 24: 1–7.

31 Waterson M J. Advertising and cigarette consumption. London, Advertising Association, 1984.

32 Godfrey C. Government policy, advertising and tobacco consumption in the UK: a critical review of the literature. British Journal of Addiction, 1986, 81: 445–452.

33 McGuinness T, Cowling K. Advertising and the aggregate demand for cigarettes. European Economic Review, 1975, 6: 311–328.

34 Radfar M. The effect of advertising on total consumption of cigarettes in the United Kingdom. Working paper no 3. City of London Polytechnic, Department of Economics, 1983.

35 Roemer R. Recent developments in legislation to combat the world smoking epidemic. WHO/SMO/HLE/86. Geneva, WHO, 1986.

36 Cox H, Smith R. Political approaches to smoking control: a comparative analysis. Applied Economics, 1984, 16: 569–582.

37 Chapman S. Cigarette advertising and smoking: a review of the evidence. London, BMA Professional Division, 1985.

38 See 37.

39 Jacobson B. Beating the ladykillers. Women and smoking. London, Gollancz, 1988.

40 Lochsen P M et al. Trends in tobacco consumption and smoking habits in Norway. A report from the Norwegian Council on smoking and health. Oslo, Norwegian Council on Smoking and Health, 1984.

41 See 15.

42 National No Smoking Day Steering Committee. How effective was national no smoking day, 1984? Health Education Journal, 1985, 44: 59–65.

43 Scottish Health Education Coordinating Committee. Health education in the prevention of smoking-related disease. Edinburgh, SHEG, 1983.

44 Brotherston K G (ed). The Scottish epidemic. Edinburgh, Scottish Committee ASH, 1985.

45 Roberts J, Graveling O A (eds). The big kill. Smoking epidemic in England and Wales. For HEC and BMA. Manchester, North West Regional Health Authority, 1985.

46 Castle P, Jacobson B. The health of our regions. An analysis of the strategies and policies of regional health authorities for promoting health and preventing disease. A report for the Health Education Council. Birmingham, NHS Regions Health Promotion Group, 1988.

47 Greenoak J. A survey of district policies and initiatives on food and health. Health Education Council, 1985. Unpublished.

48 Crofton J. Health Education in the prevention of smoking related diseases. Scottish Health Boards. Forthcoming.

49 ASH. Local authority policy on smoking – a survey of councils in England and Wales. London, ASH, 1985.

50 Scottish Health Education Coordinating Committee. Health education in the prevention of smoking-related disease: the local authority response. April 1985.

Unpublished.

51 Royal College of General Practitioners. Prevention of arterial disease in general practice. Report no 19. London, RCGP, 1981.

52 Weaver R. Fluoride and wartime diet. British Dental Journal, 1985, 88, 9: 231–239.

53 World Health Organization. Prevention of coronary heart disease. Report of a WHO expert committee. Technical report series no 678. Geneva, WHO, 1982.

54 World Health Organization. Community prevention and control of cardiovascular diseases. Report of a WHO expert committee. Geneva, WHO/DVD85.2, 1984.

55 World Health Organization. Primary prevention of coronary heart disease. Report of a WHO meeting, Anacapri. Reports and studies no 98. Geneva, WHO, 1985. Forthcoming.

56 British Cardiac Society. Report of British Cardiac Society working group on coronary disease prevention. London, British Cardiac Society, 1987.

57 European Atherosclerosis Society. Strategies for the prevention of coronary heart disease. European Heart Journal, 1987, 8: 77–88.

58 Anon (editorial). European plan for heart disease prevention. British Medical Journal, 1987, 294: 449.

59 Tudor Hart J. Coronary prevention in Britain: action at last? British Medical Journal, 1987, 294: 225–226

60 Committee on Medical Aspects of Food Policy. Panel on diet in relation to cardiovascular disease. Diet and cardiovascular disease. London, Department of Health and Social Security, 1984.

61 Anon. Coronary heart disease prevention – plans for action. A report based on an interdisciplinary workshop conference at Canterbury. 28–30 September 1983. London, Pitman Medical, 1984.

62 British Medical Association. Diet, nutrition and health. London, BMA, 1986.

63 Winkler J T, Sanderson M. Strategies for implementing NACNE recommendations. The Lancet, 1983: 1353–1354.

64 Fullard E, Fowler G et al. Facilitating prevention in primary care. British Medical Journal, 1984, 289: 1585–1587.

65 Fullard E, Fowler G et al. Promoting prevention in primary care: controlled trial of low technology, low cost approach. British Medical Journal, 1987, 294: 1080–1082.

66 Cottrell R. Eating in the early 1980s. London, British Nutrition Foundation, 1984.

67 Anon. Consumer attitudes to understanding of nutrition labelling. London, Ministry of Agriculture, Fisheries and Food, 1986.

68 Anon (editorial). Nutritional labelling of foods: a rational approach to banding. A document prepared by Nutrition Advisory Committee of Coronary Prevention Group. The Lancet, 1986, i: 469.

69 Luba A. The food labelling debate. London, London Food Commission, 1985.

70 Anon. Britain needs a food and health policy: the government must face its duty. The Lancet, 23 August 1986: 434–436.

71 Montague S. Healthy eating and the NHS. A review of the development and implementation of local food and health policies in Britain. University of Bradford, 1985.

72 Gibson L, Winkler J. Local food health policies in the UK. 1987. Forthcoming.

73 Cole-Hamilton I. Diet and Health. Nutrition – a negotiating issue. In: Bargaining Report, October 1985, 44: 13–15.

74 See 51.

75 Directorate of the Welsh Heart Programme. Pulse of Wales. Preliminary report of the Welsh heart survey. Heartbeat report no 4. Cardiff, Heartbeat Wales, 1986.

76 Harding J, Price L. Preventing coronary heart disease: a report of policies and initiatives in the UK. London National Coordinating Committee on Coronary Heart Disease Prevention, London.

77 Directorate of the Welsh Heart Programme. Take Heart. A consultative document on the development of community-based heart health initiatives in Wales. Report no 1. Cardiff, Heartbeat Wales, 1985.

78 World Health Organization. Problems related to alcohol consumption. Report of a WHO expert committee. Technical report series no 650. Geneva, WHO, 1980.

79 Central Policy Review Staff. Alcohol policies in the United Kingdom. Stockholm University, 1982.

80 Royal College of Psychiatrists. Alcohol and alcoholism. London, Tavistock, 1979.

81 Royal College of Psychiatrists. Alcohol our favourite drug. London, Tavistock, 1986.

82 Royal College of Physicians. The medical consequences of alcohol: a great and growing evil. London, Pitman, 1987.

83 Royal College of General Practitioners. Alcohol – a balanced view. London, RCGP, 1986.

84 British Medical Association. Young people and alcohol. London, BMA, 1986.

85 Scottish Health Education Coordinating Committee. Health education in the prevention of alcohol-related problems. Edinburgh, SHECC, 1985.

86 Health Education Advisory Committee for Wales. Dealing with alcohol problems in Wales. Cardiff, HEAW, 1986.

87 Action on Alcohol Abuse. An agenda for action on alcohol. London. Action on Alcohol Abuse, 1986.

88 Breeze E. Differences in drinking patterns between selected regions. OPCS Social Survey. London, HMSO, 1985.

89 See 81.

90 See 85.

91 Kendell R E, de Roumanie M et al. Effect of economic changes on Scottish drinking habits 1978–82. British Journal of Addiction, 1983, 78: 365–379.

92 Maynard A. Social costs of alcohol use. In: Alcohol: preventing the harm. Conference proceedings. London, Institute of Alcohol studies, 1984.

93 Hansen A. The portayal of alcohol to television. Health Education Journal, 1986, 45, 3: 127–131.

94 See 78.

95 Wood D. Beliefs about alcohol. Research report no 5: London, Health Education Council, 1986.

96 Anderson P. Managing alcohol in general practice. British Medical Journal, 22 June 1985: 1873–1875.

97 Wallace P, Cremona A et al. Safe limits of drinking: general practitioners' views. British Medical Journal, 1985, 290: 1875–1876.

98 Budd J et al. Tyne Tees alcohol education campaign: an evaluation. Centre for Mass Communication Research. Unpublished.

99 Lambert D. The north east England project on alcohol misuse. Health Education Council. Unpublished.

100 Simnett I, Corder J. Understanding alcohol. A programme in south west England to promote sensible drinking by stimulating informed debate. London, Health Education Council, 1985.

101 Plant M A. Drugs in perspective. London, Tavistock, 1987.

102 Saunders B. Help for problem drinkers. In: Plant M A (ed) Drinking and problem drinking. London, Junction Books, 1982.

103 Potamianos G, North W R S et al. Randomised controlled trial of conventional hospital management in the treatment of alcoholism. The Lancet, 4 October 1986: 797–799.

104 Robertson I, Heather N. So you want to cut down on your drinking? Edinburgh, Scottish Health Education Group, 1986.

105 Glen I, Henery J et al. A pilot study of controlled drinking in individuals with alcohol abuse presenting to general practitioners in the Highlands and Islands. Scottish Health Education Group, 1986. Unpublished.

106 Duffy J C, Plant M A. Scotland's liquor licensing changes: an assessment. British Medical Journal, 1986, 292: 36–39.

107 Smith R. Time, gentlemen, please. British Medical Journal, 24 January 1987: 202.

108 Jeffs B W, Saunders W M. Minimising alcohol-related offences by enforcement of existing licensing legislation. British Journal of Addiction, 1983, 78: 67–77.

109 Gofton L, Douglas S. Drink and the city. New Society, 20 December 1985: 502.

110 Smith R. Government hypocrisy on drugs. British Medical Journal, 15 March 1986: 712–713.

111 Department of Health and Social Security. Prevention and health: drinking sensibly. London, HMSO, 1981.

112 Department of Health and Social Security. Voluntary organisations and alcohol misuse. London, DHSS, 1982.

113 Tether P, Robinson D. Preventing alcohol problems: a guide to local action. London, Tavistock, 1986.

114 Wallace P, Haines A. Use of a questionnaire in general practice to increase the recognition of patients with excessive alcohol consumptions. British Medical Journal, 29 June, 1985: 1949–1953.

115 Ashton L. Sensible drinking survey. London, Health Education Council, 1985.

116 Romelsjo A, Agren G. Has mortality related to alcohol decreased in Sweden? British Medical Journal, 20 July 1985: 167–169.

117 Adams J. The efficiency of seat belt legislation. Occasional paper. London, University College, 1981.

118 Ashton S J, Thomas P D et al. The effects of mandatory seat belt use in Great Britain. Paper presented at Tenth International Conference of Experimental Safety Vehicles. July, 1985.

119 Mackay M. Seat belts and risk compensation. British Medical Journal, 21 September 1985: 757–758.

120 See 119.

121 Rutherford W H. The medical effects of seat belt legislation in the United Kingdom. Office of the Chief Scientist. Research report no 13. London, HMSO, 1985.

122 Lynham D A. The effect of local traffic safety measures in United Kingdom. Presented to the Evaluation 85 international meeting traffic safety measures. Crowthorne, TRRL, 1985.

123 Plowden S, Hillman M. Danger on the road: the needless scourge. London, Policy Studies Institute, 1984.

124 Dunbar J A. A quiet massacre. A review of drinking and driving in the United Kingdom. Occasional Paper no 7. London, Institute of Alcohol Studies, 1985.

125 See 81.

126 Blennerhassett committee. Drinking and driving. Report. Department of the Environment. London, HMSO, 1976.

127 Department of Transport. Road accidents in Great Britain 1985. London, Department of Transport, 1986.

128 Sabey B E, Everest J T. Prevention against drinking and driving. Presented to the tenth international conference on alcohol. Drugs and traffic safety. Crowthorne, TRRL, 1986.

129 Sabey B E. Planning perspectives on traffic safety in the United Kingdom. Presented to the Symposium '85 Individual Responsibility. Joint responsibility, Crowthorne, TRRL, 1985.

130 See 129.

131 Plowden S. Reducing motorcycle accidents. In: Road safety what next? Proceedings of a conference held at Policy Studies Institute October 1985. PSI Occasional Paper, 86/3. London, PSI, 1986.
132 See 129.
133 House of Commons Transport Committee. First report: road safety. London, HMSO, 1985.
134 See 127.
135 See 123.
136 See 127.
137 MacKay M. Vehicle characteristics, growth rates and crash performance. Birmingham, Department of Transport and Highways, 1986.
138 See 119.
139 Paciullo G. Random breath testing in New South Wales, December 1982 to February 1983. Medical Journal of Australia, 25 June 1983: 620–621.
140 Homel R. The impact of random breath testing in New South Wales December 1982 to February 1983. Medical Journal of Australia, 25 June 1983: 616–617.
141 See 79.
142 See 126.
143 See 84.
144 See 81.
145 Havard J. Drunken driving among the young. British Medical Journal, 1986, 293: 774.
146 Wellings K. AIDS and the condom. British Medical Journal, 1986, 293: 1259–1260.
147 See 146.
148 Richardson A C, Lyon J B. The effect of condom use on squamous cell intraepithelial neoplasia. American Journal of Obstetrics and Gynaecology, 1981, 140, 8: 909–913.
149 Anon. AIDS – a public health crisis. Population Reports, Series L, no 6. Baltimore, Johns Hopkins University, July/August 1986.
150 See 149.
151 Kelly J A, St. Lawrence J S. Cautions about condoms in prevention of AIDS. The Lancet, 1987, i: 323.
152 Wright N H, Vessey M P et al. Neoplasia and dysplasia of the cervix uteri and contraception: a possible protective effect of the diaphragm. British Journal of Cancer, 1978, 38: 273–279.
153 Wigersma L, Oud R. Safety and acceptibility of condoms for use by homosexual men as a prophylactic against transmission of HIV during anogenital sexual intercourse. British Medical Journal, 1987, 295: 11.
154 Wells N. The AIDS virus: forecasting its impact. London, Office of Health Economics, 1986.
155 Chapman S, Hodgson J. Showers in raincoats: attitudinal barriers to prophylactic condom use in high-risk heterosexuals. Adelaide, South Australian Health Commission, 1986.
156 Winkelstein W, Samuel M et al. The San Francisco men's health study III. Reduction in human immunodeficiency virus transmission among homosexual/bisexual men. American Journal of Public Health 1987, 77, 6: 685–689.
157 Martin J L. The impact of AIDS on gay male sexual behaviour patterns in New York City. American Journal of Public Health, 1987, 77, 5: 580–581.
158 Carne C A, Johnson A M et al. Prevalence of antibodies to HIV, gonorrhoea rates, and changed sexual behaviour in homosexual men in London. The Lancet, 1987, 21: 656–658.
159 See 158.
160 Gellan M C A, Ison C A. Declining incidence of gonorrhoea in London: a response to fear of AIDS? The Lancet, 18 October 1986, 920–921.

288

161 Anderson R, May R. Plotting the spread of AIDS. New Scientist, 26 March 1987: 54–59.

162 Laara E, Day N et al. Trends in mortality from cervical cancer in the Nordic countries: organised screening programmes. The Lancet, 30 May 1987: 1247–1249.

163 Anon. (editorial). Cancer of the cervix: death by incompetence. The Lancet, 17 August 1985, 363–367.

164 Chamberlain J. (editorial). Failures of the cervical cytology screening. Organisation of a programme for cervical cancer screening. British Medical Journal, 1984, 6 October: 853–854.

165 Committee of Public Accounts. House of Commons Committee of Public Accounts 44th report: preventive medicine. Session 1985–86. London, HMSO, 1986.

166 Macgregor J E, Moss S M et al. A case-control study of cervical cancer screening in north east Scotland. British Medical Journal, 1985, 290: 1543–1546.

167 Duguid H L, Duncan I D et al. Screening for cervical intraepithelial neoplasia in Dundee and Angus 1962/81 and its relation with invasive cervical cancer. The Lancet, 9 November 1985: 1053–1056.

168 Savage W, Schwartz M. (letter). Cervical smear policy, The Lancet, 1985, ii: 1305.

169 Parkin D M et al. The impact of screening on the incidence of cervical cancer in England and Wales. British Journal of Obstetrics and Gynaecology, 1985, 92: 150–157.

170 Anon (editorial). Screening strategies for cervical cancer. The Lancet, 27 September 1986: 725–726.

171 ICRF Coordinating Committee on Cervical Screening. Organisation of a programme for cervical cancer screening. British Medical Journal, 1984, 289: 894–895.

172 IARC Working Group on Evaluation of Cervical Cancer Screening programme. Screening for squamous cervical cancer: duration of low risk after negative results of cervical cytology and its implication for screening policy. British Medical Journal, 1986, 293: 659.

173 ICRF Coordinating Committee on Cervical Screening. The management of a cervical screening programme: a statement (October 1985). Community Medicine, 1986, 8, 3: 179–184.

174 British Medical Association. Cervical cancer and screening in Great Britain. London, BMA, 1986.

175 Association of Scientific, Technical and Managerial Staffs. Behind the screen. London, ASTMS, 1985.

176 Singer A. Genital wart virus infections: nuisance or potentially lethal? British Medical Journal, 1984, 288, 6419: 735–737.

177 Anon. (editorial). Genital warts, human papilloma viruses and cervical cancer. The Lancet, 1985, ii: 1045–1046.

178 Roberts C J, Farrow S C et al. How much can the NHS afford to spend to save a life or avoid a severe disability? The Lancet, 12 January 1985: 89–91.

179 Parkin D M, Moss S M. An evaluation of screening policies for cervical cancer in England and Wales using a computer-simulated model. Journal of Epidemiology and Community Health 1986, 40: 143–153.

180 Smith A, Chamberlain J. Managing cervical screening. In: Information technology in health care. Institute of Health Services Management. London, Kluwer Publications, 1987.

181 Department of Health and Social Security and Welsh Office. AIDS: monitoring the response to the public education campaign. London, HMSO, 1987.

182 Beck E J, Cunningham D G et al. HIV testing: changing trends at a clinic for sexually transmitted diseases in London. British Medical Journal, 1987, 295: 191–193.

183 Sonnex C, Petherick A et al. HIV infection: increase in public awareness and

anxiety. British Medical Journal, 1987, 295: 193–195.

184 Hastings G B, Leathar D S et al. AIDS publicity: some experience from Scotland. British Medical Journal, 1987, 294: 48–49.

185 Social Services Committee. Third report: problems associated with AIDS. Third Session 1986–1987. London, HMSO, 1987.

186 Ashton L. AIDS survey. Initiatives and plans for public education. London, Health Education Council, 1987.

187 Forrest Sir Patrick (chair). Breast cancer screening. Report to the health ministers of England, Wales, Scotland and Northern Ireland. London, HMSO, 1986.

188 See 187.

Chapter 8

1 Black Sir Douglas (chair). Inequalities in health. Report of a research working group. London, Department of Health and Social Security, 1980.

2 Whitehead M. The health divide. In: Inequalities in health. London, Penguin, 1988.

3 Office of Population Censuses and Surveys. Occupational Mortality 1970-2, Series DS1, with allowances made for wider differentials in 1981. London, HMSO, 1978.

4 Office of Population Censuses and Surveys. Occupational Mortality 1979–80 and 1982–83 Series DS2. London, HMSO, 1986.

5 Preston S H et al. Effects of industralisation and urbanisation on mortality in developed countries. IUSSP Solicited Papers. IUSSP Conference 19. Liege, IUSSP, 1981.

6 Pamuk E. Social class inequalities in mortality from 1921 to 1972 in England and Wales. Population Studies, 1985, 39: 17–31.

7 Marmot M G. Mortality decline and widening social inequalities. The Lancet, 1986, ii: 274–276.

8 Koskinen S. Time trends in cause-specific mortality by occupational class in England and Wales. Paper presented to IUSSP 20th general conference, Florence, 1985. Unpublished.

9 See 8.

10 Le Grand J. Inequalities in health, the human capital approach. Welfare state programme no 1. London, London School of Economics, 1985.

11 See 1.

12 See 2.

13 Wadsworth M E J. Serious illness in childhood and its association with later life achievement. In: Wilkinson R G (ed). Class and health: research and longitudinal data. London, Tavistock, 1986.

14 Illsley R. Occupational class, selection and inequalities in health. Quarterly Journal of Social Affairs 1986, 2, 2: 151–161.

15 Wilkinson R G. Occupational class, selection and inequalities in health: a reply to Raymond Illsley. Quarterly Journal of Social Affairs 1986, 2, 4: 415–422.

16 Fox A J et al. Social class mortality differentials: artefact, selection or life circumstances? Journal of Epidemiology and Community Health, 1985, 39: 8.

17 Wilkinson R G. Socioeconomic differences in mortality: interpreting the data on their size and trends. In Wilkinson R G (ed). Class and health: research and longitudinal data. London, Tavistock, 1986.

18 See 5.

19 See 6.

20 See 6.

21 Leon D A and Wilkinson R G. Inequalities in prognosis: socioeconomic differences in cancer and heart disease survival. Paper presented at European Foundation

meeting, inequalities in health. June 1986.

22 Blaxter M A. A comparison of measures of inequality in morbidity. Papers presented at European Science Foundation meeting inequalities in health. June 1986.

23 Fox A J, Goldblatt P O. Longitudinal study: sociodemographic mortality differentials 1971–1975. LS series no 1. London, HMSO, 1982.

24 OPCS. OPCS longitudinal study: Unpublished data provided by Social Statistical Research Unit, City University.

25 See 7.

26 Jacobson B. Beating the ladykillers. Women and smoking. London, Gollancz, 1988.

27 Roman E et al. Occupational mortality among women in England and Wales. British Medical Journal, 1985, 291: 194–196.

28 McIntyre S. The patterning of health by social position in contemporary Britain: direction for sociological research. Social Science and Medicine, 1986, 23: 393–415.

29 See 28.

30 Marmot M G et al. Lessons from the study of immigrant mortality. The Lancet, 1984, i: 1455–1457.

31 Gillies D R H et al. Analysis of the ethnic influences on still births and infant mortality in Bradford 1975–81. Journal of Epidemiology and Community Health, 1984, 58, 3: 214–217.

32 Marmot M G. Social inequalities in mortality: the social environment. In: Wilkinson R G (ed). Class and health: research and longitudinal data. London, Tavistock, 1986.

33 Townsend P. The geography of poverty and ill-health. Paper presented to a meeting of the British Association for the Advancement of Science. University of Bristol, 1986.

34 See 2.

35 Martini C J et al. Health indices sensitive to medical care variation. International Journal of Health Services, 1977, 7, 2: 293–309.

36 Carr-Hill R, Hardmann G F et al. Variations in avoidable mortality and variations in health care resources. The Lancet, 4 April 1987: 789–791.

37 See 8.

38 Fox A J, Adelstein A M. Occupational mortality: work or way of life? Journal of Epidemiology and Community Health, 1978, 33: 73–78.

39 Crombie D L. Social class and health status: inequality or difference? Royal College of General Practitioners Occasional Paper no 25. London, RCGP, 1984.

40 Himsworth H. Epidemiology, genetics and sociology. Journal of the Biosocial Society 1984, 16: 159–176.

41 See 2.

42 Wilkinson R G. Income and mortality. In: Wilkinson R G (ed). Class and health: research and longitudinal data. London, Tavistock, 1986.

43 See 42.

44 Wastaff A. The demand for health: theory and implications. Journal of Epidemiology and Community Health, 1986, 40: 1–11.

45 Smith R. Unemployment and health. Oxford, Oxford University Press, 1987.

46 Moser K A et al. Unemployment and mortality in the OPCS longitudinal study. In: Wilkinson R G (ed). Class and health research and longitudinal data. London, Tavistock, 1986.

47 Moser K A. Unemployment and mortality 1981–83: follow-up of the 1981 longitudinal study census sample. Working paper 43, Social Statistics Research Unit. London, City University, 1986.

48 Scott-Samuel A. Unemployment and health. The Lancet, 1984, ii: 1464–1465.

49 See 47.

50 See 45.

51 Marsh A, Matheson J. Smoking attitudes and behaviour. OPCS Social Survey

Division. London, HMSO, 1983.

52 See 26.

53 See 51.

54 Ministry of Agriculture, Fisheries and Food. Household Food and Expenditure. Report of the National Food Survey Committee. London, HMSO, 1986.

55 Rona R J et al. Social factors and height of primary school children in England and Scotland. Journal of Epidemiology and Community Health, 1978, 32: 147–154.

56 Cole-Hamilton I, Lang T. Tightening belts: a report on the impact of poverty on food. London, London Food Commission, 1986.

57 Haines F A, De Looy A E. Can I afford the diet? Birmingham, British Dietetic Association, 1986.

58 London Food Commission. Food retailing in London: a pilot study of the three largest retailers and Londoners access to food. London, LFC, 1985.

59 Department of Health and Social Security. Family expenditure survey 1985. London, HMSO, 1986.

60 Wenlock R W, Düsselduff M M. The diets of British school-children. London, DHSS, 1986.

61 Department of Health and Social Security. Nutrition and health in old age. Reports on health and social subjects no 16. London, HMSO, 1979.

62 Graham H. Caring for the family: a short report on the study of the organisation of the health resources and responsibilities of 102 families. Milton Keynes, Open University, 1985.

63 Lang T et al. Jam tomorrow. Manchester, Manchester Polytechnic, 1984.

64 Marmot M G et al. Changing social class distribution of heart disease. British Medical Journal, 1978, 2: 1109–1112.

65 See 64.

66 Wilkinson R G. Socioeconomic factors in mortality differentials. M.med.sci. thesis. Nottingham University, 1976.

67 Duval D and Booth A. The housing environment and women's health. Journal of Health and Social Behaviour, 1978, 19: 410–417.

68 Wilner D M and Walkley R P. The effects of housing on health and performance. In: Dahl L J (ed). The Urban Condition, New York, 1963.

69 Booth A. Urban crowding and its problems. New York, Praeger, 1976.

70 Robertson I. In: Donnison D and Middleton A (eds). Renewing the city. London, Routledge and Kegan Paul, 1987.

71 See 28.

72 Berkman L F, Syme S L. Social networks, host resistance and mortality: a nine-year follow-up study of Almeda County residents. American Journal of Epidemiology, 1979, 109: 186–204.

73 Medalie J H, Goldbout U. Angina pectoris among 1,000 men II: psychosocial and other factors as evidenced by a multivariate analysis of a 5 year incidence study. American Journal of Medicine, 1976, 6: 910–921.

74 See 32.

75 Young M, Willmott P. Family and kinship in East London. London, Penguin, 1962.

76 World Health Organization. Targets for health for all – targets in support of the European regional strategy for health for all. Copenhagen, WHO, 1985.

77 McKeown T, Lowe C R. An Introduction to social medicine. Oxford, Blackwell, 1974.

78 Scottish Health Education Co-ordinating Committee. Health education in areas of multiple deprivation. Edinburgh, SHECC, 1984.

79 See 2.

80 Veenhoven R. Conditions of happiness. Dordrecht, D Radel Publishing, 1984.

81 Rogers, G B. Income and inequality as a determinant of mortality: an international

cross sectional analysis. Population Studies, 1979, 33: 343–351.

82 See 42.

83 See 42.

84 See 81.

85 Central Statistical Office. Social Trends. London, HMSO, 1986.

86 See 81.

87 See 42.

88 See 44.

89 Winter J M. Public health and the extension of life expectancy in England and Wales 1901–60. In M Keynes (ed). The Political Economy of Health and Welfare. 1985 Eugenics Society Symposium. Forthcoming.

90 See 89.

91 See 2.

92 See 2.

93 Parliamentary debates. House of Commons, 1982, vol 34, cols 245–246.

94 British Medical Association. Deprivation and ill-health. London, BMA Professional Division, 1987.

95 Archbishop's Commission. Faith in the City. A call for action by church and nation. London, Church House Publishing, 1985.

96 Smith R. Whatever happened to the Black report. British Medical Journal, 1986, 293: 91–92.

97 See 2.

98 Castle P, Jacobson B. The health of our regions: an analysis of the strategies and policies of regional health authorities for promoting health and preventing disease. A report for the Health Education Council. Birmingham, NHS Regions Health promotion Group, 1988.

Chapter 9

1 The Sports Council. Exercise, health, medicine. A symposium proceedings. London, The Sports Council, 1983.

2 Fentem P H, Bassey E J. The case for exercise. London, The Sports Council, 1977.

3 Shepherd R. The value of physical fitness in preventive medicine. In: Evered D, Whelan J (eds). The value of preventive medicine. CIBA Foundation Symposium 110. London, Pitman Medical, 1985.

4 Centres for Disease Control. Public health aspects of physical activity and exercise. Special Section. Public health reports, 1985, 100, 2: 118–212.

5 Anon. (editorial). Physical activity in old age. The Lancet, 20/27 December 1986: 1431.

6 Muir Gray J A, Bassey E J, Young A. The risks of inactivity. In: Muir Gray J A (ed). Prevention of disease in the elderly. Edinburgh, Churchill Livingstone, 1985.

7 See 3.

8 See 6.

9 Barr C et al. The relationship of physical activity and exercise to mental health. Public Health Reports, 1985, 100, 2: 195–202.

10 Paffenberger R S et al. Physical activity, all-cause mortality, and longevity of college alumni. New England Journal of Medicine, 1986, 314, 10: 605–613.

11 Paffenberger R S, Hale W E. Work activity and coronary heart mortality. New England Journal of Medicine, 1975, 292: 545–550.

12 Siscovick D S et al. Physical activity and primary cardiac arrest. Journal of the American Medical Association, 1982, 243: 3113–3117.

13 Paffenberger R S et al. Physical activity as an index of heart attack risk in college

alumni. American Journal of Epidemiology, 1978, 108: 161–175.

14 Morris J N et al. Vigorous exercise in leisure time: protection against heart disease. The Lancet, 1980, 8206: 1207–1210.

15 Lindsay R. Prevention of osteoporosis. In Muir Gray J A (ed). Prevention of disease in the elderly. Edinburgh, Churchill Livingstone, 1985.

16 Koplan J P, Siscovick D S et al. The risks of exercise: a public health view of injuries and hazards. Public Health Reports, 1985, 100, 2: 189–195.

17 See 14.

18 See 10.

19 Department of Education and Science. Young people in the 80s. A survey. London, HMSO, 1983.

20 The Sports Council. Sport in the community – the next 10 years. London, The Sports Council, 1982.

21 Directorate of the Welsh Heart Programme. Pulse of Wales. Preliminary report of the Welsh heart health survey. Heartbeat report no 4. Cardiff, Heartbeat Wales, 1986.

22 MORI. Public attitudes towards fitness: research study conducted for Fitness Magazine, No. 2391. London, MORI, 1984.

23 Dishman R K, Sallis J F et al. The determinants of physical activity and exercise. Public Health Reports, 1985, 100, 2: 158–171.

24 McIntosh P, Charlton V. The impact of sport for all policy 1966–1984 and a way forward. London, The Sports Council, 1985.

25 The Sports Council. Provision for sport. London, The Sports Council, 1972.

26 See 24.

27 Crew V. Research and evaluation of the HEC's Look After Yourself! programme. London, Health Education Council, 1986.

28 Brown G et al. Final report to the HEC on the LAY tutor training programme. Department of Adult Education, University of Nottingham, 1984.

29 Health Education Council. The Great British Fun Run. Evaluation report parts I, II and III. London, HEC, 1985.

30 See 24.

31 Faculty of Community Medicine. Promoting exercise in the community: guidelines for health promotion no 7. London, Faculty of Community Medicine.

32 Haskell W Z, Montoye H J et al. Physical activity and exercise to achieve health-related physical fitness components. Public Health Reports, 1985, 100, 2: 202–212.

33 Brown G, Harris T. The social origins of depression. London, Tavistock, 1978.

34 Paykel E S. The contribution of life events to causation of psychiatric illness. Psychological Medicine, 1978, 8: 245–254.

35 Lloyd C. Life events and depressive disorder reviewed: II events as precipitating factors. Archives of General Psychiatry, 1980, 37: 541–548.

36 Andrews G, Tennant C. Life events, stress and psychiatric illness. Psychological Medicine, 1978, 8: 545–549.

37 Totman R. Social causes of illness. London, Souvenir Press, 1979.

38 Rutter M. Stress, coping and developments: some issues and some questions. Journal of Child Psychiatry, 1981, 22, 4: 323–356.

39 Haggerty R J. Life stress, illness and social supports. Development Medicine and Child Neurology, 1980, 22: 391–400.

40 Kessler R C. Stress, social status and psychological distress. Journal of Health and Social Behaviour, 1979, 20: 259–272.

41 See 37.

42 See 37.

43 Jones D R et al. Bereavement and cancer: some data on deaths and spouses from the longitudinal study of Office of Population Censuses and Surveys. British Medical Journal, 1984, 289: 461–464.

44 Parkes C M. Benjamin B et al. Broken heart: a statistical study of increased mortality among widowers. British Medical Journal, 1969, 1: 740–743.
45 Helsing K H, Szklo M et al. Factors associated with mortality after widowhood. American Journal of Public Health, 1981, 71: 802–809.
46 See 38.
47 See 34.
48 Berkman L F. Assessing the physical health effects of social networks and social support. Annual Reviews of Public Health, 1984, 5: 413–432.
49 Broadhead W E et al. The epidemiologic evidence for a relationship between social support and health. American Journal of Epidemiology, 1983, 117: 521–535.
50 See 49.
51 See 49.
52 Pless I B, Satterwhite B A. Measures of family functioning and its application. Journal of Social Science and Medicine, 1973, 7: 613–621.
53 Sosa R et al. The effects of a supportive companion on perinatal problems, length of labour and mother infant interaction. New England Journal of Medicine, 1980, 303: 579–600.
54 Gottlieb B H. Preventive interventions involving social networks and social support. In: Gottlieb B H (ed). Social networks and social support. Beverley Hills, Sage Publications, 1981.
55 Berkman L, Syme S. Social networks, host resistance and mortality: a nine-year follow-up study of Alameda County residents. American Journal of Epidemiology, 1979, 109: 186–204.
56 Blazer D. Social support and mortality in an elderly community population. American Journal of Epidemiology, 1982, 115: 684–94.
57 House J, Robbins C et al. The association of social relationships and activities with mortality: prospective evidence from the Tecumseh Community Health Study. American Journal of Epidemiology, 1982, 116: 123–140.
58 See 21.

Chapter 10

1 Brown G W, Harris T. Social class and affective disorder. In: Ihsam Al-Issa (ed). Culture and psychopathology. Baltimore, University Park Press, 1982.
2 Glazer D. Psychiatric disorders. A rural/urban comparison. Archives of General Psychiatry, 1985, 42: 651–656.
3 Paykel E S. The contribution of life events to causation of psychiatric illness. Psychological Medicine, 1978, 8: 245–254.
4 Brown G W, Harris T. Stress or vulnerability and depression: a question of replication. Psychological Medicine, 1986, 16: 739–744.
5 Tennant C. Female vulnerability to depression. Psychological Medicine, 1985, 15: 733–737.
6 Wing J K, Bebbington P. Epidemiology of depressive disorders in the community. Journal of Affective Disorders, 1982, 4: 331–345.
7 Balter M B et al. A cross-national comparison of anti-anxiety/sedative drug use. Current Medical Research and Opinion, 1984, 8, supplement 4: 5–19.
8 See 7.
9 Higgett A C, Lader M et al. Clinical management of benzodiazepine dependence. British Medical Journal, 1985, 291: 688–690.
10 See 9.
11 Catalan J, Gath D H. Benzodiazepines in general practice: time for a decision. British Medical Journal, 1985, 290: 1374–1376.

12 Betts T A, Birtle J. Effect of two hypnotic drugs on actual driving performance next morning. British Medical Journal, 1982, 285: 852.

13 Skegg D C G, Richards S M et al. Minor tranquillizers and road accidents. British Medical Journal, 1979, 1: 917–919.

14 Prescott L F, Highley M S. Drugs prescribed for self poisoners. British Medical Journal, 1985, 290: 1633–1636.

15 Catalan J, Gath G et al. The effects of non-prescribing of anxiolytics in general practices – I: controlled evaluation of psychiatric and social outcome. British Journal of Psychiatry, 1984, 144: 593–602.

16 Office of Health Economics. Suicide and deliberate self-harm. London, OHE, 1981.

17 Platt S, Foster J et al. Parasuicide in Edinburgh 1984. A report on admissions to the regional poisoning treatment centre. Edinburgh, University of Edinburgh, 1985.

18 See 17.

19 See 16.

20 McClure G M G. Suicide in England and Wales, 1975–1984. British Journal of Psychiatry, 1987, 150: 309–314.

21 Kreitman N. The coal gas story: United Kingdom suicide rates, 1960–71. British Journal of Preventive and Social Medicine 1976, 30, 2: 86–93.

22 Phillips D, Carstensen L L. Clustering of teenage suicides after television news stories about suicide. New England Journal of Medicine, 1986, 315, 11: 685–689.

23 Gould M S, Shaffer D. The impact of suicide in television movies: evidence of imitation. New England Journal of Medicine, 1986, 315, 11: 690–694.

24 See 16.

25 Parkes C M. Bereavement counselling: does it work? British Medical Journal, 5 July 1980: 3–6.

26 Barraclough B, Shea M. Suicide and Samaritan clients. The Lancet, 24 October 1970: 868–870.

27 Kreitman N. How useful is the prediction of suicide following parasuicide? In: Wilmotte and Mendlewicz (eds). New trends in suicide prevention. Bibliotheca Psychiatrica, 1982, 162.

28 Murphy G. On suicide prediction and prevention. Archives of general Psychiatry, 1983, 40: 343–344.

29 Pokorny G. Prediction of suicide in psychiatric patients: report of a prospective study. Archives of General Psychiatry, 1983, 40: 249–257.

30 Alderson M R. National trends in self poisoning in women. The Lancet, 27 April 1985: 974–975.

31 See 17.

32 Chowdhury N, Hick R et al. Evaluation of an after-care service for parasuicide (attempted suicide) patients. Social Psychiatry, 1973, 8: 67–81.

33 Gibbons J, Barker P et al. Evaluation of a social work service for self-poisoning patients. British Journal of Psychiatry, 1978, 133: 111–118.

34 Hawton K, Bancroft J et al. Domiciliary and outpatient treatment of self-poisoning patients by medical and non-medical staff. Psychological Medicine, 1981, 11: 169–177.

35 See 14.

36 Office of Health Economics. Schizophrenia. London, OHE, 1979.

37 Leff J, Kuipers L et al. A controlled trial of social intervention in the families of schizophrenic patients. British Journal of Psychiatry, 1982, 141: 121–134.

38 See 37.

39 World Health Organization. Child mental health and social development. WHO Technical Report Series no 613. Geneva, WHO, 1977.

40 Royal College of General Practitioners. Prevention of psychiatric disorders in general practice. Report from general practice no 20. London, RCGP, 1981.

41 Mahaffey K R (ed). Dietary and environmental lead: human health effects. Amsterdam, Elsevier, 1985.
42 Lansdown R, Yule W (eds). The lead debate: the environment, toxicology, and child health. London, Croom Helm, 1986.
43 Taylor E. The overactive child. Clinics in Developmental Medicine no 97. The MacKeith Press, 1986.
44 Anon. Increase in abuse of children. The Lancet, 1986: 1473.
45 Jenkins J, Gray O P. Changing clinical picture of non-accidental injury to children. British Medical Journal, 10 December 1983: 1767–1770.
46 Wild N J. Sexual abuse of children in Leeds. British Medical Journal, 1986, 292: 1113–1116.
47 Bentovim A. Sexual abuse of children. British Medical Journal, 1986, 292: 1394.
48 Hobbs C J, Wynne J M. Buggery in childhood – a common syndrome of child abuse. The Lancet, 1986: 792–796.
49 See 46.
50 See 40.
51 See 40.
52 See 40.
53 See 40.
54 Rutter M. The city and the child. American Journal of Orthopsychiatry, 1981, 51, 4: 610–625.
55 Rutter M et al. Attainment and adjustment in two geographical areas – I: the prevalence of psychiatric disorders. British Journal of Psychiatry, 1975, 126: 493–509.
56 Lavik N. Urban-rural differences in rates of disorder: a comparative psychiatric population study of Norwegian adolescents. In: Graham P (ed). Epidemiological approaches in child psychiatry. London, Academic Press, 1977.
57 See 55.
58 Newman O. Defensible space. London, Architectural Press, 1973.
59 Newman O. Reactions to the 'defensible space' study and some further findings. International Journal of Mental Health, 1975, 4: 48–70.
60 Richman N. In: Child psychiatry: modern approaches. Oxford, Blackwell Scientific Publications, 1977.
61 Rutter M. Attainment and adjustment in two geographical areas. III: some factors accounting for area differences. British Journal of Psychiatry, 1975, 126: 520–533.
62 Coleman A. Utopia on trial. Vision and reality in planned housing. London, Hilary Shipman, 1985.
63 Rutter M. Changing youth in a changing society. Cambridge, Mass. Harvard University Press, 1980.
64 Office of Health Economics. Dementia in old age. London, OHE, 1979.
65 Mulley G P. Differential diagnosis of dementia. British Medical Journal, 1986, 292: 1416–1418.
66 Murphy E. Prevention is better: preventing mental illness. Geriatric Medicine, February 1984: 75–79.
67 Gurland B J, Copeland J R M et al. The mind and mood of ageing: the mental health problems of the community elderly in New York and London. London, Croom Helm, 1983.
68 See 66.
69 Parkes C M. Evaluation of a bereavement service. Journal of Preventive Psychiatry. 1981. 1: 179–88.
70 See 25.
71 See 66.

Chapter 11

1 House of Commons Social Services Committee. Second report: perinatal and neonatal mortality. London, HMSO, 1980.
2 House of Commons Social Services Committee. Third report: perinatal and neonatal mortality report: follow-up session 1983–84. London, HMSO, 1984.
3 Department of Health and Social Security. Reply to the second report from the Social Services Committee on perinatal mortality. London, HMSO, 1980.
4 Department of Health and Social Security. First report of the Maternity Services Advisory Committee. Maternity care in action. Part 1 – antenatal care. London, HMSO, 1984.
5 Department of Health and Social Security. Second report of the Maternity Services Advisory Committee. Maternity care in action. Part II – care during childbirth. London, HMSO, 1984.
6 Department of Health and Social Security. Third report of the Maternity Services Advisory Committee. Maternity care in action. Part III – postnatal and neonatal care. London, HMSO, 1985.
7 Chalmers I. The search for indices. The Lancet, 1979, ii: 1063–1065.
8 McIllwaine G M et al. The Scottish perinatal mortality survey, Scotland 1977–1981. Edinburgh, Scottish Health Service Common Services Agency, Information Services Division, 1984.
9 Chalmers I. Short, Black, Baird, Himsworth and social class differences in fetal and neonatal mortality rates. British Medical Journal, 1985, 291: 231–234.
10 Macfarlane J A. In: Chalmers I, McIlwaine G (eds). Studies of cerebral palsy in perinatal audit surveillance. London, Royal College of Obstetricians and Gynaecologists, 1980.
11 Taylor J. Mental handicap: partnership in the community. London, Office of Health Economics, 1986.
12 Office of Population Censuses and Surveys. Studies in sudden infant deaths. Studies in medical and population subjects no 45. London, HMSO, 1982.
13 Carpenter R G et al. Prevention of unexpected infant death. The Lancet, 2 April 1983: 723–727.
14 Loshak D. Sudden infant death. The Lancet, 29 March 1985: 591.
15 Pharoah P O D. Perspective and patterns. British Medical Bulletin, 1986, 42, 2: 119–126.
16 Mugford M, Stilwell J. Maternity services: how well have they done and could they do better? In: Harnson A, Grettan J (eds). Health Care UK, 1986. London, Chartered Institute of Public Finance Accounting, 1986.
17 Enkin M, Chambers I (eds). Effectiveness and satisfaction in antenatal care. London, Heinemann, 1982.
18 Dowling S. Health for a change. The provision of preventive health care in pregnancy and early childhood. London, Child Poverty Action Group, 1983.
19 See 16.
20 See 16.
21 Martin J, Monk J. Infant feeding 1980. London, OPCS, 1982.
22 Lauglo M. The Spitalfields Health Survey. Tower Hamlets Department of Community Medicine, 1984. Unpublished.
23 Watson E. Health of infants and use of health services by mothers of different ethnic groups in East London. Community Medicine, 1984, 6: 127–135.
24 Hall M et al. Antenatal care assessed. A case study of an innovation in Aberdeen. Aberdeen, Aberdeen University Press, 1985.
25 Royal College of Obstetricians and Gynaecologists. Report of the RCOG working party on routine ultrasound examination in pregnancy, 1984, London, RCOG, 1984.
26 See 15.

27 See 24.

28 Oakley A. The captured womb. A history of medical care for pregnant women. Oxford, Blackwells, 1984.

29 See 24.

30 Oakley A et al. Social class, stress and reproduction. In: Rees A R, Purcell H (eds). Disease and the environment. London, Wiley, 1982.

31 Oakley A. Social support in pregnancy: the 'soft' way to increase birthweight? Social Science and Medicine, 1985, 11: 1259–1268.

32 Oakley A, Elbourne D. Interventions to alleviate stress in pregnancy. In: Enkin M et al (eds). Effective care in pregnancy and childbirth. Oxford, Oxford University Press, 1987.

33 See 31.

34 Newton R W, Hunt L P. Psychosocial stress in pregnancy and its relation to low birthweight. British Medical Journal, 1984, 288: 1191–1194.

35 See 31.

36 Wald N H (ed). Antenatal and neonatal screening. Oxford, Oxford University Press, 1984.

37 See 36.

38 Lind T. Obstetric ultrasound: getting good vibrations. British Medical Journal, 1986, 293: 576.

39 Association for Improvements in the Maternity Services. A commentary on the report of the Royal College of Obstetricians and Gynaecologists working party on routine ultrasound examination in pregnancy. London, AIMS, 1985.

40 Wald N J, Cuckle H S. Open neural tube defects. In: Wald N J (ed). Antenatal and neonatal screening. Oxford, Oxford University Press, 1984.

41 See 40.

42 See 40.

43 Stene J, Mikkelson M. Down's syndrome and other chromosomal disorders. In: Wald N H (ed). Antenatal and neonatal screening. Oxford University Press, 1984.

44 See 43.

45 Murday V, Slack J. Screening for Down's syndrome in the North East Thames Region. British Medical Journal, 1985, 291: 1315–1318.

46 Rose G. Strategy of prevention: lessons from cardiovascular disease. British Medical Journal, 1981, 282: 1847–50.

47 Merkatz I R, Nitowsky H M et al. An association between maternal serum alpha-fetoprotein and fetal chromosome abnormalities. American Journal of Obstetrics and Gynaecology 1984, 148: 886–894.

48 Cuckle H S et al. Maternal serum alphafetoprotein measurements: a screening test for Down's syndrome. The Lancet, 1984, i: 926–927.

49 See 45.

50 Palomaki G E. Collaborative study of Down's syndrome screening using maternal serum alphafetoprotein and maternal age. The Lancet, 20 December 1986: 1460.

51 Modell B et al. Effect of fetal diagnostic testing on birth-rate of thalassaemia major in Britain. The Lancet, 15 December 1984: 1383–1386.

52 Modell B. Chorionic villus sampling: evaluating safety and efficacy. The Lancet, 30 March 1985: 737–740.

53 Sleep J et al. West Berkshire perinatal management trial. British Medical Journal, 1984, 289: 90.

54 Howie P W. Fetal monitoring in labour. British Medical Journal, 1986, 292: 427–428.

55 Grant A, Garcia J. (letter). British Medical Journal, 1986, 292: 826–27.

56 Savage W. A Savage enquiry. London, Virago Press, 1986.

57 Panel of the National Consensus Conference. Indications for Caesarean section: final statement of the panel of the National Consensus Conference on aspects of caesarean

birth. Canadian Medical Association Journal, 1986, 134: 1348–1351.
58 Macfarlane A, Mugford M (editorial). An epidemic of Caesareans? Journal of Maternal and Child Health, February 1986: 38–42.
59 Davies I M M. Perinatal and infant deaths: social and biological factors. Population Trends, 1980, 19: 19–21.
60 Murphy J F et al. Planned and unplanned deliveries at home: implications of a changing ratio. British Medical Journal, 1984, 288: 1429–1432.
61 Campbell R et al. Home births in England and Wales, 1979: perinatal mortality according to intended place of delivery. British Medical Journal, 1986, 289: 721–724.
62 Rosenblatt R A et al. Is obstetrics safe in small hospitals? The Lancet, 24 August 1985: 429–432.
63 Anon (editorial). What future for small obstetric units? The Lancet, 24 August 1985: 423–424.
64 Anon (editorial). Perinatal care: organisation and outcome. The Lancet, 5 April 1986: 777–778.
65 Department of Health and Social Security. Reducing the risk. Safer pregnancy and childbirth. London, HMSO, 1977.
66 Hagberg et al. The changing panorama of cerebral palsy in Sweden. Epidemiological trends IV 1959–78. Acta Paediatrica Scandinavica, 1984, 73: 433–40.
67 Powell T G et al. Survival and morbidity in a geographically defined population of low birthweight infants. The Lancet, 8 March 1986: 539–543.

Chapter 12

1 Romans-Clarkson S E et al. Impact of a handicapped child on mental health of parents. British Medical Journal, 1986, 293: 1395–1397.
2 Graham H. Caring for the family. Research Report no 1. London, Health Education Council, 1986.
3 Martin J, Roberts C. Women and employment – a lifetime perspective. London, HMSO, 1980.
4 See 3.
5 Bowlby J. Maternal care and mental health. Geneva, World Health Organization, 1951.
6 Rutter M. Maternal deprivation reassessed. London, Penguin Books, 1981.
7 Tizard B. The care of young children – implications of recent research. London, Thomas Coram Research Unit, 1986.
8 Moss P. The EEC's on draft on parental leave for family reasons. London, Thomas Coram Research Unit, 1985.
9 Rutter M. Fifteen thousand hours. Secondary schools and their effects on children. Cambridge, Mass., Harvard University Press, 1979.
10 Rutter M. The city and the child. American Journal of Orthopsychiatry, 1981, 51, 4: 610–625.
11 Whitehead M. Education for health: achievements of a decade. Scottish Health Education Group, 1988 (in press).
12 Department of Education and Science. Health education from 5–16. Curriculum Matters 6. An HMI Series. London, HMSO, 1986.
13 Williams T, Reid D. In: Williams T, Woesler de Panafieu C (eds). School health education in Europe. Department of Education, University of Southampton, 1985.
14 Bolam R, Medlock P. Active tutorial work training and dissemination: an evaluation. Oxford, Health Education Council/Basil Blackwell, 1985.
15 Thacker J. Extending developmental group work to junior/middle schools: an Exeter project. Pastoral Care, February 1985: 5–13.

16 Baldwin J, Wells H. Active tutorial work. Oxford, Basil Blackwell Books, 1979: 1–5.
17 The Health Visitors Association. The health visitor's role in child health surveillance: a policy statement. London, Health Visitor's Association, 1985.
18 World Health Organization European Working Group. Today's health – tomorrow's wealth, new perspectives in prevention in childhood. Summary report, Kiev. 21–25 October 1985. ICP/MCH 102/MO4(S) 698/IF. Geneva, WHO, 1985.
19 See 17.
20 Anon (editorial). Developmental surveillance. The Lancet, 26 April 1986: 950–952.
21 See 18.
22 Macfarlane J A. Child health services in the community: making them work. British Medical Journal, 1986, 293: 222–223.
23 Curtis Jenkins G H, Newton R C F. The first year of life. Edinburgh, Churchill Livingstone, 1981.
24 Chamberlain R N, Simpson R N. The prevalence of illness in childhood. London, Pitman Medical, 1979: 78–83.
25 Office of the Chief Scientist. Department of Health and Social Security. Two reports on research into services for children and adolescents. Chairmen: Morris J N, Wing J K. London, HMSO, 1980.
26 Peckham C S. Hearing impairment in childhood. British Medical Bulletin, 1986, 42: 145–149.
27 Peckham C S et al. Congenital rubella deafness: a preventable disease. The Lancet, 1979, i: 258–261.
28 See 26.
29 Tanner J M. Physical development. British Medical Bulletin, 1986, 42, 2: 131–138.
30 Alberman E. Prevention and health promotion. British Medical Bulletin, 1986, 42, 2: 212–216.
31 See 20.
32 Baird G, Hall D M B. Developmental paediatrics in primary care: what should we teach? British Medical Journal, 1985, 291: 583–586.
33 Bax M, Hart H. The health needs of the pre-school child. Archives of Disease in Childhood 1976, 51, 848–852.
34 See 20.
35 Committee on Child Health Services. The report of the Committee on Child Health Services Vol 1. Fit for the future. London, HMSO, 1976.
36 National Childrens' Bureau. Investing in the future. Child health ten years after the Court report. London, National Children's Bureau, 1987.
37 British Medical Association Child Health Forum. Appendix II, Annual Report of Council 1986/87. British Medical Journal, 28 March 1987: 34.
38 See 17.
39 Royal College of General Practitioners. Healthier children – thinking prevention. Report from General Practice no 22. London, RCGP, 1983.
40 Faculty of Community Medicine. An integrated child health service: the way forward. London, Faculty of Community Medicine, 1987.
41 Acheson E D (chair). Primary health care in inner London. Report of a study group. London, London Health Planning Consortium, 1981.
42 Gruenberg E M (ed). Vaccinating against brain syndromes: the campaign against measles and rubella. Oxford, Oxford University Press, 1986.
43 Russell L B. Is prevention better than cure? Washington DC, the Brookings Institute, 1986.
44 Begg N T. Personal communication.
45 Begg N T, Noah N D. Immunisation targets in Europe and Britain. British Medical Journal, 1985, 291: 1370.

46 See 45.

47 US Department of Health and Human Services. Promoting health, preventing disease: objectives for the nation. Washington DC, Public Health Service, 1980.

48 Committee of Public Accounts. House of Commons Forty Fourth Report, Committee of Public Accounts, Session 1985–86. Preventive Medicine. London, HMSO, 1986.

49 Report by the Comptroller and Auditor General. National Health Service: preventive medicine. London, HMSO, 1986.

50 Anon. Immunising the world's children. Population Reports March–April 1986, Series L, 5.

51 Mant D, Phillips A. Measles immunisation rates and the good practice allowance. British Medical Journal, 1986, 293: 995–997.

52 See 49.

53 Anon. Report from the PHLS, CDSC. British Medical Journal, 1986, 292: 1385–1387.

54 Carter H, Jones I G. Measles immunisation: results of a local programme to increase vaccine uptake. British Medical Journal, 1985, 290: 1717–1719.

55 Peckham C S, Martin J A M et al. Congenital rubella deafness: a preventable disease. The Lancet, 1979, i: 258–261.

56 SENSE. Rubella: the facts. London, SENSE and National Rubella Council, 1987.

57 Miller C L, Miller E et al. Effecting selective vaccination on rubella susceptibility and infection in pregnancy. British Medical Journal, 1985, 291: 1398–1402.

58 See 57.

59 Smithell R W, Sheppard S et al. National rubella surveillance programme. British Medical Journal, 1985, 291: 40–41.

60 Bart K H, Orenstein W A et al. Universal immunisation to interrupt rubella. Review of infectious diseases, March–April 1985, supplement 1; s177–s184.

61 Miller D. Pertussis vaccine and whooping cough as risk factors in acute neurological illness and death in young children, Symposium on pertussis. Geneva, 1984.

62 Nicoll A. Mythical contraindications to vaccination. The Lancet, 23 March 1985: 679.

63 Walker A, Rees L. Mythical contraindications to vaccination. The Lancet, 27 April 1985: 994.

64 Citron K M. The future of BCG vaccination in schools in England and Wales. British Medical Journal, 1986, 292: 483–484.

65 See 64.

66 Peltols H, Kurki T et al. Rapid effect on endemic measles, mumps and rubella of nationwide vaccination programme in Finland. The Lancet, 18 January 1986: 137–139.

67 Walker D, Carter H et al. Measles, mumps and rubella: the need for a change in immunisation policy. British Medical Journal 1986, 292: 1501–1502.

68 See 51.

69 Ross S K. Childhood immunoprophylaxis: achievements in a Glasgow practice. Health Bulletin 1983, 41, 5: 253–257.

70 Anon. (editorial). Failure to vaccinate. The Lancet 10 December 1983: 1343–1346.

71 James J, Clark C. Immunisation rates and the good practice allowance. British Medical Journal, 1986, 293: 1242.

72 Lingham S et al. Role of an immunisation advisory clinic. British Medical Journal, 1986, 292: 939–940.

73 Jefferson N et al. Rose of an immunisation clinic. British Medical Journal, 1986, 292: 1460.

74 See 57.

75 Hayden J et al. Measles, mumps and rubella: need for a change in immunisation policy. British Medical Journal, 1986, 293: 138–139.
76 Anon (editorial). Measles vaccine once or MMR twice. The Lancet, 20 September 1986: 671–672.
77 See 66.
78 Koplan J P et al. A benefit-cost analysis of mumps vaccine. American Journal of Diseases in Childhood, 1982, 136: 362–364.
79 White C C, Koplan J P et al. Benefits, risks and costs of immunisation for measles, mumps and rubella. American Journal of Public Health, 1985, 75, 7: 739–744.
80 See 78.
81 Cowell C R, Sheiham A. Promoting dental health. London, King Edward's Hospital Fund for London, 1981.
82 World Health Organization. Epidemiology, etiology and prevention of peridontal disease. WHO technical report series no 621. Geneva, WHO, 1978.
83 World Health Organization. Prevention methods and programmes for oral disease. WHO Technical Report Series no 713. Geneva, WHO, 1984.
84 Dental Strategy Review Group. Towards better dental health. Guidelines for the future. London, DHSS, 1981.
85 Royal College of Physicians. Fluoride, teeth and health: a report of the Royal College of Physicians. London, Pitman Medical, 1976.
86 Levine R S. The scientific basis of dental health education: London, Health Education Council, 1985.
87 See 85.
88 See 35.
89 Department of Health and Social Security. Prevention and health: everybody's business. London, HMSO, 1976.
90 Merrison Sir Alec (chair). Royal commission on the NHS. Report. London, HMSO, 1979.
91 See 84.
92 Knox E G. Fluoridation of water and cancer: a review of the epidemiological evidence. London, DHSS, 1981.
93 Jackson D, James P M C, Thomas F D. Fluoride in Anglesey 1983: a clinical study of dental caries. British Dental Journal, 1985, 158, 45–49.
94 Anderson R J, Bradnock G et al. The reduction of dental caries prevalence in English school children. Journal of Dental Research, 1982, 61 (special issue): 1311–1316.
95 Davies G N. Fluoride in the prevention of dental caries. A tentative cost-benefit analysis. The effect of fluoridation on dental caries and dental treatment. British Dental Journal, 1973, 135, 2: 79–83.
96 Kunzel W. The cost and economic consequences of water fluoridation. Caries Research, 1984, 8: 28–35.
97 Carmichael C L, French A D et al. The relationship between social class and caries experience in five year old children in Newcastle and Northumberland after 12 years fluoridation. Community Dental Health, 1984, I: 47–54.
98 National Advisory Committee on Nutrition Education. Proposals for nutritional guidelines for health education in Britain: a discussion paper. London, Health Education Council, 1983.
99 British Medical Association. Nutrition and health. London, BMA Professional Division, 1986.
100 See 98.
101 See 81.
102 Charles N, Kerr M. Attitudes towards the feeding and nutrition of young children.

York, Department of Sociology, University of York, 1984.
103 Wenlock R W, Disselduff M M et al. The diets of British school children. London, HMSO, 1986.
104 Weaver R. Fluoride and wartime diet. British Dental Journal, 1985, 88, 9: 231–239.
105 See 102.
106 See 81.
107 Arnold C, Doyle A J. Evaluation of the dental health education programme – 'natural nashers'. Community Dental Health, 1984, 1, 1: 141–147.
108 Craft M, Croucher R E, Blinkhorn A. 'Natural nashers' dental health education programme: the results of a field trial in Scotland. British Dental Journal, 1984, 156: 103–105.
109 See 84.
110 Cohen L K. Implication of findings for dental care across cultures. International Dental Journal 1978 2, 3: 383–388.
111 Anon. Routine six-monthly checks for dental disease. Drug and Therapeutics Bulletin, 1985, 24: 69–72.
112 Jenkins G N. Recent change in dental caries. British Medical Journal, 1985, 291: 1297–1292.
113 See 81.

Chapter 13

1 Sanders D. The Woman Book of Love and Sex. London, Sphere Books, 1985.
2 Spencer B. Young men: their attitudes towards sexuality and birth control. British Journal of Family Planning, 1984, 10: 13–19.
3 McKeown T. The role of medicine. Dream, mirage or nemesis. Leeds, Nuffield Provincial Hospital Trust, 1976.
4 Pearce J W D. Proceedings of the Royal Society of Medicine, 1957, 50: 321.
5 Godber G E. Safety of mother and child. The Lancet, 1969, ii: 312.
6 Weir S. A study of unmarried mothers and their children in Scotland. Scottish Health Services Studies 13. Edinburgh, Scottish Home and Health Department, 1970.
7 Crellan E, Pringle M L K et al. Born illegitimate. London, National Foundation for Educational Research in England and Wales, 1971.
8 Allen Guttmacher Institute. Report for the Ford Foundation on the Findings and policy implications of a comparative study of teenage pregnancy and fertility in developed countries. New York, Allen Guttmacher Institute, 1985.
9 Bury J. Teenage pregnancy in Britain. London, Birth Control Trust, 1984.
10 Bone M. Trends in single women's sexual behaviour in Scotland. Population Trends, 1986, 43: 7–14.
11 Ashton J R. Components of delay amongst young women obtaining terminations of pregnancy. Journal of Biosocial Science, 1980, 12: 261–263.
12 Alberman E, Dennis K H (eds). The Royal College of Obstetricians and Gynaecologists report: late abortion in England and Wales. London, RCOG, 1984.
13 Communicable Disease Surveillance Centre. Sexually transmitted disease surveillance in Britain. British Medical Journal 1985, 291: 528–530.
14 Lane, The Hon Mrs Justice (chair). Report of the Committee on the Working of the Abortion Act, volume 1–11. London, HMSO 1974.
15 See 8.
16 Ermisch J F. The potential economy of demographic change. London, Heinemann, 1983.
17 Nilsson A, Olsson H et al. Stockholm, living together – a family planning and project on Gotland, Sweden 1973–76. Stockholm, National Swedish Board of Health and

Welfare Committee on Health Education, 1977.

18 Hollander G. Family planning and education about sexuality and living together in Sweden – a summary. Stockholm, National Swedish Board of Health and Welfare, 1985.

19 Wellings K. Trends in contraceptive method usage since 1970. British Journal of Family Planning, 1986, 12: 15–22.

20 Pratt W F et al. Understanding US fertility: findings from the national survey of family growth. Population Bulletin 1984, 39, 5.

21 Layde P M, Beral V. Further analyses of mortality in oral contraceptive users. The Lancet, 1981, 7: 541–546.

22 Laing W. Family planning: the benefits and costs. London, Policy Studies Institute, 1982.

23 Leathard A. District health authority family planning services in England and Wales. Family Planning Association, 1985.

24 Killikelly P. A report on family planning services for young people in the Macclesfield district. 1983. Unpublished.

25 Cossey D. Safe sex for teenagers. London, Brook Advisory Centre, 1978.

26 Farrell C. My mother said. The way young people learn about sex and birth control. London, Routledge and Kegan Paul, 1978.

27 Allen I. Education in sex and personal relationships. London, Policy Studies Institute, 1987.

28 Bhugra D, Cordle C. Sexual dysfunction in Asian couples. British Medical Journal, 1986, 292: 111–112.

29 Brettle R P, Bisset K et al. Human immunodeficiency virus and drug misuse: the Edinburgh experience. British Medical Journal, 1987, 295: 421–424.

30 Plant M A. Drugs in perspective. London, Hodder and Stoughton, 1987.

31 See 30.

32 Pearson G, Gilman M, McIver S. Young people and heroin: an examination of heroin use in the north of England. Occasional paper no 8. London, Health Education Council, 1985.

33 Hartnoll R, Lewis R et al. Estimating the prevalence of opioid dependence. The Lancet, 26 January 1985: 203–205.

34 See 33.

35 Institute for the Study of Drug Dependence. Surveys and statistics on drug taking in Britain. London, ISDD, 1984.

36 Plant M A, Peck D F, Samuel E. Alcohol, drugs and school leavers. London, Tavistock, 1985.

37 See 30.

38 Wright J D, Pearl L. Knowledge and experience of young people of drug abuse 1969–1984. British Medical Journal 1986, 292: 179–182.

39 Peck D F, Plant M A. Unemployment and illegal drug use: concordant evidence from a prospective study and national trends. British Medical Journal, 1986, 293: 929–932.

40 Institute for the Study of Drug Dependence. Drug abuse briefing. A guide to the effects of drugs and to the social and legal facts about their non-medical use in Britain. London, ISSD, 1985.

41 Parker H, Bakyx K, Newcombe R. Drug use in Wirral: the first report of the Wirral misuse of drugs project. Sub-department of social work studies, University of Liverpool, 1986.

42 Haw S. Drug problems in Greater Glasgow. London, Chamelion Press, 1985.

43 See 39.

44 Smith R. Unemployment and health. Oxford, Oxford University Press, 1987.

45 See 32.

46 Stevenson R C. The benefits of legalising heroin. The Lancet, 29 November 1986: 1269–1270.

47 Advisory Council on the Misuse of Drugs. Prevention. A report. London, HMSO, 1984.

48 See 47.

49 Gooberman L. Operation intercept: the multiple consequences of public policy. Oxford, Pergamon Press, 1974.

50 See 47.

51 See 47.

52 See 47.

53 See 47.

54 Swisher J D. Drug education: pushing or preventing? Peabody Journal of Education, 1971: 6–79.

55 Glaser D, Snow M. Public knowledge and attitudes to drug use. New York, Addiction Control Commission, 1969.

56 Goodstadt M (ed). Research on methods and programmes of drug education. Ontario, Addiction Research Foundation, 1974.

57 Hanson D J. Drug education – does it work? In: Scarpitti F, Datesma S (eds) Drugs and youth culture. Sage Annual Reviews of Drug and Alcohol Abuse, 4, 1980.

58 Kinder B N, Pape N E, Walfish S. Drug and alcohol education programmes: a review of outcome studies. International Journal of the Addictions, 1980, 15: 1035–1054.

59 Schaps E, Diabartolo R et al. A review of 127 drug abuse prevention programme evaluations. Journal of Drug Issues, 1981, 11: 17–43.

60 Bandy P, President P A. Recent literature on drug abuse prevention and mass media: focusing on youth, parents, women and the elderly. Journal of Drug Education, 1983, 13: 255–271.

61 Dorn N. Social analysis of drugs in health education and media. In: Edwards G, Busch C (eds). Drug problems in Britain. London, Academic Press, 1981.

62 Bagnall G, Plant M A. Education on drugs and alcohol: past disappointments and future challenges. Health Education Research: Theory and Practice. Forthcoming.

63 See 60.

64 See 47.

65 See 61.

66 Robins L M. The interaction of setting and pre-dispositions in explaining novel behaviour: drug initiations before and after Vietnam. In: Kandel D B (ed). Longitudinal research on drug use. New York, Halstead, 1978.

67 Stimson G V, Oppenheimer E. Heroin addiction. London, Tavistock, 1982.

68 See 30.

69 Bucknall A B V, Robertson J R, Strachan J G. Use of psychiatric drug treatment services by heroin users from general practice. British Medical Journal, 1986, 292: 997–999.

70 Glanz A, Taylor C. Findings of a survey of the role of general practitioners in the treatment of opiate misuse: extent of contact with opiate misusers. British Medical Journal, 1986, 293: 427–430.

71 Glanz A. Findings of the national survey of the role of general practitioners in the treatment of opiate misuse: views on treatment. British Medical Journal, 1986, 292: 543–546.

72 See 47.

73 House of Commons Social Services Committee. Misuse of drugs: with special reference to the treatment and rehabilitation of misusers of hard drugs. Session 1984–85. London, HMSO, 1985.

74 Marsh C. Medicine and the media. British Medical Journal, 1986, 292: 895.

75 Bagnall G, Plant M A. Medicine and media. British Medical Journal, 1987, 295: 660–661.

76 See 47.

Chapter 14

1 Nichols T. Industrial injuries in Britain manufacturing in the 1980s – a commentary on Wright's article. Sociological Review, 1986, 38: 290–306.
2 Webb T, Schilling R et al. Health at work? A report on health promotion in the workplace. Health Education Authority. Forthcoming.
3 Employment Medical Advisory Service, Health & Safety Executive. Mortality in the British rubber industry 1967–76. London, HMSO, 1980.
4 Rubber and Plastics Research Association of Great Britain. Clearing the Air. London, Rubber and Plastics Research Association, 1982.
5 World Health Organization. Occupational health. Third Report. WHO Technical report series no 135. Geneva, WHO, 1950.
6 World Health Organization. Targets for health for all – targets in support of the European regional strategy for health for all. Copenhagen, WHO, 1985.
7 Health and Safety Executive. Health at Work: 1983–85. Report by Medical Division of the Employment Medical Advisory Service. London, HMSO, 1985.
8 World Health Organization. Identification of work-related diseases. Technical Report Series no 714. Geneva, WHO, 1985.
9 Schilling R D F. More effective prevention in occupational health practices. Journal of the Society of Occupational Medicine, 1984, 34: 71–79.
10 Sweetman P M, Taylor S W C et al. Exposure to carbon disulphide and ischaemic heart disease in a viscose rayon factory. British Journal of Industrial Medicine, 1987, 44: 220–227.
11 Nurinnen M, Hernberg S A. Effect of intervention on the cardiovascular mortality of workers exposed to carbon disulphide: a 15 year follow-up. British Journal of Industrial Medicine, 1985, 42: 32–35.
12 Russek H I, Zhoman B L. Relative significance of heredity diet and occupational stress in coronary heart disease of young adults. American Journal of Medical Sciences, 1958, 235: 266–277.
13 Theorell T, Floderus-Myrhed B. Workload and risk of myocardial infarction – a progressive psychosocial analysis. International Journal of Epidemiology, 1977, 6: 17–21.
14 Knutsson A, Akerstedt T et al. Increased risk of ischaemic heart disease in shift workers. The Lancet, 12 July 1986: 89–91.
15 Haynes S G. Low personal/job control and high heart attack rates. Paper to American Heart Association Forum. Monterrey, California, January 1985.
16 Office of Population Censuses and Surveys. Occupational mortality. In: The Registrar General's decennial supplement 1970–1972. London, HMSO, 1976.
17 Harrington J M, Oakes D. Mortality study of British pathologists. British Journal of Industrial Medicine, 1984, 41: 188–191.
18 Morris J N. Epidemiology and prevention. Opening Address. IXth Scientific Meeting, International Epidemiological Association. Edinburgh, 23 August 1981. Health and Society (Millbank Memorial Fund), 1982, 60, 1.
19 See 8.
20 Edstrom R. Quality of working life: a Scandinavian view. In: McDonald J C (ed). Recent advances in occupational health. Edinburgh, Churchill Livingstone, 1981.
21 Smith M H, Cohen B G F et al. An investigation of health complaints and job stress in video display operations. Human Factors, 1981, 23: 387–400.
22 See 2.
23 See 2.

24 See 2.
25 Health and Safety Commission. Occupational health services: the way ahead. London, Health and Safety Commission, 1978.
26 See 7.
27 Select Committee on Science and Technology. Occupational health and hygiene services. A report. Session 1983–84. London, HMSO 1983.
28 See 2.
29 Ingledew D. Workplace health promotion in the US: implications for the UK. A report to the Health Education Council, 1986. Unpublished.
30 Addenbrookes Hospital Medical School. Action on smoking and health. Paper for conference on Health Promotion in the Workplace – what's in it for business. Cambridge, Addenbrooks Hospital Medical School, 1986.
31 World Health Organization European Collaborative Group. European collaborative trial of multifactorial prevention of coronary heart disease: final report on the 6 year results. The Lancet, 19 April 1986: 869–872.
32 Department of Health and Human Services. The health consequences of smoking. Cancer and chronic lung disease in the workplace. A report from the Surgeon General. Washington DC, US DHHS, 1987.
33 See 30.
34 Harris J, Seymour L. No smoking still not a sign of the times. Occupational Health, 1983, 35: 308.
35 Moreton W J, East R. Smoking cessation programmes in the workplace. London, Health Education Council, 1982.
36 Health Education Council. Action on smoking at work: a guide to good practice. London, HEC, 1985.
37 World Health Organization. The uses of epidemiology in the study of the elderly. Technical Report Series 706. Geneva, WHO, 1984.
38 Fillenbaum G G. The wellbeing of the elderly. Approaches to multidimensional assessment. Offset Publication no 84. Geneva, WHO, 1984.
39 Fries J F, Crapo L M. Vitality and ageing: implications of the rectangular curve. San Francisco, W H Freeman & Co, 1981.
40 Alderson M, Ashwood F. Projection of mortality rates for the elderly. Population Trends, 1985, 42: 22–29.
41 Bond J, Carstairs V. Services for the elderly: a survey of the character and needs of a population of 5000 old people. Scottish Health Service Study no 42. Edinburgh, Scottish Home and Health Department, 1982.
42 Office of Population Censuses and Surveys. Elderly people in private households. Supplement to General Household Survey 1980. London, HMSO, 1981.
43 See 41.
44 Finch H. Health and older people. Research report no 6. London, Health Education Council, 1986.
45 Mossey J, Shapiro E. Self-rated health: a predictor of mortality among the elderly. American Journal of Public Health, 1982, 72: 800–808.
46 Grundy E. Mortality and morbidity among old people. British Medical Journal, 1984, 288: 663–664.
47 Department of Health and Social Security. Growing older. Lonon, HMSO, 1981.
48 World Health Organization. Objectives of health promotion in the elderly. Copenhagen, European Regional Planning Group, WHO, 1983.
49 Williams A. Economics of coronary artery bypass grafting. British Medical Journal, 1985, 291: 326–329.
50 British Medical Association. All our tomorrows: growing old in Britain. London, BMA, 1986.
51 See 41.

52 See 42.

53 Evans J G. Prevention of age-associated loss of autonomy: epidemiological approaches. Journal of Chronic Disease, 1984, 37, 5: 353–363.

54 Fox R H, Woodward P M et al. Body temperatures in the elderly: a national study of physiological, social and environmental conditions. British Medical Journal, 1973, 1: 200–6.

55 Alderson M R. Season and mortality. Health Trends, 1985, 17: 87–96.

56 Collins K J. Low indoor temperatures and morbidity in the elderly. Age and Ageing, 1986, 15: 212–220.

57 Grut M. Cold-related deaths in some developed countries. The Lancet, 24 January 1987: 212.

58 See 57.

59 Tillett H E, Smith J W G et al. Excess deaths attributable to influenza in England and Wales: age at death and certified cause. International Journal of Epidemiology, 1983, 12: 344–352.

60 See 55.

61 See 54.

62 Sakamoto-Momiyama M. Seasonality in human mortality. Tokyo, Tokyo University Press, 1977.

63 World Health Organization. The effects of the indoor housing climate on the health of the elderly. Geneva, WHO, 1982.

64 See 54.

65 See 56.

66 Norton A et al. Councils of care: planning a local government strategy for older people. Policy Studies in Ageing no 5. London, Centre for Policy on Ageing, 1986.

67 Rinder L et al. Seventy-year-old people in Gothenburg. A population study in an industrialised Swedish city. Acta Medica Scandinavica, 1975, 198: 397–407.

68 Sekular R, Hutmen L P. Spatial vision and ageing. Journal of Gerontology, 1980, 35: 692–699.

69 See 66.

70 Vetter N J. Health promotion and ageing: attitudes of the elderly to health promotion topics. Paper presented at Harrowgate Seminar on Health Promotion in Old Age, Feburary 1987. Unpublished.

71 Jajich C L, Adrian M et al. Smoking and coronary heart disease mortality in the elderly. Journal of the American Medical Association, 1984, 252, 20: 2831–2834.

72 MacLennan W J. Subnutrition in the elderly. British Medical Journal, 1986, 293: 1189–1190.

73 See 72.

74 Lindsay R. Prevention of osteoporosis. In: Muir Gray J A (ed). Prevention of disease in the elderly. Edinburgh, Churchill Livingstone, 1986.

75 Christiansen C et al. Prevention of early postmenopausal bone loss: controlled two year study in 315 normal females. European Journal of Clinical Investigation 1980, 10: 273–279.

76 Vessey M, Hunt K. The menopause, hormone replacement therapy and cardiovascular disease: epidemiological aspects. In: Studd J (ed). Hormone replacement therapy. London, MTP Press, 1987.

77 See 66.

78 Phillipson C, Strang P. Training and education for an ageing society: new perspectives for the health and social services. Working paper on health of the elderly no 3. London, Health Education Council, 1986.

79 Phillipson C, Strang P. Health education and older people: the role of paid carers. London, Health Education Council, 1984.

80 See 41.

81 Anon (editorial). Caring for the elderly. The Lancet, 4 October 1986: 821.
82 Jones D, Vetter N J. Formal and informal support received by carers of elderly dependents. British Medical Journal, 1985, 291: 643–645.
83 Brody E M. Women in the middle and family help to older people. The Gerontologist 1981, 21, 5: 471–480.
84 Estes C L et al. Women and the economics of ageing. International Journal of Health Services, 1984, 14, 1: 55–68.
85 Brody E M et al. Women's changing roles and help to elderly parents: attitudes of three generations of women. Journal of Gerontology, 1983, 38, 5: 597–607.
86 Weir F, Pinchen I. Action research with informal carers of elderly people. A study of local services and current issues. London, Health Education Council, 1985.
87 Sandford J R A. Tolerance of debility in elderly dependents by supporters at home: its significance for hospital practice. British Medical Journal, 1975, 3: 471–473.
88 Jones D A, Vetter N J. A survey of those who care for the elderly at home: their problems and their needs. Social Science and Medicine, 1984, 19, 5: 511–514.
89 See 82.
90 Association of Crossroads Care Attendant Schemes. Cause for concern. Rugby, Rugby Association of Crossroads Care Attendant Schemes, 1986.
91 Dunn R, MacBeath L et al. Respite admissions and the disabled. Journal of the American Geriatrics Society, 1983, 31: 613.
92 Challis D et al. Cost-effectiveness in social care. In: Lishman J (ed). Research highlights no 8: University of Aberdeen, Department of Social Work, 1984.
93 Bliss M R. Prescribing for the elderly. British Medical Journal, 1981, 283: 203–206.
94 Williamson J, Chopin J M. Adverse reaction to prescribed drugs in the elderly: a multi-centre investigation. Age and Ageing, 1980, 9: 73–80.
95 Age Concern. Profiles of the Elderly – their health and health services. Age Concern Research Publication no 2. Surrey, Age Concern, 1977.
96 Knox J D E. Prevention of iatrogenic disease. In: Muir Gray J A (ed). Prevention of disease in the elderly. Edinburgh, Churchill Livingstone, 1986.
97 Royal College of Physicians. Medication for the elderly. A report. Journal of the Royal College of Physicians of London, 1984, 18, 1: 7–17.
98 Knox J D E. Prescribing for the elderly in general practice. A review of the current literature. Journal of the Royal College of General Practitioners, 1980, supplement no 1, vol. 30.
99 Freer C B. Geriatric screening: a reappraisal of preventive strategies in the care of the elderly. Journal of the Royal College of General Practitioners, June 1985: 288–290.
100 Taylor R, Ford et al. The elderly at risk. A critical review of problems and progress in screening and casefinding. Age Concern research perspective monograph no 6. Surrey, Age Concern, 1983.
101 Amery A et al. Mortality and morbidity results from the European working party on high blood pressure in the elderly trial. The Lancet, 15 June 1985: 1349–1354.
102 Anon (editorial). Treatment of hypertension: the 1985 results. The Lancet, 21 September 1985: 645–648.
103 Coope J, Warrender T S. Randomised trial of treatment of hypertension in elderly patients in primary care. British Medical Journal, 1 November 1986: 1145–1151.
104 Canadian Task Force on the periodic Health examination. The periodic health examination, 2. 1984 update. The Canadian Medical Association Journal, 1984, 130: 1278–1292.
105 The Working Group on Hypertension in the Elderly. Statement on hypertension in the elderly. Journal of the American Medical Association, 1986, 256: 70–74.
106 Hendriksen C et al. Consequences of assessment and intervention among elderly people: a three year randomised controlled trial. British Medical Journal, 1984, 289: 1522–1524.

107 Vetter N J. Effect of health visitors working with elderly patients in general practice – a randomised controlled trial. British Medical Journal, 1984, 288: 369–372.

108 Kennie D C. Health maintenance of the elderly. Geriatric medicine and social policy. Clinics in geriatric medicine, 1986, 2, 1: 53–83.

109 Barber J H, Wallis J B. The effects of a system of geriatric screening and assessment on general practice workload. Health Bulletin, Edinburgh, 1982, 40: 125–132.

110 Ebrahim S, Hedley R et al. Low levels of ill health among elderly non-consulters in general practice. British Medical Journal, 1984, 289: 1273–1275.

111 Williams E. Characteristics of patients over 75 not seen during one year in general practice. British Medical Journal, 1984, 288: 119–121.

112 Freer C. Personal communication.

113 Age Concern. General practitioners and the needs of older people: a policy paper. Surrey, Age Concern, 1986.

114 Haines A, Booroff A. Terminal care at home: perspective from general practice. British Medical Journal, 1986, 292: 1051–53.

115 See 114.

Index